Cardiology

Editor

SONDRA DEPALMA

PHYSICIAN ASSISTANT CLINICS

www.physicianassistant.theclinics.com

Consulting Editor
GERALD KAYINGO

April 2025 • Volume 10 • Number 2

ELSEVIER

1600 John F. Kennedy Boulevard • Suite 1800 • Philadelphia, Pennsylvania, 19103-2899

http://www.theclinics.com

PHYSICIAN ASSISTANT CLINICS Volume 10, Number 2
April 2025 ISSN 2405-7991, ISBN-13: 978-0-443-24702-6

Editor: Taylor Hayes
Developmental Editor: Anirban Mukherjee

Physician Assistant Clinics (ISSN: 2405–7991) is published quarterly by Elsevier Inc., 360 Park Avenue South, New York, NY 10010-1710. Months of issue are January, April, July, and October. Periodicals postage paid at New York, NY and additional mailing offices. Subscription prices are $155.00 per year (US individuals), $100.00 (US students), $150.00 (Canadian individuals), $100.00 (Canadian students), $150.00 (international individuals), and $100.00 (international students). For institutional access pricing please contact Customer Service via the contact information below. Foreign air speed delivery is included in all *Clinics* subscription prices. All prices are subject to change without notice. Orders, claims, and journal inquiries: Please visit our Support Hub page https://service.elsevier.com for assistance.

Reprints. For copies of 100 or more, of articles in this publication, please contact the Commercial Reprints Department, Elsevier Inc., 360 Park Avenue South, New York, NY 10010-1710. Tel. 212-633-3874; Fax: 212-633-3820; E-mail: reprints@elsevier.com.

Physician Assistant Clinics is covered in *EMBASE/Excerpta Medica and ESCI.*

JOURNAL TITLE: Physician Assistant Clinics
ISSUE: 10.2

PROGRAM OBJECTIVE
The goal of the *Physician Assistant Clinics* is to keep practicing physician assistants up to date with current clinical practice by providing timely articles reviewing the state of the art in patient care.

TARGET AUDIENCE
Physician Assistants and other healthcare professionals

LEARNING OBJECTIVES
Upon completion of this activity, participants will be able to:
1. Review the primary risk factor for atherosclerotic cardiovascular disease (ASCVD) and various treatment options.
2. Discuss social determinants of health and how they affect health outcomes.
3. Recognize proficient clinical skills and judgment are paramount for cardiac complaints when presentations are unclear.

ACCREDITATION
The Elsevier Office of Continuing Medical Education (EOCME) is accredited by the Accreditation Council for Continuing Medical Education (ACCME) to provide continuing medical education for physicians.

The EOCME designates this journal-based CME activity for a maximum of 15 *AMA PRA Category 1 Credit*(s)™. Physicians should claim only the credit commensurate with the extent of their participation in the activity.

All other health care professionals requesting continuing education credit for this enduring material will be issued a certificate of participation.

DISCLOSURE OF RELEVANT FINANCIAL RELATIONSHIPS
The EOCME assesses conflict of interest with its instructors, faculty, planners, and other individuals who are in a position to control the content of CME activities. All relevant conflicts of interest that are identified are thoroughly vetted by EOCME for fair balance, scientific objectivity, and patient care recommendations. EOCME is committed to providing its learners with CME activities that promote improvements or quality in healthcare and not a specific proprietary business or a commercial interest.

The authors and editors listed below have identified no financial relationships or relationships to products or devices with commercial interest related to the content of this CME activity:
Jennifer L. Barnett, DMSc, PA-C, DFAAPA; Caleb Mychael Barrera, PA-C, UPMC; Kimberly A. Berggren, DMSc, PA-C; Ashley Black, PA-C; David J. Bunnell, MSHS, PA-C, DFAAPA; Sondra DePalma, DHSc, PA-C, CLS, CHC, FNLA, AACC, DFAAPA; Michael G. DePalma, DMSc, MHS, PA-C, DFAAPA; Jerica N. Derr, DMSc, PA-C; Nick Entsminger, DMSc, PA-C (CAQ-EM); Lauren S. Eyadiel, MMS, MS, PA-C, SLP, FHFSA; Robert Hill, DMSc, PA-C; Julie A. Jones, MS-PAS, PA-C; Marnie O'Donnell, MHS, PA-C; Catherine Roden, MHS, PA-C; Laura J. Ross, PA-C, CLS, DipACLM, AACC; Marie Shaner, MMS, PA-C; Robert S. Smith, DHSc, MS, PA-C, DFAAPA; Laura Solano, DMSc, MPAS, PA-C

The authors and editors listed below have identified financial relationships or relationships to products or devices with commercial interest related to the content of this CME activity:
Camille J. Dyer, DMSc, PA-C, AACC, DFAAPA: *Advisor*: Bayer

Amy E. Simone, PA-C, FACC: *Employee*: Edwards Lifesciences Corporation

Clay W. Walker, MSPA, PA-C, CPAAPA: *Advisor*: GSK

The Clinics staff listed below have identified no financial relationships or relationships to products or devices they have with ineligible companies related to the content of this CME activity:
Taylor Hayes; Kothainayaki Kulanthaivelu; Michelle Littlejohn; Patrick J. Manley; Anirban Mukherjee

UNAPPROVED/OFF-LABEL USE DISCLOSURE
The EOCME requires CME faculty to disclose to the participants:
1. When products or procedures being discussed are off-label, unlabelled, experimental, and/or investigational (not US Food and Drug Administration [FDA] approved); and

2. Any limitations on the information presented, such as data that are preliminary or that represent ongoing research, interim analyses, and/or unsupported opinions. Faculty may discuss information about pharmaceutical agents that is outside of FDA-approved labelling. This information is intended solely for CME and is not intended to promote off-label use of these medications. If you have any questions, contact the medical affairs department of the manufacturer for the most recent prescribing information.

TO ENROLL
The CME program is available to all *Physician Assistant Clinics* subscribers at no additional fee. To subscribe to the *Physician Assistant Clinics*, call customer service at 1-800-654-2452 or sign up online at www.physicianassistant.theclinics.com.

METHOD OF PARTICIPATION
In order to claim credit, participants must complete the following:
1. Complete enrolment as indicated above
2. Read the activity
3. Complete the CME Test and Evaluation. Participants must achieve a score of 70% on the test. All CME Tests and Evaluations must be completed online

CME INQUIRIES/SPECIAL NEEDS
For all CME inquiries or special needs, please contact elsevierCME@elsevier.com.

Contributors

CONSULTING EDITOR

GERALD KAYINGO, PhD, MBA, PA-C, DFAAPA
Assistant Dean, Executive Director and Professor, Physician Assistant Leadership and Learning Academy Graduate School, University of Maryland, Baltimore Baltimore, Maryland

EDITOR

SONDRA DEPALMA, DHSc, PA-C, CLS, CHC, FNLA, AACC, DFAAPA
Vice President, Reimbursement and Professional Practice, American Academy of Physician Associates, Alexandria, Virginia; Adjunct Assistant Professor, Doctor of Medical Science Program, A.T. Still University, Arizona School of Health Sciences, Mesa, Arizona

AUTHORS

JENNIFER L. BARNETT, DMSc, PA-C, DFAAPA, SFHM, CPHQ
Adjunct Associate Professor, Doctor of Medical Science Program, Graduate School, University of Maryland Baltimore, Baltimore, Maryland; Instructor, Doctor of Medical Science Program, College of Idaho, Caldwell, Idaho; Hospitalist, MedStar Medical Group, MedStar, Franklin Square Medical Center, Baltimore, Maryland

CALEB MYCHAEL BARRERA, MSPAP, PA-C
Physician Assistant, Cardiology, UPMC Central PA Heart and Vascular Institute, Harrisburg, Pennsylvania

KIMBERLY A. BERGGREN, DMSc, PA-C
Associate Clinical Education Director and Assistant Professor, School of Physician Assistant Practice, Florida State University College of Medicine, Tallahassee, Florida

ASHLEY BLACK, PA-C
Principal Faculty and Assistant Professor, Physician Assistant Studies Program, College of Health Science, Charleston Southern University, Charleston, South Carolina

DAVID J. BUNNELL, MSHS, PA-C, DFAAPA
Assistant Professor, Doctor of Medical Science Program, School of Graduate Studies, University of Maryland, Baltimore, Maryland

MICHAEL G. DEPALMA, DMSc, MHS, PA-C, DFAAPA
Associate Professor and Program Director, Master of Science in Biomedical Science Program, Department of Physician Assistant Studies, A.T. Still University, Arizona School of Health Sciences, Mesa, Arizona

SONDRA DEPALMA, DHSc, PA-C, CLS, CHC, FNLA, AACC, DFAAPA
Vice President, Reimbursement and Professional Practice, American Academy of Physician Associates, Alexandria, Virginia; Adjunct Assistant Professor, Doctor of Medical Science Program, A.T. Still University, Arizona School of Health Sciences, Mesa, Arizona

JERICA N. DERR, DMSc, PA-C
Director of Experiential Learning, Assistant Professor, Division of PA Education, Department of Physician Assistant Education, Oregon Health and Science University, Portland, Oregon; Associate Director of Research and Capstone Activities, Department of Physician Assistant Studies, A.T. Still University DMSc Program, Mesa, Arizona

CAMILLE J. DYER, DMSc, PA-C, AACC, DFAAPA
Immediate Past President, Constituent Organization of AAPA, African Heritage PA Caucus, Boynton Beach, Florida

NICK ENTSMINGER, DMSc, PA-C (CAQ-EM)
Guest Lecturer, Master of Science in Physician Assistant Studies Program, Dominican University of California, San Rafael, California

LAUREN S. EYADIEL, MS, MMS, PA-C, SLP, FHFSA, Heart Failure - Certified
Assistant Professor, Department of PA Studies, Wake Forest University School of Medicine; Department of Cardiovascular Medicine, Atrium Health Wake Forest Baptist, Winston-Salem, North Carolina

ROBERT HILL, DMSc, PA-C
Program Director and Assistant Professor, Department of Physician Assistant Practice, Bradly University, Peoria, Illinois

JULIE A. JONES, MS-PAS, PA-C
Physician Assistant, Department of Congenital Heart Center, Penn State Health, Hershey, Pennsylvania

MARNIE O'DONNELL, MHS, PA-C
Physician Assistant, Department of Congenital Heart Disease, Penn State Health, Hershey, Pennsylvania

CATHERINE RODEN, MHS, PA-C
Physician Assistant, Department of Congenital Heart Center, Penn State Health, Hershey, Pennsylvania

LAURA J. ROSS, PA-C, CLS, AACC, DipACLM
Director of the Heart Disease Prevention and Lipid Clinic, Department of Cardiology, Park Nicollet Heart and Vascular Center, St. Louis Park, Minnesota

MARIE SHANER, MMS, PA-C
Physician Assistant, Department of Congenital Heart Center, Penn State Health, Hershey, Pennsylvania

AMY E. SIMONE, PA-C, FACC
Senior Director, THV, Clinical Affairs, Edwards Lifesciences, Irvine, California

ROBERT S. SMITH, DHSc, MS, PA-C, DFAAPA
Regional Lead Clinician for Family Medicine, Pediatric Associates Family of Companies, Irving

LAURA SOLANO, DMSc, MPAS, PA-C, ATSU
Adjunct Faculty, Biomedical Science Program, Department of PA Studies, A.T. Still University, Texas

CLAY W. WALKER, MSPA, PA-C, CPAAPA
Assistant Professor, Department of Family Medicine, Mayo Clinic, Phoenix, Arizona; Assistant Professor, Department of Physician Assistant Studies, A.T. Still University, Mesa, Arizona

Contents

> Atherosclerotic cardiovascular disease (ASCVD) remains a major cause of global mortality. This article reviews the pathophysiology of ASCVD, focusing on endothelial dysfunction, lipid accumulation, and inflammation in plaque formation, and discusses key risk factors, including hypercholesterolemia, hypertension, and diabetes. Emphasizing the synergy of multiple risk factors, practical tools like the Framingham Risk Score and ACC/AHA calculators are presented for predicting ASCVD risk and guiding treatment. Clinicians are encouraged to use these tools to tailor preventive strategies, combining lifestyle changes and pharmacotherapy for comprehensive, personalized management of ASCVD, ultimately improving patient outcomes.

> Hypertension (HTN) is a common clinical condition contributing to the risk of all-cause mortality, atherosclerotic cardiovascular disease, kidney disease, and other sequelae. Effective blood pressure management with evidence-based interventions can reduce associated morbidity and mortality. This article provides an overview of HTN, including its definition(s), epidemiology, pathophysiology, diagnosis, and management. Common causes of secondary HTN, their presentations and recommended evaluations, and management are also summarized.

> A review of the cholesterol guidelines, statin intolerance, nonstatin treatments with clinical pearls, and a case study are presented to provide physician associates with the knowledge to effectively manage hyperlipidemia to prevent cardiovascular disease.

> This article reviews nonpharmacologic treatment modalities for cardiovascular disease and the associated pathophysiology. Therapy modalities highlighted include physical exercise, nutrition, stress reduction, and sleep optimization. Additionally, the article addresses specific care of ethnic and special populations and barriers to care and social determinants of health.

> Chest pain is a common complaint routinely assessed by physician assistants. Diagnostic accuracy requires sound clinical acumen encompassing examination findings and risk factors to determine cardiac probability. These factors include race, socioeconomics, comorbidities, and family history. Further, the inclusion of both subjective and objective red flags assists in determining patient stability or an emergent need for diagnostic testing specific to a patient's likely diagnosis. Combining clinical information with evidence-based tools, such as history, electrocardiogram findings, age, risk factors, and an initial troponin level score, PERC, Well's PE score, and others fosters rapid identification of life-threatening causes of chest pain.

> Acute coronary chest pain management focuses on diagnosing and treating acute coronary syndrome (ACS), emphasizing rapid identification and appropriate management to improve patient outcomes. It covers symptoms of ACS and diagnostic tools such as electrocardiogram and cardiac troponins. Acute management of ST-elevation myocardial infarction and non-ST elevation acute coronary syndrome (NSTE-ACS) is identified. A two-pronged approach to treating NSTE-ACS includes early invasive and ischemia-guided therapy. Treatment strategies include medication management, aspirin, anticoagulants, beta-blockers, angiotensin-converting enzyme inhibitors, and interventions like percutaneous coronary intervention.

> Heart failure is a common condition with significant morbidity and mortality that affects patients that physician assistants care for, regardless of where they practice. For patients with heart failure with reduced ejection fraction, the goal is rapid titration of the 4 pillars of guideline-directed medical therapy (GDMT): beta blockers, angiotensin receptor neprilysin inhibitors, mineralocorticoid receptor antagonist, and sodium glucose co-transporter 2 inhibitors. If left ventricular ejection fraction fails to improve with GDMT, device and advanced heart failure therapies should be considered.

Hispanic populations. Cardiovascular disease remains the leading cause of morbidity and mortality worldwide among these groups, highlighting the profound impact of social injustices and racial inequities on all aspects of health. Achieving health equity means addressing the systemic barriers that prevent certain populations from achieving the same health outcomes and requires a societal approach to address both historical and current injustices.

PHYSICIAN ASSISTANT CLINICS

SERIES OF RELATED INTEREST

Primary Care: Clinics in Office Practice
https://www.primarycare.theclinics.com/
Medical Clinics
https://www.medical.theclinics.com/

THE CLINICS ARE AVAILABLE ONLINE!
Access your subscription at:
www.theclinics.com

Foreword

From Knowledge to Practice: Your Path to Excellence in Cardiovascular Medicine

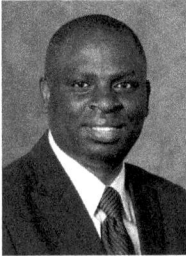

Gerald Kayingo, PhD, MBA, PA-C, DFAAPA
Consulting Editor

Heart diseases are the leading cause of death in America and a huge burden on national health expenditures. Despite technological advancements, the mortality, morbidity, and costs associated with heart diseases are projected to increase substantially. Minority racial and ethnic groups are likely to be disproportionally impacted. More than ever before, continuing medical education is critical to keep health care providers informed on latest science, effective prevention strategies, and up-to-date treatment options. In this issue, Sondra DePalma has curated a marvelous collection of cardiovascular topics for clinicians of all stages and settings. Anchored on groundbreaking science, the issue is succinctly organized to cover etiologies, epidemiology, disease presentations, differential diagnosis, prevention, and pharmacologic and nonpharmacologic interventions. New knowledge, such as the effect of COVID-19 on cardiovascular health, has been woven in. The authors have pulled together the latest practice guidelines, making this issue a one-stop shop on what a clinician needs to know in Cardiology. The issue not only covers theoretical and practical approaches to cardiovascular disease but also emphasizes the intersectionality with lifestyle factors, health systems science, and social determinants of health. The future of cardiovascular medicine is ripened for disruption with advances in precision medicine and artificial intelligence. This issue lays the foundation upon which practitioners will adapt to these rapidly growing technologies. Kudos to the editor and contributors, you have

Physician Assist Clin 10 (2025) xv–xvi
https://doi.org/10.1016/j.cpha.2024.12.003
2405-7991/25/© 2024 Published by Elsevier Inc.

set the standard for cardiovascular disease management. This issue should be in every PA's pocket tools.

Gerald Kayingo, PhD, MBA, PA-C, DFAAPA
Assistant Dean, Executive Director and Professor
Physician Assistant Leadership and Learning Academy
Graduate School, University of Maryland
Baltimore 520 West. Fayette Street, Suite #130
Baltimore, MD 21201, USA

E-mail address:
gkayingo@umaryland.edu

Website:
http://www.umaryland.edu/

Preface

Cardiology

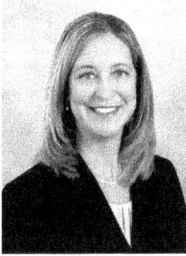

Sondra DePalma, DHSc, PA-C, CLS, CHC, AACC, FNLA, DFAAPA
Editor

The severity of cardiovascular disease (CVD) and its effects cannot be overstated. According to the Centers for Disease Control and Prevention, heart disease is the leading cause of death for men and women, accounting for one death every 33 seconds and one in five deaths in the United States. CVD is also a significant cause of disability and decreased quality of life and leads to increased health care utilization and spending. The burden of CVD is not distributed equally, with certain racial and ethnic groups experiencing higher rates of disease. People in some geographic regions and with exposure to more adverse social determinants of health also experience a disproportionate risk of CVD and associated morbidity and mortality.

Physician assistants/physician associates (PAs) are integral to identifying, preventing, treating, and managing CVD. Whether in primary care or specialty medicine, PAs regularly encounter patients with CVD or its risk factors. This makes knowledge of evidence-based management of heart and vascular disease, hypertension, and dyslipidemia essential.

Thank you to all the authors of this issue, who are experts in cardiology, medical education, or other focus areas and contributed articles relevant to clinical practice. The articles reflect current, evidence-based evaluation, diagnosis, pharmacologic management, interventions, and prevention of CVD. The articles also explore new and emerging topics in cardiology. The articles in this issue provide PAs with relevant

Physician Assist Clin 10 (2025) xvii–xviii
https://doi.org/10.1016/j.cpha.2024.12.002
2405-7991/25/© 2024 Published by Elsevier Inc.

physicianassistant.theclinics.com

information to reduce CVD, minimize its sequelae, and improve the health and well-being of millions of Americans.

Sondra DePalma, DHSc, PA-C, CLS, CHC, AACC, FNLA, DFAAPA
Reimbursement and
Professional Practice
American Academy of
Physician Associates
2318 Mill Road, Suite 1300
Alexandria, VA 22314, USA

Doctor of Medical Science Program
A.T. Still University
Arizona School of Health Sciences
5850 East Still Circle
Mesa, AZ 85206, USA

E-mail address:
sdepalma@aapa.org

Atherosclerotic Cardiovascular Disease

Epidemiology, Pathophysiology, and Practical Risk Assessment

Jerica N. Derr, DMSc, PA-C[a,b,*], Ashley Black, PA-C[c,1]

KEYWORDS

- Atherosclerosis • ASCVD • Cardiovascular risk • Endothelial dysfunction
- Plaque formation • Lifestyle modification • Risk assessment tools

KEY POINTS

- Atherosclerotic cardiovascular disease (ASCVD), a leading global cause of mortality, arises from progressive vascular changes, including lipid accumulation and inflammation.
- Endothelial dysfunction initiates the cascade of ASCVD by enabling lipid infiltration into the subendothelial space, fostering plaque formation.
- Practical risk assessment tools, including the Framingham Risk Score and ACC/AHA Risk Calculator, help identify high-risk patients and guide interventions.
- Managing ASCVD risk involves lifestyle modifications and pharmacotherapy, supported by early detection and tailored patient education.

INTRODUCTION

Atherosclerotic cardiovascular disease (ASCVD) is characterized by the buildup of cholesterol-rich plaques within arterial walls, leading to vessel narrowing and increased cardiovascular event risks such as heart attacks and strokes.[1] Historically, ASCVD has been one of the most significant health challenges worldwide. Risk factors—both modifiable, like lifestyle habits, and nonmodifiable, such as age and genetics—accelerate the development of endothelial dysfunction and lipid deposition in the arteries. These processes create a proinflammatory environment conducive

[a] Division of PA Education, Department of Physician Assistant Education, Oregon Health and Science University, 2730 South Moody Avenue, CL5PA, Portland, OR 97201, USA; [b] Department of Physician Assistant Studies, A.T. Still University DMSc Program, Mesa, AZ, USA; [c] Physician Assistant Studies Program, College of Health Science, Charleston Southern University, Health Science Building 9200 University Boulevard, Charleston, SC 29406, USA
[1] Present address: 117 Moon Shadow Lane, Summerville, SC 29485.
* Corresponding author. 1483 Gator Trak, Charleston, SC 29414.
E-mail address: derr@ohsu.edu

Physician Assist Clin 10 (2025) 189–199
https://doi.org/10.1016/j.cpha.2024.11.003
physicianassistant.theclinics.com
2405-7991/25/© 2024 Elsevier Inc. All rights are reserved, including those for text and data mining, AI training, and similar technologies.

Abbreviations	
ASCVD	atherosclerotic cardiovascular disease
BP	blood pressure
CAD	coronary artery disease
CVDs	cardiovascular diseases
EC	endothelial cell
FH	hypercholesterolemia
HTN	hypertension
LDL	low-density lipoprotein
LDL-C	low-density lipoprotein cholesterol
oxLDL	oxidation of LDL
TG	triglyceride
VSMCs	vascular smooth muscle cells

to plaque formation and progression, often resulting in severe vascular complications if untreated.

DEFINITIONS

- *ASCVD*: A condition characterized by the accumulation of cholesterol-rich plaque in the arteries, leading to narrowing and hardening of these vessels. This can impede blood flow and increase the risk of cardiovascular events such as heart attack, stroke, and peripheral artery disease.[1]
- *Endothelial dysfunction*: A condition where the inner lining of blood vessels loses its normal function. This dysfunction is marked by a reduced ability of the endothelium to produce vasodilators such as nitric oxide, which helps in the relaxation of blood vessels. It also involves an increased production of vasoconstrictors, proinflammatory markers, and prothrombotic factors. This shift in balance leads to impaired blood vessel dilation, increased vascular inflammation, and a higher tendency for clot formation, contributing to the development of cardiovascular diseases (CVDs).[2]
- *Plaque rupture*: A critical event in the pathogenesis of most acute coronary syndromes. It occurs when the fibrous cap of an atherosclerotic plaque within an artery wall breaks or tears, exposing the underlying core of lipids and necrotic tissue to the bloodstream. This exposure can lead to rapid thrombosis, which can obstruct blood flow and result in myocardial infarction or stroke.[3]
- *Ischemia*: A condition where there is a reduction in blood flow to a part of the body, usually due to a blockage in one or more arteries. This reduced blood flow limits the oxygen supply to the tissues, which can cause cells to function improperly or die. Ischemia is a critical factor in various medical conditions, including heart attacks, strokes, and peripheral artery disease.[4]
- *Coronary artery disease (CAD)*: A condition characterized by the narrowing of the coronary arteries due to the buildup of plaque—a mix of fat, cholesterol, and other substances. This process is known as atherosclerosis. The narrowing can reduce blood flow to the heart muscle, causing chest pain, shortness of breath, and other cardiac symptoms. If a plaque ruptures, it can lead to a complete blockage of the artery, resulting in a myocardial infarction or sudden cardiac death.[5]

DISCUSSION
Epidemiology of Atherosclerotic Cardiovascular Disease

ASCVD is among the leading global causes of mortality. Data from the World Health Organization indicate that CVDs are responsible for approximately 17.9 million deaths each year, accounting for 32% of all global deaths, with a significant portion attributed to ASCVD, particularly CAD and stroke.[6] In the United States, ASCVD affects around 18.2 million adults, or 7.6% of the population aged 20 years and older, and is responsible for about one in four deaths.[7–9] The incidence of ASCVD worldwide varies by geographic region, lifestyle, and access to health care. High-income nations have seen declines in ASCVD rates due to advancements in health care and preventive interventions,[10] whereas low-income and middle-income countries are experiencing rising ASCVD rates.[11] The Global Burden of Cardiovascular Diseases and Risk Factors Study highlights that ischemic heart disease, a primary form of ASCVD, results in 9.1 million cases annually.[12] Certain demographic factors also affect ASCVD prevalence; for instance, men in the United States have a higher ASCVD prevalence than women in most age groups, although this gap narrows postmenopause.[13] Additionally, Black adults are at a greater ASCVD risk compared to White, Hispanic, and Asian populations,[9,13] and the American Heart Association notes that ASCVD prevalence rises significantly after the age of 45 years in men and the age of 55 years in women.[13]

Recent epidemiologic trends illustrate how lifestyle factors like poor diet, physical inactivity, and smoking significantly contribute to ASCVD prevalence, particularly in developing countries.[11,13] Obesity and diabetes, which are rising globally, further increase ASCVD risk. In contrast, certain high-income countries have managed to curb ASCVD rates through public health initiatives promoting healthier diets, smoking cessation, and physical activity.[11,13] Medical advancements, including statins for cholesterol control,[14] antiplatelet therapy,[15] and revascularization procedures,[16] have also led to lower mortality rates and improved patient outcomes.[17] Comprehensive health care systems have seen significant reductions in ASCVD incidence and mortality over the past several decades.[11,13] Policies targeting ASCVD risk factors, such as smoking bans in the United States[18] and regulations to reduce trans fats and sodium in processed foods,[19] have been effective in lowering ASCVD risk, especially in high-income regions.

For practicing physician assistants, the practical implications of these trends emphasize the importance of early detection and risk factor management to reduce ASCVD morbidity and mortality.[20] Tools like the ASCVD Risk Calculator, which assesses 10 year cardiovascular event risk based on factors such as age, cholesterol levels, blood pressure, smoking status, and diabetes, are recommended for routine use in clinical practice.[1] Patient education should prioritize modifiable lifestyle risk factors, including adopting a heart-healthy diet, engaging in regular physical activity, and smoking cessation.[1] Additionally, health care providers should stress the importance of medication adherence, particularly for patients prescribed statins or antihypertensives, as it is critical to long-term ASCVD prevention. Education on recognizing early cardiovascular event signs can further enable timely medical interventions.[1] Broad public health approaches, such as campaigns to reduce obesity and community initiatives promoting physical activity, are essential to alleviating ASCVD's population-level burden. Policies supporting healthier food options in schools, workplaces, and community settings could further assist in ASCVD prevention efforts.

Pathophysiology of Atherosclerosis

ASCVD is characterized by dysfunction across multiple aspects of the coronary vasculature. Central to this dysfunction is chronic lipid accumulation and the activation of inflammatory pathways, which drive the disease's progression.[21] Unlike the passive deposition of lipids in the arterial wall, atherosclerotic plaque formation is an active and chronic process.[22] This process initiates with endothelial cell (EC) dysfunction, subsequently leading to the formation of fatty streaks, the development of fibroatheromas, and ultimately the emergence of complex atherosclerotic lesions.

Endothelial dysfunction

Atherosclerosis begins with EC dysfunction,[23] a process central to ASCVD development. ECs are integral to the vascular endothelial lining and maintain vascular homeostasis by interacting with blood components, including lipids, red and white blood cells, inflammatory mediators, and platelets.[22] ECs release nitric oxide, a critical vasodilator, and express adhesion molecules that influence platelet aggregation.[22] When endothelial dysfunction occurs, lipids infiltrate the subendothelial space, initiating the accumulation of lipids within the arterial wall.[22] Additionally, EC dysfunction leads to increased vasoconstriction, further narrowing the lumen and increasing ischemic risk. It also initiates a proinflammatory and prothrombotic state in the vascular intima, marked by an increased cytokine release, platelet activation, and oxidative stress.[22] Areas with turbulent blood flow, such as coronary artery bifurcations, are especially prone to endothelial injury.[22]

Fatty streak formation

Fatty streak formation follows the migration of lipid particles from the vascular lumen into the subendothelial space.[24] This process often begins in childhood[25] and occurs mainly in areas of low and oscillatory shear stress, notably at arterial bifurcations.[21,25] Lipid infiltration occurs due to the compromised ECs, setting the stage for atherogenesis.[21] Fatty streaks advance to fibroatheroma as circulating low-density lipoprotein (LDL) particles increase, underscoring the importance of lipid accumulation in atherosclerosis progression.[21,24] The presence of inflammatory cells within early atherosclerotic lesions highlights the persistent inflammatory response triggered by lipid deposits.[22]

Fibroatheroma

The subendothelial lipid particles undergo enzymatic transformations that promote a proinflammatory environment in the arterial wall, with LDL identified as a particularly atherogenic particle.[21] In this phase, the primary subendothelial reaction that drives plaque formation is the oxidation of LDL (oxLDL), which occurs through interactions with cytokines and chemokines.[22] OxLDL stimulates macrophage migration into the subendothelial layer, perpetuating inflammation.[26] In addition, foam cells, derived from macrophages, accumulate lipids, leading to cytoplasmic foamy appearances and contributing to further lipid retention and inflammatory responses.[23] These foam cells eventually undergo apoptosis, adding cellular debris to the developing lesion.[27] Vascular smooth muscle cells (VSMCs) migrate into the subendothelial space, further contributing to lesion development by proliferating in response to local inflammatory mediators.[21] As the plaque thickens, hypoxia develops, triggering angiogenesis, which increases plaque size and inflammation, leading to the formation of a necrotic core.[22]

Plaque rupture

Plaque progression ultimately leads to a stage where rupture may occur, although the mechanisms behind this are not fully understood. Vulnerable plaques, prone to rupture, generally contain large lipid cores and necrotic centers.[26] The fibrous cap, which separates the vessel lumen from the necrotic core, is susceptible to injury and degradation. ECs within the fibrous cap are often thin and fragile, making them more vulnerable to damage, which can expose proinflammatory and prothrombotic materials, encouraging platelet and red blood cell deposition that increases thrombus formation. When the fibrous cap degrades due to macrophage activity, plaque stability declines, raising the risk of rupture and adverse cardiovascular events. Studies indicate that intact fibrous caps are less associated with lipid-rich plaque and that ruptured plaques correlate with poorer Major Adverse Cardiovascular Events (MACE)-free survival outcomes compared to intact caps.[26]

Atherosclerosis is a multifocal, slowly progressive process characterized by multiple pathologic mechanisms that disrupt vascular homeostasis, ultimately leading to vessel dysfunction and potential occlusion. This progression from endothelial dysfunction to plaque formation and eventual rupture underscores the complex interplay of lipid accumulation, chronic inflammation, and cellular changes within the arterial wall. Understanding these stages is crucial for developing targeted interventions, as each phase presents unique opportunities for clinical management aimed at preventing lesion growth, stabilizing vulnerable plaques, and reducing the risk of cardiovascular events associated with atherosclerotic disease.

Risk Factors and Their Interactions

ASCVD is a complex, multifactorial condition driven by multiple established risk factors. These factors include hypercholesterolemia, smoking, hypertension (HTN), diabetes mellitus, age, male gender, and family history, each contributing uniquely to ASCVD risk.[28] These risk factors are known to accelerate vascular damage and promote lipid infiltration into the arterial wall, ultimately fostering an environment conducive to ASCVD progression.[21]

Hypercholesterolemia is the most prevalent risk factor among patients diagnosed with ASCVD, and it significantly elevates the risk for both subclinical and clinical disease progression.[21] Both elevated low-density lipoprotein cholesterol (LDL-C) and elevated triglyceride (TG) levels are implicated in an increased ASCVD risk, although LDL-C is recognized as the most significant causal factor over decades of research.[29] Studies indicate that LDL-C-lowering therapies can reduce ASCVD risk by up to 80%, regardless of a patient's gender, smoking status, or insulin resistance.[29] The sedentary lifestyle and obesity associated with modern living also contribute to hypercholesterolemia, further emphasizing its role in ASCVD risk.[25]

Smoking has long been established as a critical risk factor for ASCVD, doubling an individual's risk and amplifying it further when combined with conditions like HTN, diabetes, and hyperlipidemia.[28] Studies show that smokers, regardless of gender, face a higher likelihood of developing clinical or subclinical ASCVD than nonsmokers.[30] Notably, smoking cessation has been shown to reduce plaque burden, underscoring the benefit of cessation interventions for patients with ASCVD.[30] The combination of smoking with comorbid obesity results in an especially poor prognosis, adding to the complexity of managing ASCVD in this population.[31]

HTN is another well-recognized ASCVD risk factor, associated with significant vascular changes that exacerbate disease progression.[32] Mechanistically, HTN induces EC dysfunction and impairs vasodilation, resulting in increased vascular wall stress and frictional forces.[22] Improved blood pressure control across the population has correlated with a decline in ASCVD-related morbidity and mortality, highlighting the importance of early and sustained blood pressure management.[33] Cardioprotective medications, including beta-blockers, provide additional benefits in patients with HTN, further reducing ASCVD risks.[32]

Diabetes mellitus contributes to ASCVD risk by promoting insulin resistance and fostering a proinflammatory, prothrombotic environment within the vascular system.[34] These conditions accelerate endothelial dysfunction and create dyslipidemia, which contributes to plaque formation and progression.[24] Intensive glucose control in patients with diabetes has shown a reduction in ASCVD event rates, underlining the critical importance of diabetes management in ASCVD prevention.[27]

Advancing age is one of the most prominent risk factors for ASCVD, reflecting the chronic and cumulative nature of atherosclerotic plaque formation.[24] With age, individuals experience increased VSMC proliferation and hematopoietic changes, which contribute to endothelial injury and ASCVD risk.[22] The likelihood of ASCVD-related conditions such as hyperlipidemia, HTN, and diabetes also increases with age, further compounding the risk.[28]

Men are at higher risk for ASCVD than women, often presenting with the disease at an earlier age despite comparable lipid levels.[35] Women, however, generally present with ASCVD later in life, partially due to the protective effects of estrogen before menopause.[36] This gender disparity underscores the role of sex hormones in ASCVD pathogenesis and the importance of personalized prevention strategies.[35]

Genetic predisposition plays a significant role in ASCVD, with family history often correlating with an increased disease incidence (**Table 1**). Genetics affect lipid metabolism, which can lead to an early onset of ASCVD, particularly in cases of familial hypercholesterolemia (FH).[29] FH, one of the most common hereditary lipid disorders, is associated with an 18 fold increased ASCVD risk, with homozygous individuals potentially showing symptoms as early as childhood.[28]

Practical Risk Assessment Tools

A variety of tools and models for ASCVD risk assessment are available to clinicians, each offering distinct advantages for patient evaluation. The Framingham Risk Score, derived from data from the Framingham Heart Study,[36,37] is a widely recognized tool that estimates the 10 year risk of coronary heart disease based on factors such as age, sex, total and high-density lipoprotein (HDL) cholesterol, smoking status, and systolic blood pressure.[38] Another prominent tool introduced by the American College of Cardiology/American Heart Association (ACC/AHA) guidelines[39] provides a broader calculation of 10 year ASCVD risk, estimating risks for coronary death, nonfatal

Table 1
Key atherosclerotic cardiovascular disease risk factors, impacts, and clinical considerations

Risk Factor	Impact on ASCVD	Clinical Considerations
Hypercholesterolemia	Increases LDL-C/TG, accelerates plaque formation	Monitor LDL-C; consider statins for high-risk patients
Smoking	Doubles ASCVD risk; worsens with obesity, HTN, and diabetes	Encourage cessation; highlight elevated risk in all smokers
HTN	Heightens vascular stress, endothelial dysfunction	Regular blood pressure (BP) checks; use beta-blockers if indicated
Diabetes mellitus	Causes insulin resistance, proinflammatory/prothrombotic states	Promote glucose control, lifestyle changes
Age	Elevates ASCVD risk with vascular changes over time	Screen men >45 y, women >55 y; manage age-related factors
Male gender	Higher ASCVD risk, earlier onset	Emphasize early screening and prevention
Genetics and family history	FH raises early ASCVD risk	Screen for family history; consider genetic counseling

Table 2
Comparison of atherosclerotic cardiovascular disease risk assessment tools

Risk Assessment Tool	Framingham Risk Score	ACC/AHA ASCVD Risk Calculator	ACC ASCVD Risk Estimator Plus
Description	10 y CHD risk based on traditional factors	Broader 10 y ASCVD risk, including coronary death and myocardial infarction (MI)	Estimates both 10 y and lifetime ASCVD risk
Key features	Age, sex, cholesterol, smoking, and BP	Adds diabetes and race	Comprehensive, supports both short-term and long-term risks
Strengths	Simple, primary care-friendly	Inclusive of diverse populations	Patient-centered, supports personalized discussions
Limitations	May underestimate non-White risk	Possible overestimation for some groups	Complex input, challenging for routine use

myocardial infarction, and stroke while including additional factors like diabetes and race.[40] The most recent addition, the ACC ASCVD Risk Estimator Plus, builds on these models by offering both 10 year and lifetime risk estimates, incorporating the latest research findings to support more personalized patient consultations.[41]

These tools are essential in clinical practice as they enable health care providers to accurately predict cardiovascular risk and identify individuals at high risk who may benefit from preventive interventions. Using such risk assessment models allows clinicians to personalize treatment approaches, ranging from lifestyle modifications to pharmacotherapy, which can significantly reduce ASCVD morbidity and mortality among high-risk patients. By assessing each patient's unique risk profile, health care providers can initiate tailored preventive strategies, enhancing overall outcomes in cardiovascular health.

When comparing the available tools, each has specific strengths and limitations that make it suitable for different clinical contexts. The Framingham Risk Score is particularly valuable in primary care, yet it may underestimate risk in certain populations, particularly among non-White individuals.[40,42] The ACC/AHA risk calculator, however, provides a more inclusive evaluation, especially for African American patients and others from diverse backgrounds, making it more relevant in heterogeneous populations. The ACC Risk Estimator Plus is particularly beneficial in patient-centered care, offering both short-term and long-term risk assessments, though its complexity and need for detailed input can be challenging for routine use.[40,42]

Integrating risk assessment tools into patient consultations involves effectively communicating risk results to ensure patients understand their implications (**Table 2**). Utilizing visual aids such as charts or risk percentages can enhance comprehension, while discussing relatable concepts, like "risk age" or comparisons to population averages, helps patients grasp their individual risk levels.[43] After communicating these results, it is essential to engage patients in their health management plans by discussing preventive measures and their benefits. Involving patients in goal setting and encouraging them to select achievable lifestyle changes fosters active participation, increasing the likelihood of sustained behavior modifications that contribute to long-term ASCVD risk reduction.[44]

SUMMARY

In summary, ASCVD is a chronic condition driven by endothelial dysfunction and lipid accumulation, leading to plaque development and potential cardiovascular events. This article discusses key risk factors, including hypercholesterolemia, HTN, smoking, diabetes, and age, which collectively contribute to ASCVD progression. Understanding the pathophysiology of plaque formation—beginning with endothelial dysfunction and advancing to plaque rupture—is critical for clinical management. The use of risk assessment tools, such as the Framingham Risk Score and ACC/AHA Risk Estimator, provides clinicians with methods to evaluate and manage patient risk. This personalized approach can guide lifestyle and pharmacologic interventions that effectively mitigate ASCVD-related morbidity and mortality.

CLINICS CARE POINTS

- *Early identification*: Utilize ASCVD risk assessment tools, such as the ACC/AHA Risk Calculator, to identify high-risk patients early and personalize intervention strategies.
- *Targeted education*: Educate patients on the importance of managing modifiable risk factors like diet, exercise, and smoking cessation to reduce ASCVD risk.

- *Pharmacologic management*: For patients with elevated LDL and TGs, consider lipid-lowering therapies, such as statins, to reduce plaque buildup and prevent disease progression.

- *Addressing comorbidities*: Monitor and manage HTN, diabetes, and obesity as they significantly increase ASCVD risk.

- *Patient engagement*: Use visual aids to communicate risk and engage patients actively in setting realistic health goals to foster long-term adherence.

DISCLOSURE

The authors have nothing to disclose.

REFERENCES

1. Arnett DK, Blumenthal RS, Albert MA, et al. 2019 ACC/AHA guideline on the primary prevention of cardiovascular disease: a report of the American college of cardiology/American heart association task force on clinical practice guidelines. Circulation 2019;140(11). https://doi.org/10.1161/CIR.0000000000000678.
2. Herrera MD, Mingorance C, Rodríguez-Rodríguez R, et al. Endothelial dysfunction and aging: an update. Ageing Res Rev 2010;9(2):142–52.
3. Falk E, Shah PK, Fuster V. Coronary plaque disruption. Circulation 1995;92(3): 657–71.
4. Yellon DM, Hausenloy DJ. Myocardial reperfusion injury. N Engl J Med 2007; 357(11):1121–35.
5. Boden WE, O'Rourke RA, Teo KK, et al. Optimal medical therapy with or without PCI for stable coronary disease. N Engl J Med 2007;356(15):1503–16.
6. Cardiovascular diseases (cvds). World Health Organization; 2021. Available at: https://www.who.int/news-room/fact-sheets/detail/cardiovascular-diseases-(cvds). Accessed October 14, 2024.
7. Alanaeme CJ, Bittner V, Brown TM, et al. Estimated number and percentage of US adults with atherosclerotic cardiovascular disease recommended add-on lipid-lowering therapy by the 2018 AHA/ACC multi-society cholesterol guideline. Am Heart J 2022;21:100201.
8. Brown JC, Gerhardt TE, Kwon E. Risk factors for coronary artery disease. StatPearls 2023. Available at: https://www.ncbi.nlm.nih.gov/books/NBK554410/. Accessed October 14, 2024.
9. Martin SS, Aday AW, Almarzooq ZI, et al. 2024 heart disease and stroke statistics: a report of US and global data from the American heart association. Circulation (New York, N.Y.) 2024;149:e347.
10. Rikhi R, Shapiro MD. Assessment of atherosclerotic cardiovascular disease risk in primary prevention. J Cardiopulm Rehabil Prev 2022;42(6):397–403.
11. Ray KK, Ference BA, Séverin T, et al. World heart federation cholesterol roadmap 2022. Global heart 2022;17:75.
12. Roth GA, Mensah GA, Johnson CO, et al. Global burden of cardiovascular diseases and risk factors, 1990-2019: update from the GBD 2019 study. J Am Coll Cardiol 2020;76:2982–3021.
13. Tsao CW, Aday AW, Almarzooq ZI, et al. Heart disease and stroke statistics-2022 update: a report from the American heart association. Circulation (New York, N.Y.) 2022;145:e153.

14. Collins R, Reith C, Emberson J, et al. Interpretation of the evidence for the efficacy and safety of statin therapy. Lancet 2016;388(10059):2532–61.

15. Capodanno D, Alfonso F, Levine GN, et al. ACC/AHA versus ESC guidelines on dual antiplatelet therapy: JACC guideline comparison. J Am Coll Cardiol 2018; 72(23):2915–31.

16. Fihn SD, Gardin JM, Abrams J, et al. 2012 ACCF/AHA/ACP/AATS/PCNA/SCAI/STS guideline for the diagnosis and management of patients with stable ischemic heart disease. J Am Coll Cardiol 2012;60(24). https://doi.org/10.1016/j.jacc.2012.07.013.

17. Ford ES, Ajani UA, Croft JB, et al. Explaining the decrease in U.S. deaths from coronary disease, 1980-2000. N Engl J Med 2007;356(23):2388–98.

18. Meyers DG, Neuberger JS, He J. Cardiovascular effect of bans on smoking in public places. J Am Coll Cardiol 2009;54:1249–55.

19. He FJ, MacGregor GA. Role of salt intake in prevention of cardiovascular disease: controversies and challenges. Nat Rev Cardiol 2018;15:371–7.

20. Yusuf S, Hawken S, Ounpuu S, et al. Effect of potentially modifiable risk factors associated with myocardial infarction in 52 countries (the INTERHEART study): case-control study. Lancet 2004;364(9438):937–52.

21. Summerhill VI, Grechko AV, Yet SF, et al. The atherogenic role of circulating modified lipids in atherosclerosis. Int J Mol Sci 2019;20(14):3561.

22. Wojtasińska A, Frąk W, Lisińska W, et al. Novel insights into the molecular mechanisms of atherosclerosis. Int J Mol Sci 2023;24(17):13434.

23. Wang Y, Chen Z, Zhu Q, et al. Aiming at early-stage vulnerable plaques: a nano-platform with dual-mode imaging and lipid-inflammation integrated regulation for atherosclerotic theranostics. Bioact Mater 2024;37:94–105.

24. Ala-Korpela M. The culprit is the carrier, not the loads: cholesterol, triglycerides and apolipoprotein B in atherosclerosis and coronary heart disease. Int J Epidemiol 2019;48(5):1389–92.

25. Pahwa R, Ishwarlal J. Atherosclerosis. StatPearls. 2023. Available at: https://www.ncbi.nlm.nih.gov/books/NBK507799/. Accessed October 30, 2024.

26. Hoshino M, Yonetsu T, Usui E, et al. Clinical significance of the presence or absence of lipid-rich plaque underneath intact fibrous cap plaque in acute coronary syndrome. J Am Heart Assoc 2019;8(9). https://doi.org/10.1161/jaha.118.011820.

27. Doodnauth SA, Grinstein S, Maxson ME. Constitutive and stimulated macropinocytosis in macrophages: roles in immunity and in the pathogenesis of atherosclerosis. Philos Trans R Soc Lond Ser B Biol Sci 2019;374(1765):20180147.

28. Stone NJ, Smith J, Orringer CE, et al. Managing atherosclerotic cardiovascular risk in young adults: JACC state-of-the-art review. J Am Coll Cardiol 2022; 79(8):819–36.

29. Ferhatbegović L, Mršić D, Kušljugić S, et al. LDL-C: the only causal risk factor for ASCVD. Why is it still overlooked and underestimated? Curr Atheroscler Rep 2022;24(8):635–42.

30. Katz B, Dwivedi A, Achenbach S, et al. Impact of sex and smoking on coronary artery disease extent and severity by coronary CT angiography: results from the CONFIRM (coronary CT angiography evaluation for clinical outcomes: an international multicenter) registry. J Am Coll Cardiol 2018;71(11). https://doi.org/10.1016/S0735-1097(18)32175-2.

31. Tsioufis KP, Kasiakogias A, Konstantinidis D, et al. Combined patterns of obesity and smoking status for prediction of coronary artery disease: a follow-up study on

treated hypertensive patients. J Am Coll Cardiol 2018;71(11). https://doi.org/10.1016/S0735-1097(18)32397-0.

32. Vrablik M, Corsini A, Tůmová E. Beta-blockers for atherosclerosis prevention: a missed opportunity? Curr Atheroscler Rep 2022;24(3):161–9.

33. Rubin JB, Borden WB. Coronary heart disease in young adults. Curr Atheroscler Rep 2012;14(2):140–9.

34. Di Pino A, DeFronzo RA. Insulin resistance and atherosclerosis: implications for insulin-sensitizing agents. Endocr Rev 2019;40(6):1447–67.

35. Dharmayat KI, Watts GF, Aguilar-Salinas CA, et al. Global perspective of familial hypercholesterolaemia: a cross-sectional study from the EAS Familial Hypercholesterolaemia Studies Collaboration (FHSC). Lancet 2021;398(10312):1713–25.

36. Bigeh A, Shekar C, Gulati M. Sex differences in coronary artery calcium and long-term CV mortality. Curr Cardiol Rep 2020;22(4):21.

37. Framingham heart study. Available at: https://www.framinghamheartstudy.org/. Accessed October 14, 2024.

38. American Heart Association. ASCVD risk estimator Plus. Available at: https://static.heart.org/riskcalc/app/index.html#!/baseline-risk. Accessed October 3, 2024.

39. Goff D, Lloyd-Jones D, Bennett G, et al. 2013 ACC/AHA guideline on the assessment of cardiovascular risk: a report of the American college of cardiology/American heart association task force on practice guidelines. J Am Coll Cardiol 2014; 63(25_Part_B):2935–59.

40. Lloyd-Jones DM, Braun LT, Ndumele CE, et al. Use of risk assessment tools to guide decision-making in the primary prevention of atherosclerotic cardiovascular disease: a special report from the American heart association and American college of cardiology. Circulation (New York, N.Y.) 2019;139:e1162–77.

41. American College of Cardiology. ASCVD risk estimator Plus. Available at: https://tools.acc.org/ASCVD-Risk-Estimator-Plus. Accessed October 3, 2024.

42. Wong ND, Budoff MJ, Ferdinand K, et al. Atherosclerotic cardiovascular disease risk assessment: an American Society for Preventive Cardiology clinical practice statement. Am J Prev Cardiol 2022;10:100335.

43. Andersson EM, Liv P, Nordin S, et al. Does a multi-component intervention including pictorial risk communication about subclinical atherosclerosis improve perceptions of cardiovascular disease risk without deteriorating efficacy beliefs? Soc Sci Med 2024;341:116530.

44. Davidson KW, Mangione CM, Barry MJ, et al. Collaboration and shared decision-making between patients and clinicians in preventive health care decisions and US preventive services task force recommendations. JAMA 2022;327:1171–6.

Hypertension
A Primer on Primary and Secondary Hypertension

Sondra DePalma, DHSc, PA-C, CLS, CHC, FNLA, AACC, DFAAPA[a,b,*]

KEYWORDS

• Hypertension • Blood pressure • Cardiology • Cardiovascular

KEY POINTS

- Hypertension (HTN) is a prevalent condition affecting nearly half (48.1%) of all adults in the United States (119.9 million).
- More than 3 in 4 adults with HTN (77.5%, 92.9 million) do not have their blood pressure adequately controlled.
- Effective treatment of HTN reduces the risk of all-cause mortality, morbidity, disability, and decreased quality of life.

INTRODUCTION

Hypertension (HTN) is associated with a considerably increased risk of cardiovascular disease (CVD), including atherosclerotic cardiovascular disease (ASCVD), peripheral artery disease, myocardial infarction, stroke, heart failure, and atrial fibrillation; chronic kidney disease (CKD); and cognitive impairment. HTN is the most significant modifiable risk factor for all-cause morbidity and mortality.[1] Nearly half (48.1%) of all adults in the United States (119.9 million) have HTN but more than 3 in 4 adults with HTN (77.5%, 92.9 million) do not have their blood pressure (BP) controlled, contributing to avoidable morbidity and mortality, decreased quality of life, and increased disability–adjusted life years and economic costs.[2,3]

CLASSIFICATIONS OF HYPERTENSION

There is no definitive threshold at which a given BP presents the absence or presence of risk; however, definitions of elevated BP and HTN are helpful for assessing population health, making decisions about nonpharmacologic and pharmacologic

[a] Reimbursement and Professional Advocacy, American Academy of Physician Associates, 2318 Mill Road, Suite 1300, Alexandria, VA 22314, USA; [b] Doctor of Medical Science Program, A.T. Still University, Arizona School of Health Sciences, 5850 E Still Circle, Mesa, AZ 85206, USA
* Corresponding author.
E-mail address: sdepalma@aapa.org

Physician Assist Clin 10 (2025) 201–212
https://doi.org/10.1016/j.cpha.2024.11.001   **physicianassistant.theclinics.com**

interventions, and monitoring the effectiveness of therapies. Definitions of HTN are based on estimates of risks versus treatment benefits and vary depending on different guidelines. One of the more widely used classifications of HTN in the United States is the multi-organization 2017 guideline for high BP in adults.[4,5] According to the 2017 ACC/AHA/AAPA/ABC/ACPM/AGS/APhA/ASH/ASPC/NMA/PCNA guideline for the prevention, detection, evaluation, and management of high BP in adults, normal, elevated, stage 1 HTN, and stage 2 HTN should be classified according to **Table 1**.

Primary and Secondary Hypertension

HTN is also classified as primary versus secondary. Primary HTN is the most common form of high BP and is categorized as such when there is no definitive cause. It usually occurs because of a combination of any of the following factors: genetics, age, lifestyle, and/or physiologic and environmental factors. Secondary HTN can be attributed to an underlying condition or cause and should be suspected in younger patients (<30 years) when there is a sudden onset of elevated BP or increased BP in patients who were previously controlled on medications, with resistant HTN (RH), and when target organ damage is disproportionate to the duration or severity of the HTN.[4,6] Causes (with prevalence) of secondary HTN include obstructive sleep apnea (25%–50%), renovascular disease (5%–34%), primary aldosteronism (8%–20%), drug or alcohol-induced (2%–4%), renal parenchymal disease (1%–2%), and other causes (>1%).[4]

Resistant Hypertension

RH is defined as BP above the treatment goal on 3 maximally tolerated antihypertensives from different drug classes or BP treated to goal on 4 agents. A diagnosis of RH requires assurance of patient adherence to prescribed medications, proper BP measurement technique, and confirmation of HTN outside the office setting with either 24-h ambulatory BP monitoring or self-measured home BP measurement with a validated digital device. Practitioner awareness of RH is important because patients with RH are at increased risk of death, CVD, myocardial infarction, stroke, heart failure, CKD, and end-stage renal disease.[6,7]

EVALUATION

It is essential to measure BP accurately and an average of 2 to 3 BP measurements should be used on 2 to 3 separate occasions. A validated BP measurement device and a properly fitting cuff are needed. The patient should quietly sit in a chair for

Table 1
Blood pressure categories in adults

BP Category	Systolic Blood Pressure		Diastolic Blood Pressure
Normal	<120 mm Hg	and	<80 mm Hg
Elevated	120–129 mm Hg	and	<80 mm Hg
Stage 1 HTN	130–139 mm Hg	or	80–90 mm Hg
Stage 2 HTN	≥140 mm Hg	or	≥90 mm Hg

Adapted from Whelton PK, Carey RM, Aronow WS et al. 2017 ACC/AHA/AAPA/ABC/ACPM/AGS/APhA/ASH/ASPC/NMA/PCNA guideline for the prevention, detection, evaluation, and management of high blood pressure in adults. *J Am Coll Cardiol*. 2018; 71(19): e127-e248. https://doi.org/10.1016/j.jacc.2017.11.006.

5 minutes and have their arm supported. The patient should avoid caffeine, exercise, and smoking for at least 30 minutes before BP measurement and have an empty bladder. At the first visit, it is recommended that BP be measured in both arms, with the arm that gives the higher reading used for subsequent measurement.[4]

Specific laboratory measurements and diagnostic tests should be obtained when HTN is newly diagnosed to estimate CVD risk, establish a baseline for medication use, and screen for secondary causes of HTN. Basic recommended testing includes fasting blood glucose, complete blood count, lipid profile, serum creatinine with estimated glomerular filtration rate, thyroid stimulating hormone, serum sodium/potassium/calcium, urinalysis, and electrocardiogram. An echocardiogram, uric acid, and urinary albumin to creatine ratio may also be used to assess the secondary causes of HTN and/or target-organ damage. CVD risk should be assessed using the American College of Cardiology/American Heart Association Pooled Cohort Equations (http://tools.acc.org/ASCVD-Risk-Estimator/) to estimate the 10-year risk of ASCVD and establish the BP threshold for treatment.[4]

Screening for secondary HTN is recommended in patients with resistant HTN, abrupt onset with age less than 30 years, onset of diastolic HTN in older adults (ie, age $\geq$ 65 years), excessive target organ damage (eg, CVD, peripheral artery disease, cerebrovascular disease, left ventricular hypertrophy, heart failure with preserved or reduced ejection fraction, retinopathy, CKD, or albuminuria), or in the presence of unprovoked or excessive hypokalemia. Screening for drug-induced HTN should occur, and identified substances (eg, nonsteroidal anti-inflammatory drugs, sympathomimetics, stimulants, oral contraceptives) ought to be discontinued or minimized.[4]

Many of the causes of secondary HTN are associated with clinical examination findings that suggest the etiology, and additional diagnostic tests are recommended based on those findings. For example, polysomnography is indicated in patients with RH, symptoms of obstructive sleep apnea, and physical findings of obesity and Mallampati class III–IV. Patients with an abdominal bruit and RH, HTN of abrupt onset or worsening/increasingly challenging to control, or early onset may have renovascular disease and assessment with a renal Duplex Doppler ultrasound, abdominal computed tomography, or magnetic resonance imaging should be considered. Another prevalent cause of secondary HTN, primary aldosteronism, should be suspected when RH is associated with spontaneous or diuretic-induced hypokalemia, and the plasma aldosterone/renin ratio under standardized conditions should be evaluated. Other screening tests should be performed based on signs, symptoms, and clinical indications.[4] See **Table 2** for a complete list of secondary causes of HTN, their prevalence, clinical indications and physical examination findings, screening tests, and additional and/or confirmatory tests.

MANAGEMENT

Most patients with HTN should be treated with evidence-based nonpharmacologic and pharmacologic interventions, when appropriate, to a goal systolic BP of less than 130/80 mm Hg. Pharmacologic therapy is recommended for ambulatory, community-dwelling adults with stage 1 HTN (BP 130–139/80–89 mm Hg) and clinical ASCVD, diabetes, CKD, or an estimated 10-year CVD risk greater than or equal to 10% and in stage 2 HTN (BP $\geq$ 140/90 mm Hg). Less aggressive management may be warranted in older adults ($\geq$65 years of age) with a high burden of comorbidity and/or limited life expectancy, institutionalized individuals with poor prognosis, or based on clinical judgment or patient preference.[4]

Table 2
Causes of secondary hypertension with clinical indications and diagnostic screening tests

	Prevalence	Clinical Indications	Physical Examination	Screening Tests	Additional/Confirmatory Tests
Common causes					
Renal parenchymal disease	1%–2%	Urinary tract infections; obstruction, hematuria; urinary frequency and nocturia; analgesic abuse; family history of polycystic kidney disease; elevated serum creatinine; abnormal urinalysis	Abdominal mass (polycystic kidney disease); skin pallor	Renal ultrasound	Tests to evaluate cause of renal disease
Renovascular disease	5%–34%[a]	RH; HTN of abrupt onset or worsening or increasingly difficult to control; flash pulmonary edema (atherosclerotic); early-onset HTN, especially in women (fibromuscular hyperplasia)	Abdominal systolic-diastolic bruit; bruits over other arteries (carotid – atherosclerotic or fibromuscular dysplasia), femoral	Renal Duplex Doppler ultrasound; MRA; abdominal CT	Bilateral selective renal intra-arterial angiography
Primary aldosteronism	8%–20%[b]	RH; HTN with hypokalemia (spontaneous or diuretic induced); HTN and muscle cramps or weakness; HTN and incidentally discovered adrenal mass; HTN and obstructive sleep apnea; HTN and family history of early-onset HTN or stroke	Arrhythmias (with hypokalemia); especially atrial fibrillation	Plasma aldosterone/renin ratio under standardized conditions (correction of hypokalemia and withdrawal of aldosterone antagonists for 4–6 wk)	Oral sodium loading test (with 24-h urine aldosterone) or IV saline infusion test with plasma aldosterone at 4 h of infusion Adrenal CT scan, adrenal vein sampling.

Obstructive sleep apnea[c]	25%–50%	RH; snoring; fitful sleep; breathing pauses during sleep; daytime sleepiness	Obesity, Mallampati class III–IV; loss of normal nocturnal BP fall	Berlin Questionnaire Epworth Sleepiness Score overnight oximetry	Polysomnography
Drug or alcohol induced[d]	2%–4%	Sodium-containing antacids; caffeine; nicotine (smoking); alcohol; NSAIDs; oral contraceptives; cyclosporine or tacrolimus; sympathomimetics (decongestants, anorectics); cocaine, amphetamines and other illicit drugs; neuropsychiatric agents; erythropoiesis-stimulating agents; clonidine withdrawal; herbal agents (Ma Huang, ephedra)	Fine tremor, tachycardia, sweating (cocaine, ephedrine, MAO inhibitors); acute abdominal pain (cocaine)	Urinary drug screen (illicit drugs)	Response to withdrawal of suspected agent
Uncommon causes					
Pheochromocytoma/ paraganglioma	0.1%–0.6%	RH; paroxysmal HTN or crisis superimposed on sustained HTN; "spells," BP lability, headache, sweating, palpitations, pallor; positive family history of pheochromocytoma/ paraganglioma; adrenal incidentaloma	Skin stigmata of neurofibromatosis (café-au-lait spots; neurofibromas); Orthostatic hypotension	24-h urinary fractionated metanephrines or plasma metanephrines under standard conditions (supine position with indwelling IV cannula)	CT or MRI scan of abdomen/ pelvis

(continued on next page)

Table 2
(continued)

	Prevalence	Clinical Indications	Physical Examination	Screening Tests	Additional/Confirmatory Tests
Cushing's syndrome	<0.1%	Rapid weight gain, especially with central distribution; proximal muscle weakness; depression; hyperglycemia	Central obesity, "moon" face, dorsal and supraclavicular fat pads, wide (1-cm) violaceous striae, hirsutism	Overnight 1-mg dexamethasone suppression test	24-h urinary free cortisol excretion (preferably multiple); midnight salivary cortisol
Hypothyroidism	<1%	Dry skin; cold intolerance; constipation; hoarseness; weight gain	Delayed ankle reflex; periorbital puffiness; coarse skin; cold skin; slow movement; goiter	Thyroid-stimulating hormone; free thyroxine	None
Hyperthyroidism	<1%	Warm, moist skin; heat intolerance; nervousness; tremulousness; insomnia; weight loss; diarrhea; proximal muscle weakness	Lid lag; fine tremor of the outstretched hands; warm, moist skin	Thyroid-stimulating hormone; free thyroxine	Radioactive iodine uptake and scan
Aortic coarctation (undiagnosed or repaired)	0.1%	Young patient with HTN (<30 y of age)	BP higher in upper extremities than in lower extremities; absent femoral pulses; continuous murmur over patient's back, chest, or abdominal bruit; left thoracotomy scar (postoperative)	Echocardiogram	Thoracic and abdominal CT angiogram or MRA
Primary hyperparathyroidism	Rare	Hypercalcemia	Usually none	Serum calcium	Serum parathyroid hormone

	Prevalence				
Congenital adrenal hyperplasia	Rare	HTN and hypokalemia; virilization (11-beta-hydroxylase deficiency [11-beta-OH]); incomplete masculinization in males and primary amenorrhea in females (17-alpha-hydroxylase deficiency [17-alpha-OH])	Signs of virilization (11-beta-OH) or incomplete masculinization (17-alpha-OH)	HTN and hypokalemia with low or normal aldosterone and renin	11-beta-OH: elevated deoxycorticosterone (DOC), 11-deoxycortisol, and androgens17- alpha-OH; decreased androgens and estrogen; elevated deoxycorticosterone and corticosterone
Mineralocorticoid excess syndromes other than primary aldosteronism	Rare	Early-onset HTN; RH; hypokalemia or hyperkalemia	Arrhythmias (with hypokalemia)	Low aldosterone and renin	Urinary cortisol metabolites; genetic testing
Acromegaly	Rare	Acral features, enlarging shoe, glove, or hat size; headache; visual disturbances; diabetes mellitus	Acral features; large hands and feet; frontal bossing	Serum growth hormone ≥1 ng/mL during oral glucose load	Elevated age- and sex-matched IGF-1 level; MRI scan of the pituitary

Abbreviations: CT, computed tomography; DOC, 11-deoxycorticosterone; IGF-1, insulin-like growth factor-1; IV, intravenous; MAO, monamine oxidase; MRA, magnetic resonance arteriography; NSAIDs, nonsteroidal anti-inflammatory drugs; OH, hydroxylase; RCT, randomized clinical trial.

 a Depending on the clinical situation (HTN alone, 5%; HTN starting dialysis, 22%; HTN and peripheral vascular disease, 28%; HTN in the elderly with congestive heart failure, 34%).

b 8% in general population with HTN; up to 20% in patients with RH.

c Although obstructive sleep apnea is listed as a cause of secondary HTN, RCTs on the effects of continuous positive airway pressure on lowering BP in patients with HTN have produced mixed results (see Section 5.4.4 for details).

d For a list of frequently used drugs causing HTN and accompanying evidence, see Table 14.

From Whelton PK, Carey RM, Aronow WS et al. 2017 ACC/AHA/AAPA/ABC/ACPM/AGS/APhA/ASH/ASPC/NMA/PCNA guideline for the prevention, detection, evaluation, and management of high blood pressure in adults. *J Am Coll Cardiol.* 2018; 71(19): e127-e248. https://doi.org/10.1016/j.jacc.2017.11.006.

Follow-up after initial BP evaluation and initiating lifestyle or pharmacologic management is essential to assess adherence and response to interventions. Adults with elevated BP or stage I HTN who do not meet an indication for pharmacologic therapy should have a repeat BP evaluation in 3 to 6 months. Patients who start antihypertensive drug therapy should be reevaluated in 1 month. If, at follow-up, the target BP has not been achieved, adherence to recommended therapies should be assessed and intensification of therapy should be considered. A repeat evaluation every year is reasonable for adults with a normal BP.[4]

Lifestyle modification

Nonpharmacologic interventions are important for the prevention and management of HTN. The most important lifestyle modifications to reduce BP include a heart-healthy diet, avoidance of overweight/obesity, appropriate physical activity via a structured exercise program, sodium reduction, potassium supplementation, and alcohol moderation. All patients with elevated BP or HTN, whether on pharmacologic therapy, should be encouraged to implement the nonpharmacologic interventions listed in **Table 3** to reduce BP.[4]

Pharmacologic treatment

Antihypertensive medication, along with lifestyle modification, is an essential component of the treatment of many patients with HTN to lower BP and reduce the risk of adverse effects of high BP, including ASCVD, kidney disease, and death. Patients with stage 1 HTN and clinical ASCVD, diabetes, CKD, or estimated 10-year CVD risk greater than or equal to 10% may be started on a single, evidence-based medication. It is recommended that patients with stage 2 HTN and an average BP more than 20/10 mm Hg above their BP target be started on 2 antihypertensive drugs with different mechanisms of action.[4]

Recommended first-line agents for BP lowering include thiazide or thiazide-type diuretics, angiotensin-converting enzyme (ACE) inhibitors, angiotensin II receptor blockers (ARBs), and calcium channel blockers (CCBs). Monotherapy with a first-line agent will cause an approximate 10 to 15 mm Hg decrease in systolic BP and an 8 to 10 mm Hg decrease in diastolic BP. Dual therapy can achieve a greater than 20 mm Hg decrease in systolic BP.[8] When using combination therapy, agents with the same or similar mechanisms of action should be avoided.[4]

Diuretics

Thiazide and thiazide-type diuretics inhibit reabsorption of luminal sodium in the distal convoluted tubule of the nephron, which promotes natriuresis and diuresis.[9] Chlorthalidone is the preferred thiazide diuretic because of its prolonged half-life and favorable CVD reduction in clinical trials. Patients taking thiazide and thiazide-type diuretics should be monitored for hyponatremia, hypokalemia, hypercalcemia, and elevated uric acid levels. These agents should be used with caution in patients with a history of acute gout, unless on uric-acid lowering therapy, and are less effective in patients with moderate-to-severe CKD (eg, GFR < 30 mL/min).[4]

Although not indicated as a first-line agent for HTN in patients without specific comorbidities, loop diuretics are recommended in patients with moderate–severe CKD and symptomatic heart failure.[4] Torsemide is the preferred agent in this drug class because of it having the longest half-life compared to other loop diuretics. Agents of this class act on the sodium–potassium-chloride cotransporter along the thick ascending limb of the loop of Henle, which inhibits the reabsorption of sodium

Table 3
Evidence-based nonpharmacologic interventions, recommendations, and approximate effect on systolic BP

Intervention	Recommended Non-pharmacologic Interventions		
	Recommendation	Dose	Approximate Effect on Systolic BP in People with Hypertension
Weight Loss	Weight loss is recommended to reduce BP in adults with elevated BP or HTN who are overweight or obese.	Ideal body weight is best, but aim for at least a 1-kg reduction in body weight for most adults who are overweight/obese.	• 1 mm Hg for every 1 kg reduction
Heart-Healthy Diet	A heart-healthy diet, such as the DASH (Dietary Approaches to Stop Hypertension) diet, that facilitates achieving a desirable weight is recommended for adults with elevated BP or HTN.	Consume a diet rich in fruits, vegetables, whole grains, and low-fat dairy products, with reduced content of saturated and total fat.	• 11 mm Hg
Sodium Reduction	Sodium reduction is recommended for adults with elevated BP or HTN.	Optimal goal is <1500 mg/d, but aim for at least a 1000-mg/d reduction in most adults.	• 5/6 mm Hg
Potassium Supplementation	Potassium supplementation, preferably in dietary modification, is recommended for adults with elevated BP or HTN, unless contraindicated by the presence of CKD or use of drugs that reduce potassium excretion.	Aim for 3500–5000 mg/d, preferably by consumption of a diet rich in potassium.	• 4/5 mm Hg
Increased Physical Activity	Increased physical activity with a structured exercise program is recommended for adults with elevated BP or HTN.	Aerobic: 90–150 min/wk Dynamic Resistance: 90–150 min/wk Isometric Resistance: 3 session per week	• 5/8 mm Hg • 4 mm Hg • 5 mm Hg
Alcohol Reduction	Adult men and women with elevated BP or HTN who currently consume alcohol should be advised to drink no more than 2 and 1 standard drinks, respectively.	Men ≤ 2 drinks per day Women ≥ 1 drink per day One standard drink is equivalent to 12 oz of beer, 5 oz of wine, or 1.5 oz of distilled spirits	• 4 mm Hg

Adapted from Whelton PK, Carey RM, Aronow WS et al. 2017 ACC/AHA/AAPA/ABC/ACPM/AGS/APhA/ASH/ASPC/NMA/PCNA guideline for the prevention, detection, evaluation, and management of high blood pressure in adults. J Am Coll Cardiol. 2018; 71(19): e127-e248. https://doi.org/10.1016/j.jacc.2017.11.006.

and chloride resulting in increased freewater excretion. Loop diuretics can cause electrolyte abnormalities, skin photosensitivity, ototoxicity, and other adverse effects.[10]

Aldosterone antagonists are preferred agents in primary aldosteronism and RH. Compared to eplerenone, spironolactone is associated with a greater risk of gynecomastia and impotence.[4] These mineralocorticoid receptor antagonists decrease sodium and water retention in the distal tubules and collecting duct while increasing potassium retention.[11] Aldosterone antagonists should be avoided in patients with significant renal dysfunction and with concomitant use of potassium supplements and other potassium-sparing drugs.[4]

Angiotensin-converting enzyme inhibitors and angiotensin II receptor blockers

ACE inhibitors and ARBs are first-line agents for the treatment of HTN. ACE inhibitors interfere with the renin-angiotensin-aldosterone system and block the angiotensin-converting enzyme that converts angiotensin I to angiotensin II, the decreased production of which enhances diuresis and reduces BP.[12] The blockade of the renin-angiotensin-aldosterone system with ARBs lowers BP, reduces vascular smooth muscle contraction, systemic vascular resistance, and sympathetic activity, and decreases sodium reabsorption and water retention.[13] These agents should not be used with each other or a direct renin inhibitor. ACE inhibitors and ARBs are contraindicated in patients who are pregnant, and acute renal failure may occur with their use in people with severe bilateral renal artery stenosis. There is a risk of hyperkalemia, especially in patients with CKD or in people on potassium supplements or potassium-sparing drugs. ACE inhibitors may also cause cough and angioedema.[4]

Calcium channel blockers

CCBs are another class of first-line antihypertensive agents; however, they should be avoided in patients with heart failure with reduced ejection fraction because of their negative inotropic effects. These agents inhibit calcium ions from entering smooth muscle and cause vasodilation.[14] Nondihydropyridine CCBs reduce heart rate and should not be regularly used with beta blockers (BBs) because of the increased risk of bradycardia and heart block. Dihydropyridine CCBs do not affect heart rate but are associated with dose-dependent pedal edema, especially in women.[4]

Beta blockers

BBs are not recommended as first-line agents for the treatment of HTN unless a patient has ischemic heart disease or heart failure. Carvedilol is the preferred BB for patients with heart failure with reduced ejection fraction. Cardioselective BBs (eg, metoprolol and atenolol) should be used in patients with bronchospastic airway disease requiring beta blockade, as noncardioselective BBs (eg, propranolol and nebivolol) are contraindicated in people with reactive airway disease. Regardless of the specific BB used, abrupt cessation should be avoided.[4]

Other treatments and considerations

Several strategies beyond pharmacologic and nonpharmacologic management should be considered. Team-based care, which may include nurses, pharmacists, community health workers, and others, can be useful in improving medication adherence, facilitating behavior change and lifestyle management, improving health literacy, promoting self-management, and improving BP control. The use of telehealth, registries, electronic health records, and emerging technologies may also help achieve BP goals. Patients with RH may also benefit from treatment by a HTN specialist.[6] Ultimately, shared decision-making between a patient and clinician, informed by evidence and clinical judgment, should direct HTN management.[4]

Another treatment strategy in patients with uncontrolled BP, despite lifestyle modifications and antihypertensive medications, is renal artery denervation.[15,16] Sympathetic denervation of the renal arteries is achieved via percutaneous, endovascular technique through the femoral artery with radiofrequency or ultrasound energy applied through the renal artery wall to ablate adjacent sympathetic nerve fibers. Denervation inhibits central sympathetic activation, reduces renin-angiotensin-aldosterone activity, decreases salt and water retention and lowers BP by approximately 10 mm Hg.[17]

Race-based treatment

Although many guidelines, including the 2017 multisociety BP guideline, have race-based treatment recommendations, there has since been recognition of the limited accuracy of evidence and appropriateness of treatment based on race and ethnicity. Race and ethnicity, which can be influenced by structural racism, social determinants of health, and other factors, should not be used as a proxy for biological differences. These factors, along with the erroneous extrapolation of findings from underrepresented minorities in clinical trials to larger populations, confound evidence demonstrating race-based differences.[18] Furthermore, the treatment of HTN based on race is associated with worsened BP control and can contribute to disparities in health.[18,19]

SUMMARY

Elevated BP and HTN are prevalent and often undertreated in the United States. BP above goal is associated with significantly increased morbidity and mortality. However, effective treatment with evidence-based interventions reduces sequelae and improves quality of life. Clinicians should treat elevated BP and HTN based on evidence, clinical judgment, and shared decision-making to achieve optimal patient-centered outcomes.

CLINICS CARE POINTS

- The diagnosis of hypertension should be made based on blood pressure measurements taken properly on separate occasions and based on evidence-based guideline recommendations.
- The management of elevated blood pressure and hypertension should include lifestyle modification and, when appropriate, pharmacologic treatment.
- Evidence-based, first line pharmacologic agents should be used preferentially in the management of hypertension.

DISCLOSURE

The author has no commercial or financial conflicts of interest.

REFERENCES

1. Oparil S, Acelajado MC, Bakris GL, et al. Hypertension. Nat Rev Dis Primers 2018;4:18014.
2. Centers for Disease Control and Prevention, Hypertension cascade: hypertension prevalence, treatment and control estimates among US adults aged 18 years and older applying the criteria from the American College of Cardiology and American Heart Association's 2017 hypertension guideline – NHANES 2017-2020, Atlanta (GA). Available at: https://millionhearts.hhs.gov/data-reports/hypertension-prevalence.html, 2023.

3. Lu Y, Lan T. Global, regional, and national burden of hypertensive heart disease during 1990-2019: an analysis of the global burden of disease study 2019. BMC Publ Health 2022;22(1):841.

4. Whelton PK, Carey RM, Aronow WS, et al. 2017 ACC/AHA/AAPA/ABC/ACPM/AGS/APhA/ASH/ASPC/NMA/PCNA guideline for the prevention, detection, evaluation, and management of high blood pressure in adults. J Am Coll Cardiol 2018; 71(19):e127–248.

5. DePalma SM, Himmelfarb CD, MacLaughlin EJ, et al. Hypertension guideline update: a new guideline for a new era. JAAPA 2018;31(6):16–22.

6. Carey RM, Calhoun DA, Bakris GL, et al. Resistant hypertension: detection, evaluation, and management: a scientific statement from the American Heart Association. Hypertension 2018;72(5):e53–90.

7. Bachinsky A, Jones EL, Thompson T, et al. Understanding resistant hypertension. JAAPA 2021;34(12):15–20.

8. Paz MA, de-La-Sierra A, Saez M, et al. Treatment efficacy of anti-hypertensive drugs in monotherapy or combination. Medicine 2016;95(30):e4071.

9. Akbari P, Khorasani-Zadeh A. Thiazide diuretics. Treasure Island (FL): StatPearls publishing; 2023. Available at: https://www.ncbi.nlm.nih.gov/books/NBK532918/.

10. Huxel C, Raja A, Ollivierre-Lawrence MD. Loop diuretics. Treasure Island (FL): StatPearls publishing; 2023. Available at: https://www.ncbi.nlm.nih.gov/books/NBK546656/.

11. Patabinadla S, Heaton J, Kyaw H. Spironolactone. Treasure Island (FL): StatPearls publishing; 2023. Available at: https://www.ncbi.nlm.nih.gov/books/NBK554421/.

12. Herman LL, Padala SA, Ahmed I, et al. Angiotensin-converting enzyme inhibitors (ACEI). Treasure Island (FL): StatPearls publishing; 2023. Available at: https://www.ncbi.nlm.nih.gov/books/NBK431051/.

13. Hill RD, Vaidya PN. Angiotensin II receptor blockers (ARB). Treasure Island (FL): StatPearls publishing; 2023. Available at: https://www.ncbi.nlm.nih.gov/books/NBK537027/.

14. McKeever RG, Hamilton RJ. Calcium channel blockers. Treasure Island (FL): StatPearls publishing; 2022. Available at: https://www.ncbi.nlm.nih.gov/books/NBK482473/.

15. Food and Drug Administration. Pma P220026: FDA summary of safety and effectiveness data, Silver Spring (MD). 2023. Available at: https://www.accessdata.fda.gov/cdrh_docs/pdf22/P220026B.pdf.

16. Food and Drug Administration. Pma P220023: FDA summary of safety and effectiveness data, Silver Spring (MD). 2023. Available at: https://www.accessdata.fda.gov/cdrh_docs/pdf22/P220023B.pdf.

17. Fengler K. Renal denervation for resistant hypertension: a concise update on treatment options and the latest clinical evidence. Cardiol Ther 2022;11(3):385–92.

18. Hernandez-Boussard T, Siddique SM, Bierman AS, et al. Promoting equity in clinical decision making: dismantling race-based medicine. Health Aff 2023;42(10):1369–73.

19. Holt HK, Gildengorin G, Karliner L, et al. Differences in hypertension medication prescribing for Black Americans and their association with hypertension outcomes. J Am Board Fam Med 2022;35(1):26–34.

Dyslipidemia

Laura J. Ross, PA-C, CLS, DipACLM, AACC

KEYWORDS

- Hyperlipidemia • Dyslipidemia • Familial hypercholesterolemia • Lifestyle medicine
- Statin • Non-statin treatment

KEY POINTS

- Dyslipidemia is a primary risk factor for atherosclerotic cardiovascular disease, and there are several treatment options to lower cholesterol and decrease the risk of mortality and morbidity.
- Lifestyle changes and medications can help decrease the risk of heart attacks, strokes, and limb ischemia.
- Statins have been proven to be effective, but are not always tolerated. Additional medications can be used if cholesterol goals are not achieved.

INTRODUCTION

Atherosclerotic cardiovascular disease (ASCVD) is a leading cause of premature mortality and morbidity worldwide in the twenty-first century.[1] ASCVD includes coronary artery disease, stroke, and peripheral artery disease. Individual factors such as smoking, hypertension, diabetes, dyslipidemia, social determinants of health, and genetics all play a role. Several case-control studies have demonstrated the role of common major ASCVD factors in determining the risk of myocardial infarction. The INTER-HEART study showed that 9 common risk factors accounted for >90% of the risk of myocardial infarction.[2] Almost 50% of the risk has been found to be related to elevated lipids (**Fig. 1**). This article will focus on treatment options for dyslipidemia.

CURRENT EVIDENCE

Cholesterol particle transportation in the plasma depends on lipoproteins since cholesterol is insoluble in water/blood. The low-density lipoprotein (LDL) brings approximately 90% of the cholesterol toward the artery wall, and the high-density lipoprotein (HDL) brings cholesterol away from the wall. Chylomicrons are composed of a main central lipid core that contains primarily triglycerides. The transportation of fatty acids is regulated by triglycerides. Lipid-lowering therapies have been shown to reduce subsequent morbidity and mortality. Leading health organizations such as

Park Nicollet Heart and Vascular Center/Methodist Hospital, Cardiology, 6500 Excelsior Boulevard, St Louis Park, MN 55426, USA
E-mail address: Laura.ross@parknicollet.com

Physician Assist Clin 10 (2025) 213–225
https://doi.org/10.1016/j.cpha.2024.11.011
2405-7991/25/© 2024 Elsevier Inc. All rights are reserved, including those for text and data mining, AI training, and similar technologies.

physicianassistant.theclinics.com

Abbreviations	
ACC	American College of Cardiology
ApoB-100	apolipoprotein B-100
CK	creatinine kinase
FH	familial hypercholesterolemia
HDL	high-density lipoprotein
Hs-CRP	high-sensitivity C-reactive protein
LDL	low-density lipoprotein
NLA	National Lipid Association
PCSK9 mAB	proprotein convertase subtilisin/kexin type 9 monoclonal antibody

the American College of Cardiology (ACC), National Lipid Association (NLA), and American Heart Association have published guidelines that are updated regularly to guide the implementation and management of risk factors.[3] Prior to considering a medication to treat dyslipidemia, it is important to evaluate secondary causes such as nephrotic syndrome, liver disease, thyroid disorders, extreme dietary patterns like the Keto diet high in saturated fat, or anorexia. Pregnancy, menopause, and acute illness can also affect lipid levels.

THERAPEUTIC OPTIONS TO TREAT CHOLESTEROL

Lifestyle modifications are the first recommendation to treat ASCVD risk factors. The pillars of lifestyle medicine also improve cholesterol.

- Whole food plant predominant diet (eg, dietary approach to stop hypertension [DASH], Mediterranean, Vegetarian, Vegan)
- 150 minutes of moderate or 75 minutes of high-intensity exercise weekly, weight resistance training 2 days a week
- Sleep 7 to 8 hours a night
- Avoid smoking and alcohol misuse (2 servings of alcohol or less daily for men and 1 or less for women).

Describing the Harvard Plate can make it easier to visualize for patients: half of the plate should be more vegetables than fruit, one-fourth of the plate whole grains, and one-fourth of the plate lean protein.[4] A healthy lifestyle and medication management can be difficult to adhere to. Patients with chronic diseases such as diabetes, hypertension, and dyslipidemia have been shown to have a 50% to 60% medication

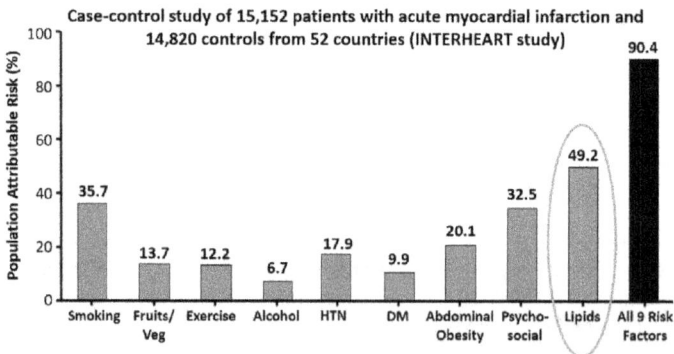

Fig. 1. Modifiable risk factors that contribute to population attributable risk. Printed with permission from Clinical Education Alliance.[2]

compliance rate.[5] The cause of poor compliance is multifactorial and includes cost, pill burden, and barriers to care. Addressing social determinants of health such as food and housing insecurity, affordability of medications, racism, walkable neighborhoods, clean air, and access to health care are all variables that can affect cardiovascular outcomes in the setting of dyslipidemia. Regular activity, smoking cessation, alcohol use in moderation, and maintaining a healthy weight are all cornerstones of lifestyle medicine.[6] These can be implemented without significant side effects or cost to improve cardiovascular risk. Clinicians can make a heart-healthy food recommendation at each visit, such as encouraging the increase of fiber to lower cholesterol. Some patients with significant risk factors benefit the most from a combination of statins and lifestyle changes regardless of the LDL goal.

First-Line Medication

Statins have been a treatment option since the 1980s and are the first-line pharmaceutical treatment for decreasing the risk related to high cholesterol in higher risk primary (no ASCVD) and secondary prevention (ASCVD) patients. There have been several clinical trials with statins in patients with ASCVD that have demonstrated a decreased risk of heart attacks and strokes.[7,8] There are 7 statin medications that vary in potency and tolerability (**Fig. 2**). A meta-analysis of statin studies shows that the lower the LDL, the lower the risk of cardiovascular disease.[10] Statins also lower inflammatory markers like the high-sensitivity C-reactive protein (hs-CRP).[11] Statins can contribute to plaque stabilization, reversal of endothelial dysfunction, and decreased thrombogenicity.[12]

STATIN TREATMENT BENEFIT GROUPS

There are 4 categories of patients at higher ASCVD risk who would benefit from LDL lowering with statin medications outlined later: Secondary prevention for patients who already had a cardiovascular event, LDL >190, patients living with diabetes, primary patients with an elevated 10 year ASCVD score of >7.5%. Repeat testing of cholesterol fractionation, glucose, and alanine transaminase a liver function test (ALT) is recommended 6 to 12 weeks after any medication or lifestyle modification.

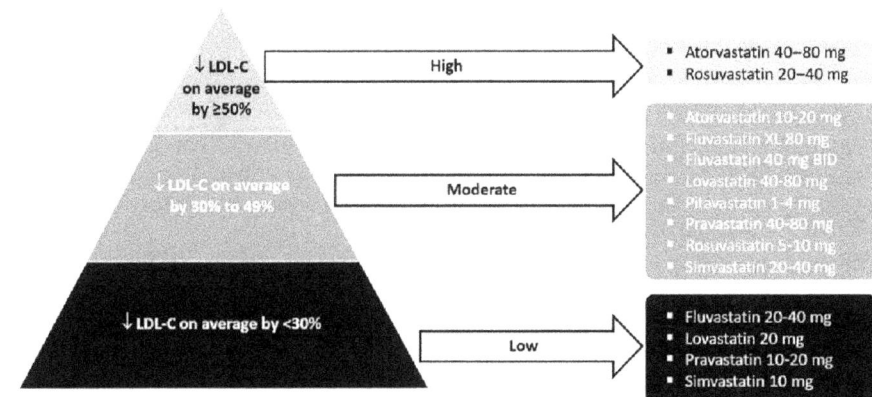

Fig. 2. Statin intensity and low-density lipoprotein cholesterol reduction. Permission granted from Clinical Education Alliance.[9]

Secondary Prevention

The ACC/AHA guidelines recommend high-intensity statin therapy for secondary prevention in patients aged 40 to 75 years, but continuing statins or initiating moderate-intensity doses is reasonable at ages outside that range with shared decision-making.[13] A meta-analysis of patients with ASCVD demonstrated a 22% risk reduction of major events for each 1 mmol/L (38 mg/dL) of LDL lowering, even if the baseline LDL is near the goal of <70 mg/dL.[14] There does not appear to be an LDL level that is too low or at which treatment benefit stops. More recent evidence shows that very low lifelong LDL levels between 15 and 30 mg/dL are associated with lower incidence of ASCVD without adverse effects.[15]

LDL goals vary based on the patient's risk factors. Adults with clinical ASCVD who are *very high risk* have an LDL goal of <55 mg/dL, and if not at *very high risk* the LDL goal is <70 mg/dL (**Table 1**). *Very high-risk* is defined by 2 major events or 1 major and 2 or more high-risk conditions (**Table 2**).

Nonstatin treatment options

If LDL is not to goal on statins, or statins are not tolerable, clinicians can consider the addition of nonstatin therapy such as ezetimibe, a proprotein convertase subtilisin/kexin type 9 monoclonal antibody (PCSK9 mAB), bempedoic acid, or inclisiran siRNA molecule treatments (however, the coadministration of PCSK9mAB and inclisiran is not recommended because they both work on the same pathway). The mechanisms of action, expected LDL lowering, and evidence to lower ASCVD events of these agents are outlined later and in **Table 2**.

- Ezetimibe was shown to improve cardiovascular outcomes in the IMPROVE-IT trial and lowers LDL by decreasing the absorption of cholesterol at the intestinal border (**Table 3**).[17]
- PCSK9 mABs inhibit LDL receptor degradation and have been shown to lower the LDL by 50% to 60%.[18,19]
- The findings of the CLEAR Outcomes tiral showed that for patients who could not tolerate statins or high doses of statins. Depending on concurrent lipid lowering therapies, it lowered the LDL an additional 18-25%..[20] There is a combination pill with ezetimibe and bempedoic acid that has the benefit of decreasing the pill burden and can lower the LDL approximately 40%.[21]
- Inclisiran is a small interfering mRNA molecule that silences the production of the PCSK9 protein, with an effect of lowering the LDL 50%.[22] Cardiovascular outcome trial results are ongoing for primary and secondary prevention.

Table 1
Secondary prevention low-density lipoprotein goals.Criteria for defining patients as "Very High-Risk" for future atherosclerotic cardiovascular disease events and low-density lipoprotein goal <55

Patient Population	Low-Density Lipoprotein Cholesterol, Mg/dL	Non-high Density Lipoprotein Cholesterol, Mg/dL
Adults with atherosclerotic cardiovascular disease (ASCVD) at very high risk	<55	<85
Adults with ASCVD not at very high risk	<70	<100

Adapted from Ref.[16]

Table 2
Major atherosclerotic cardiovascular disease events and high-risk conditions

2 Major Events or 1 Major and 2 High-Risk Conditions	
Major Atherosclerotic Cardiovascular Disease (ASCVD) Events	**High-Risk Condition**

• ACS within past 12 mo
• History of myocardial infarction
  (other than recent ACS event above)
• History of ischemic stroke
• Symptomatic PAD
	• Age ≥65 yr
	• Chronic kidney disease
	  (eGFR 15–59 mL/min/1.73 m^2)
	• Coronary bypass or percutaneous
	  intervention outside of major ASCVD events
	• Current smoker
	• Diabetes
	• Heterozygous familial hypercholesterolemia (HeFH)
	• History of congestive HF
	• Hypertension
	• Low-density lipoprotein cholesterol
	  (LDL-C) ≥100 mg/dL despite maximally
	  tolerated statin + exetimibe

Adapted from Ref.[16]

Patients can also be referred to a lipid specialist and registered dietician if LDL is not to goal on maximally titrated statins.

- Secondary Prevention add on therapy for High (LDL goal <70) or Very High Risk (LDL goal <55) patients:
  o If <25% LDL lowering is indicated to get the LDL to goal, ezetimibe is a cost-effective choice due to the generic price. If a patient has risk factors of heart failure, hypertension, age >75 years, diabetes, stroke, coronary artery bypass graft surgery, peripheral arterial disease, estimated glomerular filtration rate (eGFR) <60, or smoking, the number needed to treat to prevent an event is significantly lower than if those are not present. If ezetimibe is not tolerated or effective, the addition of bempedoic acid may be considered.
  o If >25% LDL lowering is indicated to get the LDL to goal, then inhibiting PCSK9 would offer a 50% to 60% LDL reduction. However, the potential cost should be part of shared decision-making. If PCSK9 mAB are not tolerated or there are barriers to compliance, inclisiran has the ease of twice a year dosing in the clinic. Inclisiran reimbursement is unique because coverage typically comes out of the medical benefit compared to the pharmacy benefit, and this can make the deductible more reasonable for some patients. The medication is not detectable after 48 hours, so longer term side effects are uncommon.[23]

Low-Density Lipoprotein >190

If the LDL is >190 mg/dL, the diagnosis of familial hypercholesterolemia (FH) should be considered. The criteria for FH are outlined in **Table 4**. Genetic testing will confirm but does not exclude a causative mutation.

Heterozygous FH affects 1:250 people and, if untreated, confers a 50% risk of a cardiovascular event for men in their fifth decade of life and a 30% risk for females by the time they are in their sixth decade of life.[25]

Homozygous FH (HoFH) is rarer, affecting 1:300,000 individuals worldwide.[26] This diagnosis should be considered if the LDL is >150 mg/dL on 3 different lipid-lowering agents. Patients with HoFH often have a loss of function of the LDL receptor so

Table 3
Summary of nonstatin medication expected low-density lipoprotein reduction and Cardiovascular outcome trials

Drug	MoA	Route, Frequency	Mean LDL-C Reduction	CV Outcomes
Ezetimibe	Cholesterol absorption inhibitor	Oral, daily	18%	*IMPROVE-IT*: CVD reduction (ARR: 2%; RRR: 6%) when added to moderate-intensity statin and ezetimibe combination therapy in patients with ACS and LDL-C ≥50 mg/dL
Bempedoic acid	ATP citrate lyase inhibitor	Oral, daily	17%–18%	*CLEAR Outcomes*: Reduced MACE in statin intolerant primary prevention patients with LDL-C ≥100 mg/dL and secondary prevention patients with LDL-C between 100 and 190 mg/dL (ARR: 1.6%; RRR 13%)
Alirocumab Evolocumab	PCSK9 inhibitor monoclonal antibody	Subcutaneous, every 2 wk or once/mo	45%–58%	*ODYSSEY Outcomes and FOURIER*: Reduced MACE (ARR: 1.5%–1.6%; RRR: 15%) in patients with LDL-C ≥70 mg/dL on maximally tolerated statins
Inclisiran	PCSK9 RNA synthesis inhibitor	Subcutaneous, at baseline, 3 mo, twice per yr	48%–52%	*ORION-4* expected to complete in 2026 *VICTORIAN-2P* expected to complete in 2027 *VICTORIAN-1P* primary prevention enrollment 2023

Permission granted from Clinical Education Alliance.

Abbreviations: ACS, acture coronary syndrome; ARR, absolute risk reduction; CVD, cardiovascular disease; MACE, major adverse cardiac events; MoA, mechanism of action, RRR, relative risk reduction

Data from acc.org/latest-in-cardiology/articles/2014/12/18/11/57/improve-it-how-much-really-is-the-improvement. Cannon. NEJM. 2015; 372:2387. Lloydjones. J Am Coll Cardiol. 2022; 80:1366. Nissen. NEJM. 2023; 388:1353. Sabatine. NEJM. 2017; 376:1713. Schwartz. NEJM. 2018; 379:2097. NCT03705234. NCT05030428.

Table 4
Diagnostic criteria for familial hypercholesterolemia

International Classification of Diseases, 10th revision (ICD-10)	Clinical Criteria	With Genetic Testing
Family history of familial hypercholesterolemia (FH)	LDL not applicable if a first-degree relative has confirmed FH	Genetic testing not performed
Homozygous FH	LDL >400 mg/dL and 1 or both parents have clinically diagnosed FH, positive genetic testing	Two identical or nonidentical defects. Occasionally homozygotes will have LDL <400 mg/dL.
Heterozygous FH	LDL >160 mg/dL for children and >190 mg/dL for adults with 1 first-degree relative affected or with premature coronary artery disease (CAD) or positive genetic testing	One abnormal LDL defect. If >400 mg/dL and only 1 defect, treat as homozygous.

Adapted from Ref.[24]

PCSK9 inhibition may not be as effective. The LDL goal for patients with FH is <100 mg/dL. Patients who have HoFH have additional treatment options including evinacumab, which is a fully human monoclonal antibody inhibitor of ANGPTL3, given in the clinic as a monthly infusion. It results in an LDL reduction of approximately 50%.[24] Lomitapide and LDL apheresis are other treatment options.

Patients Living with Diabetes

Patients without ASCVD but with diabetes also benefit from statins to lower their ASCVD risk due to this high-risk condition.

- If the 10-year ASCVD risk is <7.5%, the goal is a 30% to 49% reduction of LDL to an LDL goal <100 mg/dL with a moderate-intensity statin. However, clinicians may consider increasing to a high-intensity statin if the goal is not met or there are diabetes risk enhancers such as a duration of >10 years, albuminuria, eGFR <60 mL/min, retinopathy, neuropathy, or ankle-brachial index (ABI) <0.9.
- If the 10-year ASCVD risk is >20%, the goal is a >50% reduction of LDL to an LDL goal <70 mg/dL with a high-intensity statin and, if not to goal, the addition of ezetimibe can be considered.[16]

Patients with an Elevated 10-Year Atherosclerotic Cardiovascular Disease Risk According to the American College of Cardiology/American Heart Association Risk Calculator

Primary prevention patients with a risk for ASCVD have been found to benefit from statin therapy, which reduces the risk of all-cause mortality and ASCVD events.[27] The benefits of statin therapy appear to be present across diverse populations,[13] and it may be reasonable to add ezetimibe to reach the goals based on the following recommendations:

- If the 10-year risk is 5% to 7.5% with risk-enhancing factors and/or an elevated CT coronary calcium score, statin treatment can be considered.

- If the 10-year risk is 7.5% to 19%, a 30% to 49% reduction in LDL and an LDL goal <100 mg/dL is recommended with a moderate-dose statin.
- If the 10-year ASCVD risk is >20%, a 50% reduction in LDL and an LDL goal <70 mg/dL with a high-intensity statin is recommended. It may be reasonable to add ezetimibe to reach the goals.
- Primary prevention patients with a baseline LDL of >190, a coronary calcium score >300, or positive genetic testing for familial hypercholesterolemia have a greater chance of having PCSK9mAB, proprotein convertase subtilisin kexin type 9 small interfering RNA (PCSK9 siRNA), or bempedoic acid covered by insurance.

FURTHER RISK STRATIFICATION
Computed Tomography Coronary Calcium Score

This test can be used to personalize the risk prediction of CV disease for primary prevention in the next 5 to 10 years. Consider this test for men >40 and women >50 years old who are not sure if the benefits of statins outweigh the risks. Calcium takes time to form around cholesterol plaques inside the coronary artery walls and may not show up before those ages. This test takes approximately 10 minutes, uses no contrast, and has similar radiation exposure as a mammogram. The number needed to treat to prevent 1 major adverse cardiovascular event in 10 years is >200 if the score is 0, 100 if the coronary artery calcium (CAC) score is 1 to 100, and 12 if the CAC score is >100.[28]

- If the score is zero, it is reasonable to avoid medical therapy unless the patient has diabetes, smokes, has an LDL >190 mL/d, or a significant family history of premature coronary artery disease. Those conditions make it more likely there are fatty, noncalcified cholesterol plaques that are at risk for inflammation and CV events, so medical treatment is still advised. If those conditions are absent and the score is zero, consider working on lifestyle changes and then repeating the CT coronary calcium score again in 3 to 5 years for higher risk patients and 5 to 7 years for lower risk patients.
- If the score is >100, consider also adding aspirin 81 mg daily for primary prevention.[29]
- Repeat CAC testing is not recommended unless the score is zero, and then consider repeating 5 years later to reassess risk.

Statin Intolerance

Studies suggest that 5% to 30% of patients have a statin intolerance.[30] To classify a patient with statin intolerance, the NLA recommends that at least 2 statins be tried, 1 of which is the lowest approved daily dose. Insight into intolerance has been examined in several studies. One example is a placebo-controlled trial of 60 participants, with alternating treatments each month between a bottle of statin tablets, a bottle of placebo tablets, and an empty bottle—the mean symptom score was 8.0/25.0 in no-tablet months. It was higher in statin and placebo months, with no statistically significant difference between those groups.[9] However, if patients feel they are not tolerating a medication despite an uncommon or common side effect, alternative treatment options are often necessary.

Alternative statin dosing can be considered if symptomatic. Water soluble longer acting statins such as rosuvastatin may be better tolerated at 5 mg on Mondays, Wednesdays, and Fridays, and patients may feel better "having the weekend off" statins while still achieving 20% to 30% LDL reduction.

Routine creatinine kinase (CK) levels are not recommended in the absence of symptoms. Even if CK levels are normal, changes in lipid therapy are indicated if the patient feels they are not tolerating the statin. If CK levels are >3 times the upper limit of normal with symptoms, therapy could be adjusted. Population studies have shown mild CK elevation in certain race and sex groups and is related to muscle mass.[31]

Triglycerides

The ACC 2021 expert consensus decision pathway outlines recommendations for managing patients with persistent hypertriglyceridemia, which is a risk factor for cardiovascular disease.[32] Once the LDL goal is achieved, consideration of hypertriglyceridemia management is indicated.[33]

A personalized approach with lifestyle modifications as first-line therapy is suggested, including a 10% to 15% very low-fat diet, avoidance of refined carbohydrates and alcohol, and exercise interventions. These can lower the triglycerides by up to 50%. If the triglycerides are still >500 mg/dL, there is an increased risk of pancreatitis. Therefore, consider adding prescription-grade omega-3 fatty acids, fibrates, or statins to get the LDL to goal.[32] However, avoid the combination of gemfibrozil and statins to prevent rhabdomyolysis.

The REDUCE-IT trial showed a 25% relative risk reduction in major adverse cardiovascular events in patients receiving icosapent ethyl (pure eicosapentaenoic acid ethyl ester/EPA) compared to placebo. This reduced risk included heart attacks, strokes, CV-related deaths, and other CV events. Therefore, this medication can be thought of as a CV event reducer, more than just a triglyceride medication.[34] Based on these data, the NLA 2019 scientific statement recommends icosepent ethyl 2 g twice a day to reduce cardiovascular risk for secondary prevention patients, and primary prevention patients living with diabetes and 1 additional risk factor with triglycerides >135 and <500.[35]

This same effect with omega 3s has not been seen with docosahexaenoic acid (DHA) and EPA combination medications in the VITAL and ASCEND trials.[36,37]

High-Density Lipoprotein

Current testing does not evaluate how effective high-density lipoprotein (HDL) is in carrying cholesterol away from the artery walls. Low HDL is a risk factor for ASCVD, but medications that increase HDL have not improved CV outcomes. Exercise lowers cardiovascular risk and can increase HDL and may improve the functional capacity and decrease inflammation. There is a U-shaped curve when looking at patients with very low HDL and very high HDL; both extremes carry a higher risk of CVD.[38] When levels are significantly elevated, it is postulated that the HDL is not as functional to carry cholesterol away from the arterial walls, which increases risk. High intake of alcohol, antipsychotic, and seizure medications can contribute to the elevation.

Biomarkers

- The Lipoprotein (a) protein can be attached to cholesterol particles; elevation is present in approximately 20% of the population and it has a genetic predisposition. If elevated, it increases the ASCVD risk by 3 to 4 times, depending on the elevation. It also contributes to a higher risk of aortic stenosis as it is prothrombotic and inflammatory.[39] PCSK9 mAB can lower lipoprotein (a) levels up to 20%, but currently there is no indication to use proprotein convertase subtilisin

---

Box 1
Risk-enhancing factors for shared decision-making

- Family history of premature ASCVD (men <55 and women <65 years)
- Primary hypercholesterolemia (LDL 160–189 mg/dL)
- Metabolic syndrome
- Chronic kidney disease (eGFR 15–59)
- Chronic inflammatory condition (psoriasis, rheumatoid arthritis, or human immunodeficiency virus/acquired immunodeficiency syndrome)
- History of premature menopause (<40 years) or history of preeclampsia
- High-risk ethnicity (South-Asian)
- Elevated biomarkers
- Triglycerides >150 mg/dL
- Elevated hs CRP >2.0
- Elevated lipoprotein (a) >50
- Elevated Apolipoprotein B-100 >130. Triglycerides >200 mg/dL can contribute to a discordance between LDL and ApoB.
- ABI <0.9

Adapted from Ref.[3]

---

kexin type 9 monoclonal antibody (PCSK9i) to just lower high lipoprotein (a) levels. Current trials are looking at novel therapies to lower lipoprotein (a).

- Apolipoprotein B-100 (ApoB-100) is a protein that plays a crucial role in lipid metabolism and transportation in the body. Each cholesterol particle carries 1 molecule of ApoB-100, so it is a good surrogate measure for atherogenic cholesterol particle numbers. Elevated levels of ApoB-100 are associated with an increased risk of ASCVD. There can be discordance between the LDL and apo-B100 levels in 7% to 15% of patients, which is most common with hypertriglyceridemia, diabetes, or metabolic syndrome. The apolipoprotein B-100 can help identify those people who have residual risk despite normal LDL levels.[40]
- Hs-CRP is a marker of inflammation and is associated with an increased risk of developing CVD. Patients with elevated hsCRP > 2 mg/L for 2 separate checks have been shown to be at intermediate risk.[41] If this is >10, it is likely related to other inflammation. Medications like statins and bempedoic acid have been shown to lower hs-CRP levels and ASCVD risk.

Risk Enhancing Factors

Personalization of risk assessment in primary prevention can help with shared decision-making when weighing the risks versus the benefits of adding medication to treat dyslipidemia.[3] Risk-enhancing factors are listed in **Box 1**.

CASE STUDY

Ms X is 55-year-old who has a family history of coronary artery disease but is hesitant to take medications to treat an LDL of 200 mg/dL. A CT coronary calcium (CAC) score is 301, >90th percentile. LDL improves to 180 mg/dL after switching from a keto diet to a Mediterranean one. She tries 2 different statins with side effects. Ezetimibe is considered, but this will not result in an LDL goal of <100 mg/dL, which is indicated. A PCSK9 mAB is approved in light of the high baseline LDL and CAC, and LDL decreases >50% to 90 mg/dL and is now to goal. If she was hesitant to take home injections, bempedoic acid in a combination tablet with Zetia or inclisiran could be offered.

SUMMARY

Lifestyle changes are the first-line treatment to improve dyslipidemia. If those are not effective for higher risk primary or secondary prevention, statin medications should be started. Nonstatin therapies can also be added to lower cholesterol and cardiovascular risk such as ezetimibe, bempedoic acid, PCSK9 mAB, inclisiran, and icosapent ethyl to achieve LDL goals.

CLINICS CARE POINTS

- Try 2 statins before diagnosing intolerance.
- High-risk primary or secondary prevention patients with an LDL above goal on maximally tolerated statin therapy:
  ○ <25% LDL lowering required—ezetimibe or bempedoic acid.
  ○ >25% LDL lowering required—PCSK9mAB, bempedoic acid/ezetimibe combination, or inclisiran injections every 6 months.
- Consider high-dose prescription omega 3 EPA icosapent ethyl for high-risk primary or secondary prevention patients.
- Lifestyle changes such as decreasing sweets, alcohol, sugar sweetened beverages, bakery items, and saturated fats can decrease triglycerides up to 50%.

DISCLOSURE

No disclosures.

REFERENCES

1. Teo KK, Rafiq T. Cardiovascular risk factors and prevention: a perspective from developing countries. Can J Cardiol 2021;37(5):733. Epub 2021 Feb 19.
2. Yusef S, Hawken S, Ounpuu S, et al. Effect of potentially modifiable risk factors associated with myocardial infarction in 52 countries (the INTERHEART study): case-control study. Lancet 2004;364(9438):937–952.2.
3. Arnett D, Blumenthal RS, Albert MA, et al. 2019 ACC/AHA guideline on the primary prevention of cardiovascular disease: task force on clinical practice guidelines. Circulation 2019;140:e596–646.
4. Healthy eating plate, Harvard health. Available at: https://nutritionsource.hsph.harvard.edu/healthy-eating-plate/.
5. McCarthy R. The price you pay for the drug not taken. Bus Health 1998;16(10):27–33.
6. Lichtenstein A, Appel LJ, Vadiveloo M, et al. 2021 dietary guidance to improve cardiovascular health: a scientific statement from the American heart association. Circulation 2021;144:e472–87.
7. Scandinavian simvastatin survival study group randomized trial of cholesterol lowering in 4444 patients with coronary heart disease: the scandinavian simvastatin survival study (4S). Lancet 1994;344:1383–9.

8. Mills EJ, O'Regan C, Eyawo O, et al. Intensive statin therapy compared with moderate dosing for prevention of cardiovascular events: a meta-analysis of>40 000 patients. Eur Heart J 2011;32(11):1409.

9. Howard JP, Wood FA, Finegold JA, et al. Side effect patterns in a crossover trial of statin, placebo, and No treatment. JACC 2021;78(12):1210–22.

10. Khan SU, Michos ED. Cardiovascular mortality after intensive LDL-Cholesterol lowering: Does baseline LDL-Cholesterol really matter? Am J Prev Cardiol 2020;1:100013.

11. Kandelouei T, Abbasifard M, Imani D, et al. Effect of statins on serum level of hs-CRP and CRP in patients with cardiovascular diseases: a systemic review and meta-analysis of randomized controlled trials. Mediators Inflamm 2022;2022:8732360.

12. Vaughn CJ, Gotto AM, Basson CT. The evolving role of statins in the management of atherosclerosis. JACC 2000;35(1):1.

13. Chou R, Cantor A, Dana T, et al. Statin use for the primary prevention of cardiovascular disease in adults. Updated evidence report and systematic review for the US preventive services task force. JAMA 2022;328(8):754–71.

14. Baigent C, Blackwell L, Emberson J, et al. Efficacy and safety of more intensive lowering of LDL cholesterol: a meta-analysis of data from 170,000 participants in 27 randomized trials. Lancet 2015;385:1670–81.

15. Giugliano R, Pedersen TR, Park JG, et al. Clinical efficacy and safety of achieving very low LDL-cholesterol concentrations with the PCSK9i evolocumab: a prespecified secondary analysis of the FOURIER trial. Lancet 2017;390:1962–71.

16. Lloyd-Jones DM, Lloyd-Jones DM, Morris PB, et al. 2022 ACC expert consensus decision pathway on the role of nonstatin therapies for LDL-cholesterol lowering in the management of ASCVD risk. JACC 2022;80(14):1366–418.

17. Cannon CP, Blazing MA, Giugliano RP, et al. Ezetimibe added to statin therapy after Acute3 coronary syndrome. NEJM 2015;372:238–2397.

18. Sabatine M, Giugliano RP, Keech AC, et al. Evolocumab and clinical outcomes in patients with cardiovascular disease. NEJM 2017;376:1713–22.

19. Schwartz F, Steg PG, Szarek M, et al. Aliracumab and cardiovascular outcomes after acute coronary syndrome. NEJM 2018;379:2097–107.

20. Nissen S, Lincoff AM, Brennan D, et al. Bempedoic acid and cardiovascular outcomes in statin-intolerant patients. NEJM 2023;388:1353–64.

21. Ray K, Bays HE, Catapano AL, et al. Safety and efficacy of bempedoic acid to reduce LDL cholesterol. NEJM 2019;380:1022–32.

22. Kausik R, Troquay RPT, Visseren FLJ, et al. Long-term efficacy and safety of inclisiran in patients with high cardiovascular risk and elevated LDL cholesterol (ORION-3): results from the 4 year open-label extension of the ORION-1 trial. Lancet 2023;11:109–19.

23. Kallend d, Stoekenbroek R, He Y, et al. Pharmacokinetics and pharmacodynamics of inclisiran, a small interfering RNA therapy, in patients with hepatic impairment. J Clin Lipidol 2022;16:208–19.

24. Raal F, Rosenson RS, Reeskamp LF, et al. Evinacumab for homozygous familial hypercholesterolemia. NEJM 2020;383:711.

25. Hopkins PN, Toth PP, Ballantyne CM, et al. National lipid association expert panel on familial hypercholesterolemia. Familial hypercholesterolemias: prevalence, genetics, diagnosis and screening recommendations from the national lipid association expert panel on familial hypercholesterolemia. J Clin Lipidol 2011;5(3 Suppl):S9–17.

26. Sjouke B, Kusters DM, Kindt I, et al. Homozygous autosomal dominant hypercho-lesterolaemia in The Netherlands: prevalence, genotype-phenotype relationship, and clinical outcome. Eur Heart J 2015;36(9):560.

27. Available at: https://tools.acc.org/ldl/ascvd_risk_estimator/index.html#!/calulate/estimator/ (Accessed 16 December 2024).

28. Mitchell JD, Fergestrom N, Gage BF, et al. Impact of statins on cardiovascular outcomes following coronary artery calcium scoring. J Am Coll Cardiol 2018; 72(25):3233–42.

29. Orringer C, Blaha MJ, Blankstein R, et al. The NLA scientific statement on CAC scoring to guide preventive strategies for ASCVD risk reduction. J Clin Lipidol 2021;15:33–60.

30. Cheeley M, Saseen JJ, Agarwala A, et al. NLA scientific statement on statin intol-erance: a new definition and key consideration for ASCVD risk reduction in the statin intolerant patient. J Clin Lipidol 2022;16:361–75.

31. Siamak MK, Oddis CV, Aggarwal R. Approach to asymptomatic creatinine kinase elevation. Cleve Clin J Med 2016;83(1):37–42.

32. Virani S, Morris PB, Agarwala A, et al. ACC expert consensus decision pathway on the management of ASCVD risk reduction in patients with persistent hypertri-glyceridemia: a report of the American College of cardiology solution set over-sight committee. JACC 2021;78(9):960–93.

33. Grundy S, Stone NJ, Bailey AL, et al. 2018 Guideline on the management of blood cholesterol: a Report of the ACC/AHA task force on clinical practice guidelines. Circulation 2018;139:e1082–143.

34. Bhatt D, Steg PG, Miller M, et al. Cardiovascular risk reducation with icosapent ethyl for hypertriglyceridemia. NEJM 2019;380:11–22.

35. Orringer Carl E, Jacobson TA, Maki KC. National Lipid Association Scientific Statement on the use of icosapent ethyl in statin-treated patients with elevated tri-glycerides and high or very-high ASCVD risk. J Clin Lipidol 2019;13(Issue 6): 860–72.

36. Manson J, Cook NR, Lee IM, et al. Marine n-3 fatty acids and prevention of car-diovacular disease and cancer. NEJM 2019;380:23–32.

37. Bowman L, Mafham M, Wallendszus K, et al, ASCEND Study Collaborative Group. Effects of n-3 fatty acid supplements in diabetes mellitus. NEJM 2018; 379:1540–50.

38. Madsen CM, Varbo A, Nordestgaard BG. Extreme high high-density lipoprotein cholesterol is paradoxically associated with high mortality in men and women: two prospective cohort studies. Eur Heart J 2017;38(32):2478.

39. Pia R, Benn M, Tybjaerg-Hansen A, et al. Extreme lipoprotein (a) levels and risk uof MI in the general population. Circulation 2008;117:176–84.

40. Razavi A, Bazzano LA, He J, et al. Discordantly normal ApoB relative to elevated LDL-C in persons with metabolic disorders: a marker of atherogenic heterogene-ity. Am J Prev Cardiol 2021;7:100190.

41. Ridker P, Danielson E, Fonseca FAH, et al. Rosuvatsatin to prevent vascular events in men and women with elevated CRP. NEJM 2008;359:2195–207.

Managing Lifestyle Management

Diet, Exercise, and Other Nonpharmacologic Interventions

Robert S. Smith, DHSc, MS, PA-C[a],*, Laura Solano, DMSc, MPAS, PA-C[b,1]

KEYWORDS

- Nonpharmacologic • Exercise • Sleep • Cardiovascular disease • CBT • Nutrition
- Pathophysiology of CVD

KEY POINTS

- Nonpharmacologic therapy is an effective treatment as demonstrated in the pathophysiological effects of cardiovascular disease (CVD).
- Exercise, intentional nutrition, and optimal sleep are important in treating CVD.
- Addressing modifiable and nonmodifiable risk factors can be effective by genetic and nongenetic barriers such as social determinants of health.

INTRODUCTION

Nonpharmacologic treatment of coronary heart disease has an essential role in the successful treatment of cardiovascular disease (CVD). Despite our technological advances, heart disease continues to be the leading cause of death not only in the United States but also across the westernized world.[1] Many organizations have spoken about the need for lifestyle modifications and dietary changes as an important method to prevent and treat CVD. This article reviews current evidence related to the nonpharmacologic treatment of CVD, the benefits of physical activity (PA) and the adverse effects of sedentary behavior, the pathophysiology associated with physical and dietary habits. The overall health benefits of simple nonpharmacologic treatments include exercise, diet, nutrition, stress management, contemporary technology, barriers and social determinants of health, and recommended strategies for implementation of this treatment modality.

---

[a] Pediatric Associates Family of Companies, Irving, USA; [b] ATSU Adjunct Faculty, Biomedical Science Program, Department of PA Studies, A.T. Still University, TX, USA
[1] Present address: 4200 S. Freeway, Fort Worth, TX 76115.
* Corresponding author. 506 South Nursery Road, Irving, TX 75060.
E-mail address: Rsspac1958@gmail.com

Physician Assist Clin 10 (2025) 227–244
https://doi.org/10.1016/j.cpha.2024.11.010
physicianassistant.theclinics.com
2405-7991/25/© 2024 Elsevier Inc. All rights are reserved, including those for text and data mining, AI training, and similar technologies.

Abbreviations	
ACS	acute coronary syndrome
AF	atrial fibrillation
AHA	The American Heart Association
BMI	body mass index
CAD	coronary artery disease
CBT	cognitive behavioral therapy
CI	confidence interval
CVD	cardiovascular disease
DALYs	disability-adjusted life years
DASH	dietary approaches to stop hypertension
HF	heart failure
ROS	reactive oxygen species
OSA	obstructive sleep apnea
PA	physical activity
SDOH	social determinants of health
TMA	trimethylamine
TMAO	trimethylamine N-oxide

BURDEN OF DISEASE

According to Stark, Johnson, and Roth, in 2022 there were approximately 315 million cases of coronary artery disease (CAD) globally. There has been a decrease in age-standardized prevalence of approximately 18% since 1990.[1] According to the Centers for Disease Control and Prevention, there were approximately 371,506 deaths from CAD in 2022 in the United States.[2] Tsao and colleagues discussed that approximately 5% of adults in the United States over the age of 20 have CAD.[3,4] Despite a global decrease in prevalence, CAD remains the leading cause of death in the world.[1,5] Rala-panawa and Sivakanesan commented on disability-adjusted life years (DALYs) and highlighted that CAD is the *foremost* single cause of DALYs globally. The authors specify that there is a burden of approximately 129 million DALYs annually and emphasize the great global economic cost.[5]

DEFINING NONPHARMACOLOGIC TREATMENTS

Nonpharmacologic treatment can be defined as primary prevention 2.0, or in other words, focusing on early prevention even in the face of disease process. Early recognition of risk factors decreases morbidity and mortality, and diligent application of these therapies can be successful in preventing or in most cases regressing progression.[6] In most instances, clinicians begin assessing patients for CAD in their late 20s or early 30s, which can be effective; however, these authors postulate that it is necessary to evaluate patients at much younger ages by paying attention to familial health and history by doing an early assessment that includes an evaluation of tobacco use, measurement of body mass index (BMI), blood pressure checks, and cholesterol screening for overweight patients, and further recommends that this should be completed for all patients by the age of 20.[7] The mainstays of nonpharmacologic treatments have been diet, exercise, and avoidance behavior, all of which are affected by 2 types of risk factors: nonmodifiable and modifiable.

NONMODIFIABLE RISK FACTORS

Nonmodifiable risk factors are factors that cannot be controlled. It is important to have an overarching understanding of the implications of these nonmodifiable risk factors.

AGE

Age is directly correlated to the deterioration of cardiovascular functionality over time, and older adults are at increased risk of atherosclerosis, stroke, and myocardial infarction (MI).[8] Age-related changes are associated with oxidative inflammatory stressors that affect CVD. See **Fig. 1** for diagram of age-related risk factors.

Age is associated with increased oxidative stress, which leads to an increased susceptibility for functional and electrical abnormalities that lead to CVD. These abnormalities include atrial fibrillation (AF) and heart failure (HF), which are a result of increased reactive oxygen species (ROS) due to oxidative stress and increased production of inflammatory signal molecules. Age is also associated with an increased risk for frailty, obesity, and diabetes. These conditions are also independent risk factors for CVD. Multiple risk factors result in a high incidence of CVD in aging adults. Age also affects the type of PAs patients may be able to do for preventive care.

GENDER

There are sex differences in the prevalence and effect of CVD. Gender-specific issues such as pregnancy, polycystic ovary syndrome, premature menopause, and multiparity increase the future risk of CAD.[9,10] Men and women have increased CVD with age, which corresponds to an overall decline in sex hormones with aging, primarily estrogen and testosterone, despite hormone replacement therapies that have been demonstrated not to improve outcomes.[8]

GENETICS

Genetic factors may determine cardiovascular capacity and muscular hypertrophy patterns. Several areas of interest relate to the genetics of cardiorespiratory fitness and adaptation to exercise. There are predisposing genetic factors that increase CVD, including arrhythmias, congenital heart disease, cardiomyopathy, and high blood cholesterol.[11]

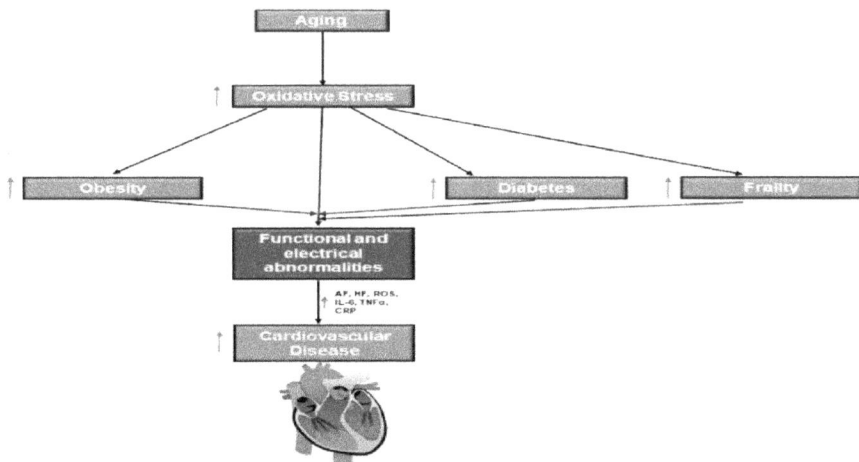

Fig. 1. Schematic diagram of age-related risk factors for CVD. CRP, C-reactive protien; IL-6, interlukin 6; TNFa, tumor necrosis factor alpha.

FAMILY HISTORY

Family history, while traditionally considered nonmodifiable, has some modifiability because environment influences deoxyribonucleic acid (DNA), and a person's lifestyle can be modified.

ETHNICITY

Racial and ethnic differences in CVD mortality persist despite a significant reduction in the CVD burden in the US general population.[11] In the United States, Black persons and other ethnic groups are at an increased risk of obesity, diabetes, and hypertension compared with White persons.[11]

MODIFIABLE RISK FACTORS
Dietary Lifestyle and Nutrition

According to Diab and colleagues, the Mediterranean diet focuses on poly and mono-unsaturated fats, nuts, and fish. The diet, dietary approaches to stop hypertension (DASH), is specific for blood pressure reduction. Plant-based diets avoid animal products and focus on reducing atherosclerosis and improving the microbiome's diversity.[12] According to Diab and colleagues, animal proteins and fats increase trimethylamine (TMA) and trimethylamine N-oxide (TMAO). TMA is a metabolite that is further metabolized to TMAO. TMAO engages in the production of atherosclerosis.

Diab and colleagues investigated the effects of different diets, for example, low carbohydrate, high protein, low fat, intermittent energy restriction, Mediterranean, Nordic, vegetarian, DASH, and others. The authors focused on anthropometric parameters and cardiometabolic risk factors relationship to the diets. The authors found that the Mediterranean diet demonstrated evidence of reducing weight, BMI, total cholesterol, glucose, and blood pressure parameters. There was also weak evidence of improvements in low density lipoprotein (LDL), high density lipoprotein (HDL), triglycerides, insulin, and glycated hemoblogin (A1c). The authors concluded that the Mediterranean diet had the strongest and most consistent evidence.

The Mediterranean diet has proven to have positive effects on cardiovascular health. Dinu and colleagues conducted an umbrella review of 80 articles reporting 495 studies that included meta-analyses of observational research, including randomized trials.[13] The Mediterranean diet consists of fish, fruits and vegetables, whole grains, olive oil, cheese, and yogurt.

The American diet consists of moderate amounts of red meats, saturated fats, and processed carbohydrates versus healthier options such unprocessed carbohydrates, extra-virgin olive oil, fish, nuts, and seeds, whole grains, vegetables, and fruits. See **Table 1** for American diet food swaps for healthier Mediterranean choices.

Onwuzo and colleagues conducted a review of the clinical research and highlighted the effectiveness and reach of the DASH diet as a nonpharmacologic approach to hypertension management.[14] The authors reviewed several studies (from 2001 to 2020) and found that the DASH diet was effective at reducing blood pressure in all the clinical evidence reviewed, including the DASH diet as an intervention in a systematic review that included 17 randomized controlled trials. The authors found positive health effects and reductions in blood pressure when the DASH diet was used in the treatment.

Further research supports the effectiveness of the DASH diet. Filippou and colleagues conducted a systematic review and meta-analysis of randomized controlled trials and concluded the DASH diet reduces BP in persons with and without hypertension and that reduction does not depend on baseline blood pressure levels or

Table 1
Simple swaps for a Mediterranean diet choice

	American Diet	Mediterranean Diet
Fats	Butter, vegetable oil, coconut oil	Extra virgin olive oil
Meats	Red Meat, hamburger, steak, meatballs	Fish, salmon, tuna, tilapia, mackerel, cod
Grain	Refined breads, pasta, macaroni and cheese, spaghetti, white rice	Whole grains, brown rice, oats, couscous, barley, quinoa
Milk	High-fat milk	1% skim or 2% whole milk
Snacks	Cereal Bars, cheese crackers, chips	Nuts and seeds, fruits. vegetables
Salad Dressings	Mayonnaise, miracle whip	Hummus, vegetable-based spreads

hypertension treatment.[15] Furthermore, Filippou and colleagues concluded that the effect of the diet is greater on younger individuals with a higher sodium intake.[15] Therefore, the author's findings support the utilization of the DASH diet to accompany the pharmacologic treatment of hypertension.

Gibbs and colleagues conducted a systematic review and meta-analysis of controlled intervention trials including 41 trials and found that the DASH diet reduced systolic blood pressure (SBP) by 5.53 mm Hg (95% confidence interval (CI): -7.95 to -3.12),Mediterranean diet reduced SBP by 0.95 mm Hg (95% CI: -1.70 to -0.20), vegan diet by 1.61 mm Hg (95% CI: -4.53–1.31), lacto-ovo vegetarian diet by 5.47 mm Hg (95% CI: -7.60 to -3.34), and nordic diet by 4.47 mm Hg (95% CI: -7.14 to -1.81).[16] According to Diab and colleagues, prebiotics and fiber (as included in the Mediterranean, DASH, and plant-based diets) have multiple cardiovascular benefits, namely improved gut homeostasis, insulin sensitivity, glycemic control, and decreased inflammation and the risk of hypertension.[12]

The DASH diet is a proven diet to decrease blood pressure and improve cardiac health. The DASH diet encourages the inclusion of foods such as vegetables, fruits, whole grains, and dairy foods low in fat. The diet recommends limiting sugar-sweetened foods/beverages, red meats, sodium, and saturated and trans-saturated fat. This diet includes foods that are high in nutrients, fiber, and minerals. The DASH diet recommends reduced sodium consumption, specifying that 2,300 mg of sodium is recommended for a 2100-calorie diet; and that 1,500 mg of sodium was more effective for lowering blood pressure.

Plant-based diets include a variety of fruits and vegetables. A vegetarian diet includes plant-based foods, eggs, and dairy; however, it does not include consumption of animal protein. The vegan diet includes plant-based foods and excludes eggs and dairy products. The Nordic diet includes fruits, primarily berries, and vegetables that are rich in fiber, as well as whole grains with a high predilection for rye, barley, and oats. One difference between the Mediterranean diet and the Nordic diet is that the Nordic diet includes canola oil instead of olive oil. The Nordic diet allows for animal protein in limited amounts and fish/seafood, poultry, and red meat are permitted; however, in smaller proportions.

Weight Management/Obesity

Obesity is a broad subject that involves a multitude of physiologic changes that adversely affect the body over time, which leads to dysmetabolic syndrome or syndrome X. This condition is a group of conditions that increase the risk of heart disease, stroke, and type 2 diabetes. Conditions include high blood pressure, high blood sugar, high triglycerides, low HDL cholesterol, and excess fat in the abdomen, waist, and

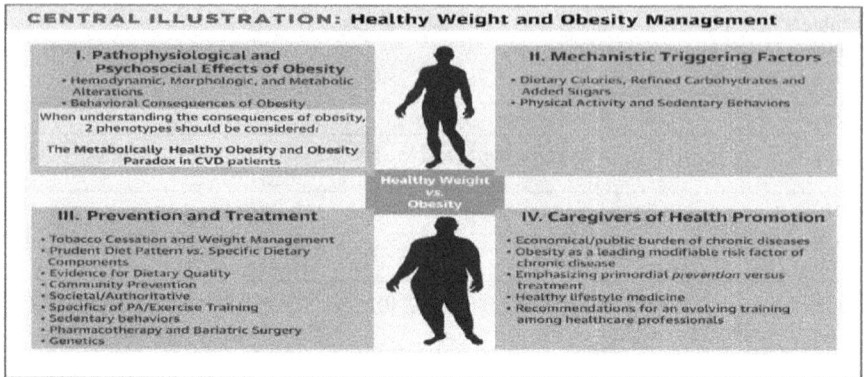

CENTRAL ILLUSTRATION: Healthy Weight and Obesity Management

I. Pathophysiological and Psychosocial Effects of Obesity
- Hemodynamic, Morphologic, and Metabolic Alterations
- Behavioral Consequences of Obesity

When understanding the consequences of obesity, 2 phenotypes should be considered:

The Metabolically Healthy Obesity and Obesity Paradox in CVD patients

II. Mechanistic Triggering Factors
- Dietary Calories, Refined Carbohydrates and Added Sugars
- Physical Activity and Sedentary Behaviors

Healthy Weight vs. Obesity

III. Prevention and Treatment
- Tobacco Cessation and Weight Management
- Prudent Diet Pattern vs. Specific Dietary Components
- Evidence for Dietary Quality
- Community Prevention
- Societal/Authoritative
- Specifics of PA/Exercise Training
- Sedentary behaviors
- Pharmacotherapy and Bariatric Surgery
- Genetics

IV. Caregivers of Health Promotion
- Economical/public burden of chronic diseases
- Obesity as a leading modifiable risk factor of chronic disease
- Emphasizing primordial prevention versus treatment
- Healthy lifestyle medicine
- Recommendations for an evolving training among healthcare professionals

Fig. 2. Healthy weight and Obesity. (Carl J. Lavie et al., Healthy Weight and Obesity Prevention: JACC Health Promotion Series, Journal of the American College of Cardiology, 72 (13), 2018, 1506-1531, https://doi.org/10.1016/j.jacc.2018.08.1037.)

hips. Overweight and obesity are the main risk factors for metabolic syndrome. The main treatments are all of the nonpharmacologic treatments discussed in this article. See **Fig. 2** for the effects of healthy weight and obesity.

Obesity is measured using the BMI as described by the National Heart, Lung, and Blood Institute.[17] See **Table 2** for BMI categories.

Exercise

Metabolic and pathophysiology are associated with nonpharmacologic treatments in CVD The pathophysiological effects of exercise have been shown to prevent psychological, antirhythmic, antithrombotic, and antiatherosclerotic negative effects and improve hemodynamics. At the cellular level, aerobic forms of exercise have been shown to have several beneficial antiatherogenic effects, including a decrease in serum triglycerides, an increase in high-density lipoprotein, and a decrease in low-density lipoprotein. Markers of inflammation decrease with routine cardio activities. Mononuclear cell production of atherogenic cytokines fell by 58.3% and the production of atheroprotective cytokines increased by 35.9% with exercise. Hemostatic factors associated with thrombosis (eg, platelet aggregation and adhesiveness) have also been shown to improve with exercise. Decreasing or discontinuing exercise training in the setting of deconditioning, have effects that revert to pretraining levels.[1] Concentrations of plasminogen antigens are lower in physically active women compared with their nonobese sedentary counterparts. Levels of fibrinogen similar to blood viscosity were shown to decrease relative to an increase in leisure-time PA. However, it is important to note these benefits could not be reproduced following a formal exercise

Table 2 Body mass index categories	
Underweight	= <18.5
Normal weight	= 18.5–24.9
Overweight	= 25–29.9
Obesity	= BMI of 30 or greater
Obese Class I	= 30.0–34.9
Obese Class II	= 35.0–39.9
Obese Class III	= $\geq$40

regimen in patients with known CVD.[1] See **Fig. 3** for the cardioprotective mechanisms of exercise.

Exercise can be subdivided into aerobic, anaerobic, and flexibility categories. Aerobics relies on oxygen to sustain movement; this type of exercise includes activities such as running, jogging, cycling, jump rope exercise, and rowing. Resistance exercise may incorporate weights or resistance training bands. Flexibility exercises may involve the practice of stretching or yoga.

Aerobic Exercise

The American Heart Association (AHA) recommends 150 minutes per week of moderate-intensity aerobic activity, 75 minutes per week of vigorous aerobic activity, or a combination.[18] The AHA describes moderate exercise as brisk walking, water aerobics, dancing, gardening, tennis, and biking at slow speeds.[18] The AHA describes vigorous exercise as hiking uphill, running, swimming laps, heavy yard work, tennis (singles), cycling 10 miles per hour or faster, and jumping rope.[17]

Resistance Training

Correira and colleagues conducted a systematic review and meta-analysis of randomized controlled trials. The review identified 14 studies and demonstrated the mean values of systolic and diastolic blood pressure decreased significantly after resistance training.[19] The authors concluded that strength training performed at least 2 to 3 times a week is a good strategy to decrease blood pressure in persons with hypertension.

To increase muscle mass, it is recommended to focus on large muscle groups with a minimum frequency of 3 times a week and to include a general increase in the weights/resistance to increase muscle mass and strength. There are gender and genetic differences that influence muscle mass development and size. Different muscle groups must be focused on at least 3 times a week to increase mass, for example, 3 times a week for quadriceps, hamstrings, and gastrocnemius and the other 3 days may

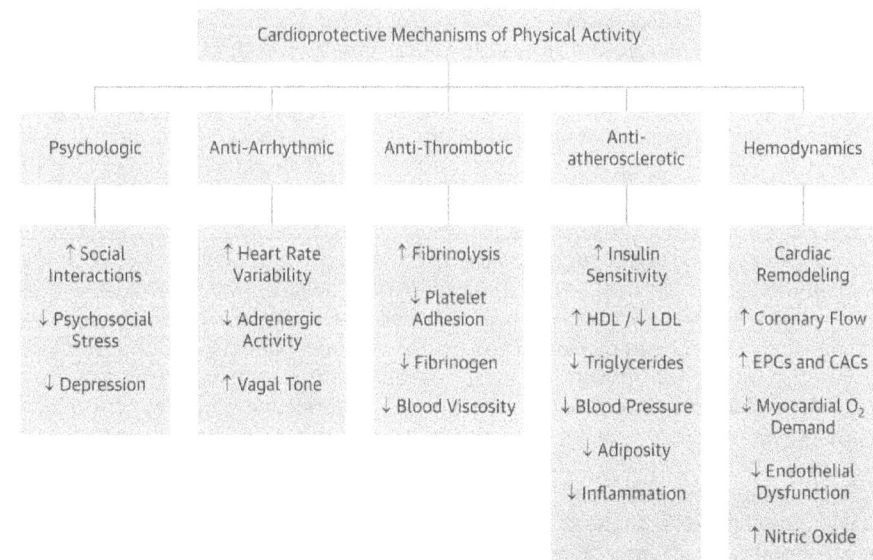

Fig. 3. Cardioprotective mechanisms of PA. (Sergey Kachur et al., Impact of cardiac rehabilitation and exercise training programs in coronary heart disease, Progress in Cardiovascular Diseases, 60 (1), 2017, 103-114, https://doi.org/10.1016/j.pcad.2017.07.002.)

be focused on abdomen/core muscles or upper body (eg, trapezius, deltoids, and bi-ceps). A fitness trainer best guides the exercise training to minimize the risk of injury by increasing weight too quickly or using incorrect biomechanics.

Flexibility

The American College of Sports Medicine recommends that healthy adults stretch at least 2 days per week, spend approximately 1 minute on each major muscle group, and that stretching sessions should have an approximate duration of 10 minutes.[20] There are many types of flexibility exercise modalities including yoga, Pilates, and Tai Chi.

Exercise Prescription

Exercise prescriptions are a useful component of nonpharmacologic management in the treatment and prevention of CVD. O'Regan and colleagues undertook a narrative review of the experiences of general practitioners and patients and introduced a pre-scriptive method, *ABC* of prescribing exercise as medicine.[21] The authors found that even though exercise is a proven method for the treatment and prevention of heart dis-ease, exercise prescription is not common. O'Regan and colleagues discussed the ABC of exercise prescription to include step A where the clinician assesses readiness to change and discusses the type of exercise the patient may enjoy.[21] The second step B includes an intervention that should include the patient's daily schedule and a written prescription. Step C describes continued support in person or by telephone. During step C, the clinician may offer support, motivation, and counseling and may renew the exercise prescription. See **Table 3** for an example of exercise prescription for a beginner. The prescription may be renewed to increase duration and intensity. For example, a person who can walk initially may progress to jogging or short sprints, and repetitions, sets, or weight may be increased in resistance training.

Health Management

Health management involves adequate blood pressure control, eulipidemia, and euglycemia. See **Tables 4–6** for recommended blood pressure targets. Eulipidemia is a precursor to optimal cardiac health. See **Table 7** for target lipid ranges. Euglyce-mia is a known component of the prevention of CVD. See **Table 8** for glycemic goals.

Family History, Social Determinants of Health, Cultural Competency, and Special Populations

Familial lifestyle and social determinants of health, including socioeconomic status, neighborhood, and physical environment such as air pollution, poor water, food qual-ity, exposure to chemicals such as carbon monoxide, and housing can contribute to the development of heart disease. The home environment affects CVD. For example, growing up with active smokers in a family that eats a steady diet of fast-food meals, or a family that has decreased literacy or economic opportunities can affect the choices made in PAs or dietary choices because of cost or availability. These factors may in-fluence blood pressure and cholesterol levels.

Social support networks and access to health care may help to explain persistent racial and ethnic differences in CVD due to increased risk factors. Cultural compe-tency is integral to understanding familial dynamics, understanding nutritional require-ments, accepting or declining care, and trusting or mistrusting the medical community. Providers must have an open approach to treating patients so as to pro-vide the care necessary to afford change. Special populations include patients who

Table 3
Exercise prescription sample

Modality	Sunday	Monday	Tuesday	Wednesday	Thursday	Friday	Saturday
Strength: 3 sets of 8 repetitions	Legs (squats)	Abdominal muscles and upper body (sit-ups, push-ups/pull-ups)	Legs (lunges)	Abdominal muscles and upper body (sit-ups, push-ups/pull-ups)	Legs (Squats)	Abdominal muscles and upper body (sit-ups, push-ups/pull-ups)	Rest
Aerobic: Duration 20–30 min	Walking	Stationary bicycle	Walking	Stationary bicycle	Jog ½ mile Walk one mile	Stationary bicycle	Rest
Flexibility	Stretching (Toe touches, Side reach, sky reach)	Yoga or Tai Chi	Stretching (Toe touches, Side reach, sky reach)	Yoga or Tai Chi	Stretching (Toe touches, Side reach, sky reach)	Yoga or Tai Chi	Rest

Table 4
Adult blood pressure targets

Categories	SBP, mm Hg	And/Or	Diastolic Blood Pressure, mm Hg
American College of Cardiology/AHA			
Normal	<120	And	<80
Elevated	120–129	And	<80
Hypertension, stage 1	130–139	Or	80–89
Hypertension, stage 2	≥140	Or	≥90
European Society of Cardiology/European Society of Hypertension			
Optimal	<120	And	<80
Normal	120–129	And/or	80–84
High Normal	130–139	And/or	85–89
Hypertension, grade 1	140–159	And/or	90–99
Hypertension, grade 2	160–179	And/or	100–109
Hypertension, grade 3	≥ 180	And/or	≥110
Isolated systolic Hypertension	≥140	And	<90

Adapted from AHA 2020 / International Society of Hypertension Global Hypertension Practice Guidelines

are older, disabled, and non-English language speakers. These groups require the provider to be vested in spending time to meet each patient's individual needs.

Stress and Stress Management

Implications of stress on metabolism and its effect on cardiovascular health have been demonstrated when evaluating patients with chronic stress, illustrating causation. It has an important role in pathologic consequences in increasing the prevalence and severity of several CVD risk factors, including hypertension, diabetes mellitus, and obesity.[1,16,22]

Although data demonstrate a correlation to CVD disease, there are no specific measures or tools to fully ascertain the effects of stress. There is, however, compelling evidence that even stress attributable CVD risk is equivalent to other risk factors, suggesting stress is a particularly potent contributor to CVD.[22]

Table 5
Simplified pediatric blood pressure targets

Age	SBP (mm Hg)	Diastolic BP (mm Hg)
Infant	<97	-
Toddler (1–2 years old)	98–101	52–58
Preschooler (3–5 years old)	101–104	58–64
Child (6–12 year old)	105–114	66–75
Adolescent (>13 year old)	120	80

Adapted AAP Guidelines 2023 / Baylor College of Medicine -Shypailo, RJ. 2018

Table 6
Definitions of blood pressure categories and stages

Category	For Children Aged 1 to <13 y	For Children Aged ≥13 y
Normal BP:	<90th percentile	<120/<80 mm Hg
Elevated BP:	≥90th to <95th percentile or 120/80 mm Hg to <95th percentile (whichever is lower)	120/<80–129/<80 mm Hg
Stage 1 HTN:	≥95th to<95th percentile + 12 mm Hg or 130/80–139/89 mm Hg (whichever is lower)	130/-139 mm Hg
Stage 2 HTN:	≥95th percentile + 12 mm Hg or >140/90 mm Hg (whichever is lower)	≥140/90

BP-for-age status categories and their related percentile ranges.
Abbreviations: BP, blood pressure, HTN, hypertension.
Adapted AAP Guidelines 2023 / Baylor College of Medicine -Shypailo, RJ. 2018

Stress has been demonstrated to increase activity in the amygdala in posttraumatic stress disorder, anxiety, and depression.[23] Cellular glycolysis shown by F-fluorodeoxyglucose positron emission tomography/computed tomography can be used to

Table 7
Recommended cholesterol levels

Age	Total Cholesterol	HDL Cholesterol	LDL Cholesterol	Triglycerides	NonHDL Cholesterol
19 and younger	Below 170	Above 45	Below 110	*Ages* 0–9 y <75 10–18 yrs. <90 19 y <150	<120
20 and older, assigned male at birth	125–200 (<185 Excellent)	40 or higher (>60 Excellent)	Below 100 (Ideally <85)	Below 150	<130
20 and older assigned female at birth	125–200 (<185 Excellent)	50 or higher (>60 Excellent)	Below 100 (Ideally <85)	Below 150	<130
Borderline to moderately elevated 19 and younger	171–199	≥40–45 Low – *Abnormal*	110–129	Ages 0–9 y 75–99 10–18 y 0–129 19 y 120–150	120–144
Borderline to moderately elevated 20 and older	201–239	<40 Low - *Abnormal*	>130	>150	>130 or higher
High Levels 19 and younger	200 or higher	<40	200 or higher	Ages 0–9 y >99 10–18 y >130 19 y > 150	145 or higher
High Levels 20 and older Extremely High	240 or higher	<40	160–189 190	>150	>130 or higher

Adapted from AHA 2024 / National Library of Medicine 2024 / US Dept. of HHS 2022

Table 8
Criteria for screening and diagnosis of prediabetes and diabetes type 1 and 2

	Prediabetes	Diabetes	Differentiating Diabetes Type 1 vs Type 2
A1C	5.7%–6.4% (39–47 mmol/mol)	≥6.5% (48 mmol/mol)	Assess Antibodies GADA, IA-2A, IAA, ZnT8A
FPG	100–125 mg/dL (5.6–6.0 mmol/L)	≥126 mg/dL (7.0 mmol/L)	
2-h plasma glucose during 76-g OGTT	104–199 mg/dL (7.8–11.0 mmol/L)	≥200 mg/dL (11.1 mmol/L)	
Random plasma glucose		≥200 mg/dL (11.1 mmol/L)	

Abbreviations: GADA, glutamic acid decarboxylase autoantibodies; IA-2A, insulinoma-associated antigen-2 autoantibodies; IAA, insulin autoantibodies; ZnT8A, zinc transporter 8 autoantibodies.

Adapted from American Diabetes Association. Diagnosis and classification of diabetes: Standards of care in diabetes—2025. Diabetes Care. 2025;48(Supplement 1):S21-S36. https://doi.org/10.2337/dc25-S002.

simultaneously quantify regional brain activity, which correlates with a higher risk of MI as demonstrated on stress testing.[24]

Stress reduction activities lead to better adaptiveness to other types of stress; however, the total amount of stress one can receive before negative health effects occur is unknown. Stress reduction activities that include regular exercise, both aerobic and resistance, are beneficial, such as.

- Aerobic exercise—walking, running, swimming, or biking.
- Weight training (light and heavy).
- Yoga, Tai Chi, and Pilates.
- Meditation, prayer, and other spiritual activities.[23]

Cognitive Behavioral Therapy

Cognitive behavioral therapy (CBT) is a psychological approach to maladaptive behaviors. The core principles of the therapy include that erroneous thought patterns cause negative behaviors and that individuals can change their behavior after changing their beliefs. CBT has applications in improving diet choices to healthier options, increasing PA, discontinuing smoking, and managing stress.

Li and colleagues conducted a meta-analysis of research interventions that included CBT in patients with coronary heart disease.[25] The authors reviewed 22 randomized controlled trials that included 4991 patients with coronary heart disease. The results demonstrated several positive outcomes including that CBT reduced symptoms of depression −2.00 (95% CI: −2.83 to −1.16, $P<.001$); anxiety, −2.07 (95% CI: −3.39 to −0.75, $P=.002$); stress, −3.33 (95% CI: −4.23 to −2.44, $P<.001$); and BMI: −0.47 (95% CI: −0.81 to −0.13, $P=.006$).[24] Therefore, CBT is a practical component of the nonpharmacologic treatment of coronary heart disease and hypertension.

Sleep Disorders and Cardiovascular Disease

Sleep, diet, and PA are the 3 pillars of health. Unlike other health behaviors, healthy sleep is not included in the American College of Cardiology/AHA CVD prevention guidelines. An unhealthy diet, a sedentary lifestyle, and poor sleep contribute to CVD.[26,27] Approximately 35% of US adults are short sleepers (<7 hours), approximately 20% report excessive daytime sleepiness, and less than 50% report having a good night of sleep every night. The presence of sleep disorders, such as insomnia and obstructive sleep apnea (OSA), has been linked to other adverse sleep exposures, such as short sleep, suggesting that multiple unhealthy sleep phenotypes may occur concurrently and potentially interact, further augmenting the risk for chronic disease.[27]

Chronic sleep disturbances are known to have a range of negative health consequences, with the relationship between OSA and hypertension being well-established through numerous studies. Numerous sleep disorders, such as narcolepsy, central sleep apnea, OSA, and insomnia, have shown different effects on CVD outcomes.[28] Increased risks of illnesses such as acute coronary syndrome, hypertension, cardiovascular mortality, and coronary artery calcification are associated with sleep disorders. See **Box 1** for strategies to improve sleep quality.

Adverse Lifestyle Issues

Adverse lifestyle choices refer to habits that are deleterious to cardiovascular health. They include smoking, cannabis use, and alcohol consumption. Smoking cigarettes, cigars, e-cigarettes, and vaping are all major causes of CVD. Smoking or inhaling tobacco and nicotine in any form increases the risk of many types of CVD, including coronary heart disease (CHD), stroke, peripheral arterial disease, and abdominal and aortic aneurysm . The mechanism by which smoking affects the cardiovascular system involves endothelial dysfunction by reducing nitrogen monoxide production, promoting prothrombotic conditions and activating inflammatory routes.[29] Cannabis use is associated with adverse cardiovascular outcomes, with heavier use (more days per month) associated with higher odds of adverse outcomes.[28]

Smoking Cessation

The benefits of quitting cannot be overstated, as smoking cessation has been associated with a reduction in cardiovascular mortality. This ranges from the reduction in the incidence of hypertension, type 2 diabetes, and HF.[30] Smoking cessation strategies include behavioral interventions such as CBT, hypnosis, and deflection alternative activities such as physical fitness, crafts, or other things to change triggers. Inclusion of nicotine replacement therapy and pharmacologic aids may also be helpful.

Alcohol Consumption

Alcohol increases the risk of hypertensive heart disease, cardiomyopathy, AF, atrial flutter, and strokes. Alcohol affects human physiology either through years of consumption, acute intoxication, or dependence. It has been linked with approximately 230 diseases (International Classification of Diseases, 10th edition), including 40 diseases that would not prevail without alcohol. Alcohol has been ascribed as a crucial

---

Box 1
Strategies for improving sleep quality

Proper screening for sleep disorders with a sleep specialist (Sleep Studies).

Initiation of continious positive airway pressure (CPAP)/ implanted mechanical/ oral devices, as necessary.

Regular sleep schedule for consistency.

Improve bedroom environment optimization removing clutter, computers, and other electronics.

Dietary restrictions of caffeine and alcohol.

factor in deaths due to infectious diseases, intentional and unintentional injuries, digestive diseases, and several noncommunicable diseases.[31]

Recommended limits are none. Alcohol consumption (100 g/week) is linearly associated with a higher risk of stroke, HF, fatal hypertensive disease, and fatal aortic aneurysm and has a borderline elevation in the risk of coronary heart disease, as compared to those consuming between 0 to 25 g/week.[31] Previously, there were some indications that there may have been a health benefit of modest use of alcohol, but that has been proven to be a myth. There is no benefit to consuming alcohol. Strategies for moderation or abstinence include patient education, CBT, and support and mentoring programs.

STRATEGIES AND IMPLEMENTATION TECHNIQUES FOR LIFESTYLE CHANGES
Motivational Interviewing

Motivational interviewing is based on resolving a person's ambivalent feelings about their deleterious health behavior. A pillar of the success of motivational interviewing is that the clinician can express empathy. Upon appropriate rapport building, the clinician may be able to collaborate with a person to set goals that are positive for the person's health. There are 4 steps: engage, direct, evoke, and plan.

According to Rodzen, the steps to the motivational interview include (1) Engaging with the patient to address fears, goals, and barriers, (2) focusing on the person's most wanted goal, which highlights the behavior they are most ready to change, (3) empowering the person with the sense they can change, and (4) setting specific goals and collaborating to achieve goals.[32] As per Misfud and colleagues, a combination approach of face-to-face sessions and telephone follow-up provided by a trained clinician may be the most effective method to support change.[33]

Social Support and Connections

Data support the idea that social support and connections improve cardiovascular health. Coyte and colleagues conducted a prospective population-based study of older men.[34] The study included 3,698 participants, and information was collected on social relations based on marital status, living situation, and social contacts with

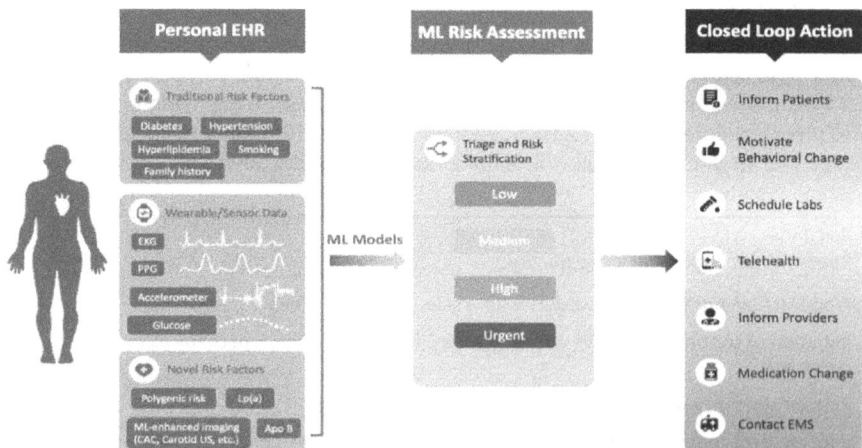

Fig. 4. Technology and digital health. Apo B, CAC, EKG, EMS, ML, PPG. (Javaid, A et al., Medicine 2032: The future of cardiovascular disease prevention with machine learning and digital health technology, AJPC, 2022;12(100379) https://doi.org/10.1016/j.ajpc.2022.100379.)

friends and family.[34] Of the 3698 participants, 33 developed HF.[34] The results of the study demonstrated that men with low social connections to friends and family had an increased risk of incident HF (hazard ratio 1.59, 95% CI 1.15 to 2.18).[34] Fostering social connections and avoiding loneliness have a role in preventing heart disease.

Technology and Digital Health

Digital health interventions, including digital health technology, digital medicine, telemedicine, mobile health, remote monitoring, wearable devices, and consumer technologies are important public health and clinical interventions for improving adherence and promoting lifestyle changes for preventing and treating CVD. The future will bring machine learning to automatically record biometric data in an electronic health record. This will allow providers to analyze real-time data and make more informed decisions on a patients' evolving health.[35] See **Fig. 4** for the technological applications to health management.

SUMMARY

CVD continues to be the leading cause of death in the United States despite medical advancements and technology that are being used to address this disease. Poor primary prevention seems to be the root cause. While global burden remains high, health care providers worldwide must apply nonpharmacologic treatments early in the disease process. CVD is a multisystemic issue that is directly affected by nonmodifiable risk factors and modifiable risk factors. While the nonmodifiable risk factors cannot be changed, understanding these factors helps clinicians identify at-risk patients. Multiple risk factors can be modified. Nonpharmacologic therapy is centered around 6 pillars.[36]

- *Nutrition:* Consuming a fiber-filled, nutrient-dense, antioxidant-rich eating pattern based predominantly on a variety of minimally processed vegetables, fruits, whole grains, legumes, nuts and seeds.
- *Physical Activity:* Engaging in regular and consistent PA.
- *Stress Management*: Incorporating stress-reducing behaviors may be difficult in modern society but is essential for whole-person health.
- *Restorative Sleep*: Striving for 7 to 9 hours of high-quality sleep, allowing the body to reset and recover.
- *Social Connection*: Strengthening and maintaining relationships and connections with others that bring meaning and purpose to life.
- *Avoidance of Risky Substances*: Reducing or eliminating the consumption of or exposure to any substances that cause harm through toxicity, addiction, physical damage, or adverse side effects.

Understanding trends of cardiovascular risk factors, variations in risk factors between racial and ethnic backgrounds, and determining patients' socioeconomic status may guide public health policies for targeted interventions aimed at eliminating health disparities and reducing CVD.

CLINICS CARE POINTS

- Knowledge of modifiable and nonmodifiable risk factors is essential for providing nonpharmacological treatment of cardiovascular disease.
- Address the 6 pillars of lifestyle medicine, which include nutrition, physical activity, stress management, restorative sleep, social connections, and avoidance of risky substances.

- Failure to implement early nonpharmacological treatment can adversely affect longevity and long-term health outcomes.

DISCLOSURE

The authors do not have any applicable disclosures or financial gain associated with this paper.

REFERENCES

1. Fletcher G, Landolfo C, Niebauer J, et al. Promoting physical activity and exercise: JACC health promotion series. J Am Coll Cardiol 2018;72(14):1622–39.
2. Stark B, Johnson C, Roth G. Global prevalence of coronary artery disease: an update from the global burden of disease study. J Am Coll Cardiol 2024; 83(13_Supplement):2320.
3. CDC. National Center for Health Statistics. Multiple cause of death 2018–2022 on CDC WONDER database. Available at: https://wonder.cdc.gov/mcd.html. Accessed May 3, 2024.
4. Ralapanawa U, Sivakanesan R. Epidemiology, and the magnitude of coronary artery eisease and acute coronary syndrome: a narrative review. J Epidemiol Glob Health 2021;11(2):169–77.
5. Tsao CW, Aday AW, Almarzooq ZI, et al. Heart disease and stroke statistics-2023 update: a report from the American heart association. Circulation 2023;147(8): e622.
6. Regmi M, Siccardi MA. Coronary artery disease prevention. NIH.gov. 2019. Available at: https://www.ncbi.nlm.nih.gov/books/NBK547760/. Accessed September 4, 2024.
7. Gooding HC, de Ferranti SD. Cardiovascular risk assessment and cholesterol management in adolescents: getting to the heart of the matter. Curr Opin Pediatr 2010;22(4):398–404.
8. Rodgers JL, Jones J, Bolleddu SI, et al. Cardiovascular risks associated with gender and aging. J Cardiovasc Dev and Dis 2019;6(2):19.
9. DeFilippis E, Van Spall H. Is it time for sex-specific guidelines for cardiovascular disease? J Am Coll Cardiol 2021;78(2):189–92.
10. Hajar R. Genetics in cardiovascular disease. Heart Views 2020;21(1):55–6.
11. He J, Zhu Z, Bundy JD, et al. Trends in cardiovascular risk factors in US adults by race and ethnicity and socioeconomic status, 1999-2018. JAMA 2021;326(13): 1286–98.
12. Diab A, Dastmalchi LN, Gulati M, et al. A heart-healthy diet for cardiovascular disease prevention: where are we now? Vasc Health Risk Manag 2023;19:237–53.
13. Dinu M, Pagliai G, Angelino D, et al. Effects of popular diets on anthropometric and cardiometabolic parameters: an umbrella review of meta-analyses of randomized controlled trials. Adv Nutr 2020;11(4):815–33.
14. Onwuzo C, Olukorode JO, Omokore OA, et al. DASH Diet: a review of its scientifically proven hypertension reduction and health benefits. Cureus 2023;15(9): e44692.
15. Filippou CD, Tsioufis CP, Thomopoulos CG, et al. Dietary approaches to stop hypertension (DASH) diet and blood pressure reduction in adults with and without hypertension: a systematic review and meta-analysis of randomized controlled trials. Adv Nutr 2020;11(5):1150–60.

16. Gibbs J, Gaskin E, Ji C, et al. The effect of plant-based dietary patterns on blood pressure: a systematic review and meta-analysis of controlled intervention trials. J Hypertens 2021;39(1):23–37.

17. Lavie C, Laddu D, Arena R, et al. Healthy weight and obesity prevention: JACC health promotion series. J Am Coll Cardiol 2018;72(13):1506–31.

18. National Heart, Lung and Blood Institute (NIH), Stahl JM, Malhotra S. Obesity surgery indications and contraindications. In: StatPearls [Internet]. Treasure Island (FL): StatPearls Publishing; 2024. Available at: https://www.ncbi.nlm.nih.gov/books/NBK513285/.

19. AHA. Heart Association recommendations for physical activity in adults and kids. American Heart Association 2024. Available at: https://www.heart.org/en/healthy-living/fitness/fitness-basics/aha-recs-for-physical-activity-in-adults.   Accessed September 1, 2024.

20. Correira RR, Veras ASC, Tebar WR, et al. Strength training for arterial hypertension treatment: a systematic review and meta-analysis of randomized clinical trials. Sci Rep 2023;13(1):201.

21. American College of Sports Medicine. Position stand. Quantity and quality of exercise for developing and maintaining cardiorespiratory, musculoskeletal, and neuromotor fitness in apparently healthy adults: guidance for prescribing exercise. Med Sci Sports Exerc 2011;43(7):1334–59.

22. O'Regan A, Pollock M, D'Sa S, et al. ABC of prescribing exercise as medicine: a narrative review of the experiences of general practitioners and patients. BMJ Open 2021;7:e001050.

23. Osborne MT, Shin LM, Mehta NN, et al. Disentangling the links between psychosocial stress and cardiovascular disease. Circ. Cardiovasc.Imaging 2020;13(8): e010931.

24. Satyjeet F, Naz S, Kumar V, et al. Psychological stress as a risk factor for cardiovascular disease: a case-control study. Cureus 2020;12(10):e10757.

25. Li YN, Buys N, Ferguson S, et al. Effectiveness of cognitive behavioral therapy-based interventions on health outcomes in patients with coronary heart disease: a meta-analysis. World J Psychiatry 2021;11(11):1147–66.

26. Popovic D, Marija B, Tesic M, et al. Defining the importance of stress reduction in managing cardiovascular disease - the role of exercise. Prog Cardiovasc Dis 2022;70:84–93.

27. Makarem N, Castro-Diehl C, St-Onge MP, et al. Redefining cardiovascular health to include sleep: prospective associations with cardiovascular disease in the MESA sleep study journal of the American Heart Association. JAHA 2022; 11(21). https://doi.org/10.1161/JAHA.122.025252.

28. Ravichandran R, Gupta L, Singh M, et al. The interplay between sleep disorders and cardiovascular diseases: a systematic review. Cureus 2023;15(9):e45898.

29. Okorare O, Evbayekha EO, Adabale OK, et al. Smoking cessation and benefits to cardiovascular health: a review of literature. Cureus 2023;15(3):e35966.

30. Jeffers AM, Stanton Glantz S, Byers ML, et al. Association of cannabis use with cardiovascular outcomes among US adults. JAHA 2024;13(5). https://doi.org/10.1161/JAHA.123.030178.

31. Arora M, ElSayed A, Beger B, et al. The impact of alcohol consumption on cardiovascular health: myths and measures. Global heart 2022;17(1):45.

32. Rodzen M. Putting in the patient in charge. Physician Assistant Clinics 2020;2: 135–42.

33. Mifsud JL, Galea J. Motivational interviewing, and outcomes in primary preventive cardiology. Br J Cardiol 2021;28(4):47.

34. Coyte A, Perry R, Papacosta AO, et al. Social relationships and the risk of incident heart failure: results from a prospective population-based study of older men. Eur Heart J Open 2021;2(1):oeab045.

35. Javaid A, Zghyer F, Kim C, et al. Medicine 2032: the future of cardiovascular disease prevention with machine learning and digital health technology. AJPC 2022; 12:100379.

36. American College of Lifestyle Medicine. 6 pillars of lifestyle medicine, Am J lifestyle med. Available at: https://lifestylemedicine.org/3. Accessed September 4, 2024.

Chest Pain Evaluation

Nick Entsminger, DMSc, PA-C (CAQ-EM)

KEYWORDS

- Physician assistant • Chest pain • Myocardial infarction • Cardiac examination
- Physical exam • Cardiac differentials

KEY POINTS

- An organized cardiac assessment combines a subjective (reported) and objective (physical assessment) examination with key risk factors to determine cardiac likelihood.
- An initial chest pain assessment focuses on red flags (eg, poor skin signs, abnormal vital signs, etc.) consistent with risk of rapid deterioration.
- Diagnostic studies add support for a differential, yet do not necessarily rule out a cardiac cause. Clinical suspicion and sound assessment skills are paramount.
- Outpatient studies may be warranted for patients complaining of intermittent symptoms, or those patients at high-risk for an impending acute coronary syndrome (ACS).
- Because there is no clinical decision-making tool to exclude ACS definitively, proficient clinical skills and judgment are required.

INTRODUCTION

A chest pain evaluation requires a focused assessment of subjective and objective findings and underlying risk factors to determine the probability of a cardiovascular (CV) cause. This assessment approach requires the optimization of key information, whether reported or identified on physical examination. Because there is no clinical decision-making reference to definitively exclude acute coronary syndrome (ACS),[1] Physician assistants (PAs) must approach cardiac evaluations through a lens of probability, as chest pain complaints invoke a myriad of differential diagnoses from the benign to detrimental. To determine risks for deterioration, PAs must have the knowledge to promptly identify high-risk findings, or red flags, that require urgent evaluation and specialty intervention. Such evaluations require organized assessments, knowledge of appropriate use and interpretation of diagnostic tests, and a thorough review of a patient's medical, social, familial, and medication history.

EPIDEMIOLOGY AND RISK FACTORS

Heart disease is endemic to the United States. It is the leading cause of death for both men and women of all racial and ethnic populations.[2] Coronary artery disease (CAD),

Master of Science in Physician Assistant Studies Program, Dominican University of California, 50 Acacia Avenue, San Rafael, CA 94901, USA
E-mail address: nentsmin@gmail.com

Physician Assist Clin 10 (2025) 245–260
https://doi.org/10.1016/j.cpha.2024.11.012
2405-7991/25/© 2024 Elsevier Inc. All rights reserved, including those for text and data mining, AI training, and similar technologies.

Abbreviations	
ACC	American College of Cardiology
ACS	acute coronary syndrome
AHA	American Heart Association
BNP	brain natriuretic peptide
CAC	coronary artery calcium
CAD	coronary artery disease
CBC	complete blood count
CMR	cardiac magnetic resonance
CT	computed tomography
CTA	computed tomography angiography
CV	cardiovascular
ECG	electrocardiogram
EF	ejection fraction
HEART	history, electrocardiogram findings, age, risk factors, and an initial troponin level
ICA	invasive coronary angiography
JVD	jugular venous distension
LAD	left anterior descending
LMCA	left main coronary artery
MACE	major adverse cardiac event
NIDDM	non-insulin-dependent diabetes
PA	Physician assistants
SPECT	single photon emission computed tomography
STEMI	ST elevation myocardial infarction

specifically, contributes to the highest cardiac mortality rates.[3] Social determinants further influence the proliferation of heart disease across populations. Primary risk factors are higher among lower socioeconomic levels and are affected by psychological, racial, and ethnic influences that increase the likelihood of CAD (**Box 1**).[4] These risk factors contribute substantial clinical information when determining the risk. Consequently, socioeconomic areas with increased disparities represent a higher rate of CV death (**Table 1**).

FOCUSED CARDIAC ASSESSMENT

PAs should always approach chest pain complaints with an initial examination focusing on findings consistent with threats to life and the probability of rapid instability. Evaluations begin upon entering the room; during this initial approach, assessing distress and appearance can quickly and efficiently provide information relating to patient stability. A subsequent focused cardiac assessment should include simultaneous questioning and physical examination to determine a red flag diagnosis. A *red flag* is defined as a descriptor or physical finding consistent with a high probability of a critical diagnosis (eg, acute myocardial infarction [AMI], aortic aneurysm, and others).

GENERAL IMPRESSION

Beginning with the patient's skin signs, mental status, and level of distress, the PA can quickly determine clinical stability, as alterations to these factors suggest a failure of the body's compensatory mechanisms. Poor perfusion, manifesting as decreased skin color, can lead to cardiogenic shock and altered mentation from inappropriate cerebral blood flow. A patient's stability is further assessed with a review of vital signs. For example, a patient presenting with altered mentation, pallor, and a weak radial

---

Box 1
Risk factors for acute coronary syndrome

- Tobacco use
- Hypertension
- Diabetes
- Hyperlipidemia
- Male sex
- Sedentary lifestyle
- Obesity
- Poor nutrition
- Family history of MI (<55 years of age)

---

pulse too rapid to count requires immediate intervention versus someone who greets you normally upon entrance. Initial assessments are a rapid and efficient means of determining the need for prompt intervention before less emergent questioning and data gathering.

SUBJECTIVE FINDINGS

PAs must pay particular attention to key words or red flags that increase the risk of cardiac likelihood during the interview (**Fig. 1**). For example, a patient describing chest pain that worsens on exertion is significant and considered a red flag for possible ACS. The likelihood of a cardiac etiology is further supported during the interview with the presence of risk factors or comorbid conditions such as hypertension, hyperlipidemia, and other risk factors.

CASE EXAMPLE 1

A 51-year-old male presents, complaining of dull substernal chest *pressure* for 3 days that he can feel in his right shoulder. He does not appear to be in acute distress and shows no signs of diaphoresis. His vital signs are not concerning. He has a history of hypertension, non-insulin-dependent diabetes (NIDDM), obesity, hyperlipidemia, and 20-year tobacco use.

Table 1
% of heart disease by race or ethnic group, 2021

Black (Non-Hispanic)	22.6
Asian	18.6
Native Hawaiian or Other Pacific Islander	18.3
White (Non-Hispanic)	18
American Indian or Alaska Native	15.5
Hispanic	11.9
AI	17.4

Data from the National Center for Health Statistics. Multiple Cause of Death 2018–2021 on CDC WONDER Database. Available at: https://wonder.cdc.gov/mcd.html. Accessed February 2, 2023.

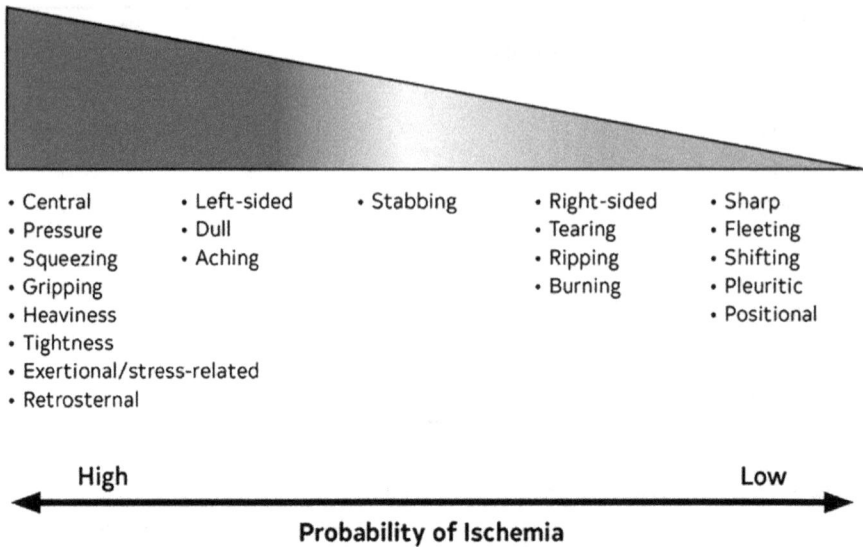

- Central
- Pressure
- Squeezing
- Gripping
- Heaviness
- Tightness
- Exertional/stress-related
- Retrosternal

- Left-sided
- Dull
- Aching

- Stabbing

- Right-sided
- Tearing
- Ripping
- Burning

- Sharp
- Fleeting
- Shifting
- Pleuritic
- Positional

High   Low

Probability of Ischemia

Fig. 1. More risk stratification of subjective complaints. The initial provided images had a citation attached with description.

Although this patient appears stable, chest pressure associated with radiation, unilateral or bilateral, suggests a high-risk for ACS. The probability of ACS is further increased by the presence of risk factors such as hypertension, diabetes, obesity, hyperlipidemia, and tobacco use. Clinicians must focus on factors, including examination findings that add to the clinical picture, that increase diagnostic probability.

OBJECTIVE FINDINGS

Physical examination red flags must be quickly recognized and evaluated in conjunction with subjective information and risk factors. Obvious physical signs of instability are most visible from a distance. These include, but are not limited to, skin pallor, diaphoresis, labored breathing, and evident pain severity cuing the PA to clinical instability and the likelihood of rapid deterioration. Less obvious findings are specific to the diagnosis: jugular venous distension (JVD), S3 gallop, lung rales, and/or peripheral edema provides evidence of heart failure, whereas abdominal pain may increase the risk of aneurysm, mesenteric ischemia, or other differential diagnoses. Building from *Case Example 1,* the clinical picture is expanded with the addition of a focused physical examination.

CASE EXAMPLE 2

A 51-year-old male presents, complaining of dull, substernal chest *pressure* for 3 days that he can feel in his right shoulder. He does not appear to be in acute distress and shows no signs of diaphoresis. His vital signs are currently stable. He has a history of hypertension, NIDDM, obesity, hyperlipidemia, and 20-year tobacco use. His skin is pink, warm, and dry, he has no respiratory distress, and his bilateral radial pulses are strong and equal. There are no signs of JVD but there is a mid-systolic murmur. He has 3/10 chest pain with radiation to the left neck, his abdomen is rotund yet soft and nontender without mass or pulsation. There is no evidence of peripheral swelling or calf tenderness.

Determination of whether this patient's murmur is acute or chronic is important; however the finding is significant either way. Often the patient is aware of the presence of a long-standing murmur. Acute murmurs are found in higher risk patients, particularly patients with a history of intravenous drug use, thoracic aneurysm, or rheumatic disease. Based on the patient's complaint, descriptors, history, risk factors, and physical findings, they appear initially stable, yet require further evaluation to identify if there is a need for rapid interventions.

VITAL SIGNS

The interpretation of vital signs during a chest pain assessment is imperative to determine patient stability. Heart rate alone during the initial assessment can provide significant patient information, from perfusion to volume status. A faint or absent radial pulse is a rapid means of identifying hypotension in a cardiac patient; because to perfuse the radial artery, systolic blood pressure must be at least 80 mm Hg. Further, a rapid or bradycardic pulse may suggest an inadequacy of cardiac output, increasing the risk for cardiogenic shock.

CASE EXAMPLE 3

A 28-year-old female presents complaining of shortness of breath and a deep *tightness* to the chest. She does not appear in distress, yet she is diaphoretic with pallor. Her radial pulse is faint, yet palpable at a regular rate that is too rapid to count.

In contrast to.

CASE EXAMPLE 4

An 84-year-old male presents with repeated syncope over the past several days. He is alert and oriented, and no distress is noted. A slow pulse is present, yet at an irregular rate of 40 beats per minute.

Both cases reveal significant findings for instability that is quickly assessed through initial findings and a rapid pulse check. Case #3 represents a high-risk for an unstable supraventricular tachycardia, while Case #4 is at risk for cardiac failure due to inadequate cardiac efficiency caused by low heart rate. These cases prompt interventions.

Blood pressure readings, respiratory status, and oral temperature further add to the clinical picture. Blood pressure measurement offers a precise indication of cardiac pump (systolic) and rest (diastolic) function during the cardiac cycle, while increased or decreased pulse pressures have been linked to heart disease or heart failure risk. A pulse pressure rise of 10 mm Hg increases the CV risk by 20%.[5] While often obvious, labored breathing is another indicator of patient stability. Observed respiratory distress focuses the cardiac assessment on potential pulmonary effects (eg, left-side heart failure) or extra-cardiac causes of chest pain, such as pulmonary embolism (PE), pneumothorax, effusion, acid-base imbalances, or infectious causes such as sepsis and pneumonia.

DIFFERENTIALS AND RISK RATIOS

Although not all chest complaints are cardiac related, PAs must begin assessments with consideration of high-risk differentials (**Box 2**), beginning with life-threatening

---

Box 2
High risk chest pain differentials

- ACS
- PE
- Pneumothorax
- Pericardial tamponade
- Aortic dissection
- Esophageal perforation
- Myocarditis

---

diagnosis (eg, MI, aneurysm, or dissection). Pain and location descriptors may increase or decrease the likelihood of ACS or other differentials. Evaluations from this standpoint also focus assessments on cardiovascular likelihood and probability of deterioration. For example, a patient complaint of sharp, left-sided chest pain provoked by chest palpation can be less concerning than sharp chest pain provoked by respiration and tachycardia on evaluation of vital signs. Subjective complaints offer subtle concerns while a focused physical examination may rapidly determine acuity. The following 2 cases provide examples of these differences.

CASE EXAMPLE 5

A 57-year-old male in mild distress complains of increasing substernal chest discomfort; the pain is described as *pressure* and is a nonradiating. This symptom is nonprovocable and not associated with any shortness of breath, dizziness, or syncope. He is mildly obese with a history of NIDDM, stage 1 hypertension, and tobacco use. His skin is normal and dry. He has no abnormal heart sounds, his lungs are clear, and he has no chest or abdominal tenderness. He has equal, strong pulses in his upper and lower extremities, and there is no noted peripheral edema. His vital signs reveal a blood pressure of 138/90 mm Hg and a radial pulse of 88 beats per minute.

This patient presentation is in contrast to Example 6 below.

CASE EXAMPLE 6

A 57-year-old, pale-appearing male in moderate distress complains of increasing substernal chest discomfort. The pain is a nonradiating pressure, nonprovocable, and not associated with any shortness of breath, dizziness, or syncope. He is mildly obese with a history of NIDDM, stage 1 hypertension, and tobacco use. His skin is pale and moist. He has cardiac auscultation findings consistent with a diastolic murmur. He has faint lower rales noted on lung auscultation, yet no chest or abdominal tenderness. He has equal, yet faint pulses to his upper and lower extremities, and there is trace peripheral edema to his feet and ankles. His vital signs reveal a blood pressure of 202/108 mm Hg and a radial pulse of 110 beats per minute.

There is a clear difference in acuity between these cases. While Case 5 should be evaluated promptly due to significant risk factors that increase the likelihood of ACS, Case 6 is clearly at higher risk for deterioration based on physical examination findings, including skin pallor, likely new-onset murmur, abnormal lung sounds, and peripheral edema separate of his medical and social history. Furthermore, elevations in his vital signs increase the possibility of underlying compensatory mechanisms caused by concerning etiologies. Case 6 supports the need for a rapid and focused cardiac assessment to identify immediate life threats.

PROGNOSTIC TOOLS

Diagnostic tools such as the history, electrocardiogram (ECG) findings, age, risk factors, and an initial troponin level (HEART) Score are frequently used to predict a major adverse cardiac event (MACE) in patients older than 21 years of age. The HEART score uses a point system assessing several factors that, if present, increase the probability of ACS. These factors include ACS suspicion based on HEART (**Table 2**). The HEART score has been externally validated and recommended for primary use in assessing ACS risk.[6] While not practical for outpatient settings due to troponin requirements, HEART scores are appropriate for emergency departments and should be documented.

Table 2 HEART score for major cardiac events	
History	**Points**
• Slightly suspicious	0
• Moderately suspicious	I
• Highly suspicious	2
ECG	
• Normal	0
• Nonspecific changes	1
• Significant ST change	2
Age	
• <45	0
• 45–64	1
• ≥65	2
Risk factor	
• None	0
• 1–2 risk factors	1
• ≤3 risk factors	2
Initial troponin	
• ≤Normal limit	0
• 1-3x normal limit	1
• >3x normal limit	2
Total Points:	
Score:	
0–3: Low risk, 0.9%-1.7% MACE risk	
4–6: Moderate risk, 12-16.6% MACE risk	
≥7: High risk, 50%–65% MACE risk	

Data from Six AJ Backus BE, Kelder JC. Chest pain in the emergency room: value of the Heart score. Neth Heart J 2008;16(6):191–6.

CHEST PAIN WORKUP

PAs should order diagnostic testing based on subjective and objective findings that indicate high probability differentials, especially when a diagnosis is unclear. Diagnostics are used to fill gaps and narrow differentials; however, unnecessary diagnostic tests, aside from an ECG, may delay care to patients with clinical instability where emergent specialist intervention is required. PAs must ensure care is specific to patient needs. The following 2 cases provide examples.

CASE EXAMPLE 7

A diaphoretic, 56-year-old obese male with a history of previous myocardial infarction (MI), hyperlipidemia, NIDDM, and chronic tobacco use presents with an acute onset of substernal chest *aching* radiating to his neck and left shoulder. He states that it, *feels exactly like my last heart attack.* His initial ECG reveals hyperacute T-waves to the anterior leads and he is hypertensive at 168/102 mm Hg with a heart rate of 92 beats per minute. This patient is clearly at high risk for ACS. While laboratory studies are collected, emergent cardiology intervention supersedes delay for further diagnostic testing.

In contrast to.

CASE EXAMPLE 8

A postmenopausal, 52-year-old female has a history of nonspecific, 3/10 chest discomfort for 3 days. She currently takes estrogen. Her initial ECG and vital signs reveal no concerns, other than a regular complex tachycardia at 110 beats per minute. Based on the reported history and physical examination, laboratory and imaging studies are ordered, including a complete blood count (CBC), complete metabolic profile, troponin, and computed tomography angiography (CTA) of the chest. While ACS is considered, this patient's history of chest pressure, hormone use, and tachycardia must be evaluated for PE, a diagnosis to assist in narrowing the differential diagnoses in this currently stable patient.

Diagnostics are tailored to address the most high-risk and likely diagnoses. Further, unstable patients requiring immediate interventions rarely benefit from the use of diagnostics. Until a patient is stabilized, superfluous testing delays care.

ELECTROCARDIOGRAM

While a normal ECG cannot fully exclude ACS during chest pain, QRS morphology changes identify the likely location of a coronary occlusion and need for urgent intervention. 12-lead ECG regions correspond to coronary arterial flows, and QRS morphologies within specific areas quickly pinpoint the area of involvement. Although any occlusion is significant, some coronary arteries supply larger areas of myocardial tissue, and thus can lead to more rapid deterioration compared to others (ie, left anterior descending [LAD] and right main coronary artery).

The acronym "Lie, Lie, ALL" or "LI, LII, AAAALL" acts as a quick reference to determine and confirm areas of significance, including ST elevation myocardial infarction (STEMI) (**Fig. 2**). Although not initially assessed in the "Lie, Lie, AALL" mnemonic, changes in lead AVR can represent an occlusion to the left main coronary artery (LMCA). Similar changes (ST depression or elevation) in any 2 leads of the same region are consistent with a positive finding. STEMI diagnosis is confirmed by ST elevation in 2 contiguous leads, yet the amount of elevation is determined by both gender and location, per the American College of Cardiology (ACC), American Heart Association

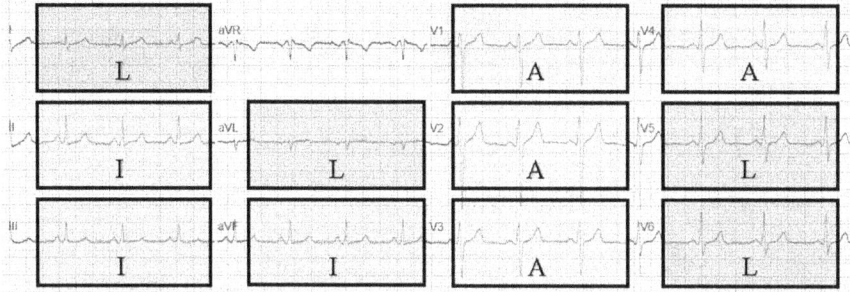

Fig. 2. 12-lead ECG with representative vantages. L, Lateral (Left circumflex), I, Inferior (right coronary artery), A, anterior (left anterior descending or LAD). AVR can represent a LMCA occlusion in the presence of ST elevation with diffuse ischemia. Reciprocal changes in leads V1-3 offer insight into potential posterior infraction.

(AHA), European Society of Cardiology, and the World Heart Federation committee guidelines (**Box 3**).[7] Evidence of a left bundle branch block, left ventricular hypertrophy, or a paced rhythm make STEMI identification difficult without access to previous ECGs or the use of scoring tools such as Sgarbossa criteria. ST depression in V1-3 is suggestive of a posterior infarction.

Knowledge of less common forms of cardiac irregularities, such as Wellen Syndrome, Brugada syndrome, hypertrophic cardiomyopathy, Wolff Parkinson White syndrome, and other conditions that require intervention also must be known. Additionally, further workups are required for high-risk patients without acute ECG findings to establish NSTEMI or noncardiac causes.

CHEST X-RAY

Chest X-rays assist in identifying structural, vascular, pulmonary, and infectious causes of chest pain complaints, and should be ordered appropriately based on differential considerations. While not as sensitive or specific as computed tomography (CT) or MRI, X-rays can be completed at the bedside, offering a rapid assessment of the lungs for infection or volume overload, as well as visualization of lung borders for evidence of pneumothorax, hemopneumothorax, and effusion. CV concerns such as cardiomegaly, an enlarged mediastinum, or the presence of suspected thoracic aneurysm can be

---

Box 3
Joint European Society of Cardiology (ESC)/American College of Cardiology (ACC)/American Heart Association (AHA)/World Heart Federation (WHF) task force ST elevation myocardial infarction criteria

- New ST-segment elevation at the J point in 2 contiguous leads with the cutoff point as greater than 0.1 mV in all leads other than V2 or V3.

- In leads V2-V3, the cutoff point is greater than 0.2 mV in men older than 40 years and greater than 0.25 in men younger than 40 years , or greater than 0.15 mV in women.

Data from Gulati M, Levy PD, Mukherjee D, et al. 2021 AHA/ACC/ASE/CHEST/SAEM/SCCT/SCMR guideline for the evaluation and diagnosis of chest pain: a report of the American College of Cardiology/American Heart Association Joint Committee on Clinical Practice Guidelines. J Am Coll Cardiol 2021;78(22):e187–e285.

identified. The AHA/ACC recommend an initial chest X-ray for heart failure patients unless its completion would delay emergent interventions such as revascularization.[8] Finally, nonchest pain complaints caused by rib fractures or large hiatal hernias can be identified.

ECHOCARDIOGRAM

Echocardiograms offer pertinent information regarding valvular compromise, ventricular wall irregularities, cardiac effusions, and evidence of heart failure with reduced ejection fraction (EF). With the increasing use of point of care ultrasound, PAs can quickly evaluate cardiac function, as well as evidence of other noncardiac chest pain causes, such as pneumothorax, pneumonia, aortic aneurysm, gallbladder disease, and others.

LABORATORY STUDIES

Laboratory studies assist in narrowing differentials during chest pain, and certain labs, such as platelet count and renal function levels, also ensure preprocedural stability before cardiac catheterization or contrast-required imaging. Although patients requiring rapid intervention do not require waiting for results, specific laboratory values offer insight into chest pain causes.

TROPONIN

Cardiac biomarkers, primarily troponin, assist in the timely identification of myocardial injury. When myocardial damage occurs, the protein troponin is released and detectable in the bloodstream. There are 3 troponin types; I and T are known as cardiac troponins. These levels are relatively specific to myocardial damage but can be influenced by extracardiac complications such as renal disease; therefore, a thorough assessment of potential factors influencing troponin elevation is required. Troponin levels elevate over time, often requiring serial assessments, as they peak at 12 to 48 hours after the onset of chest pain and slowly diminish over 4 to 10 days. Biomarkers, such as creatine kinase myocardial isoenzyme and myoglobin have no benefit in the diagnosis of ACS.[8]

COMPLETE BLOOD COUNT

CBC may offer insight into potential causes of chest pain, primarily infection, inflammation, anemia, and thrombocytopenia. Leukocytosis, especially in the presence of elevated neutrophils and bandemia, may prompt further investigation into a potential infectious process. Platelet levels are also beneficial when considering procedural risk factors.

COMPLETE METABOLIC PANEL

A complete metabolic panel assists with identifying noncardiac causes of chest pain. Abnormal electrolyte levels caused by renal disease or medications may lead to abnormal ECG morphologies and cardiac arrhythmias. Further, other values such as aspartate aminotransferase, alanine aminotransferase, and total bilirubin may indicate liver or gallbladder causes such as cholecystitis or cholangitis. Finally, renal function values offer insight into fluid volume and kidney status, which may require medication dosing changes and contrast imaging considerations, such as when using CTA and coronary CT angiography (CCTA).

OTHER LABORATORY TESTING CONSIDERATIONS
Brain Natriuretic Peptide

Brain Natriuretic Peptide (BNP) protein levels are helpful in assessing volume overload, particularly in patients with heart failure. Patients presenting with chest pain with associated shortness of breath and findings of peripheral or pulmonary edema should be assessed with a BNP. When interpreting a BNP value, PAs must be keen to other complications that cause increased levels of the protein as well, such as kidney failure and sepsis.

D-DIMER

D-dimers are formed upon the bonding of platelets during clot formation and can be measured within the bloodstream when thrombosis is suspected. D-dimer testing is highly sensitive, yet it is weakly specific due to influential factors such as age, renal disease, active cancer, pregnancy, and other factors, lending to false positive values. Consequently, D-dimer testing must be considered in the context of clinical presentation whenever PE is considered, and tools such as PERC and Well's PE criteria (**Table 3**) increase probability. Patients with a high risk for PE should undergo CTA, forgoing D-dimer.

Lipase

Lipase is produced for the digestion of fats. Lipase levels are useful in patients when pancreatitis is considered as a noncardiac cause of chest pain. Acute pancreatitis should be considered in patients with a history of long-standing hyperlipidemia (particularly hypertriglyceridemia), gallbladder disease, and alcoholism.

Table 3
PERC criteria and wells' pulmonary embolism score

PERC Criteria (yes to any, move to well's PE score)	
• Age $\geq$ 50	1
• Heart rate $\geq$ 100	1
• O_2 saturations <95%	1
• Unilateral leg swelling	1
• Hemoptysis	1
• Recent trauma/surgery $\leq$ 4 wk requiring general anesthesia	1
Well's PE Score	
• Clinical signs of deep vein thrombosis (DVT)	3
• PE #1 diagnosis OR equally likely	3
• Heart rate >100	1.5
• Immobilization for 3 wk or previous surgery within 4 wk	1.5
• Previous PE or DVT	1.5
• Hemoptysis	1
• Malignancy w/treatment within 6 mo or palliative	1
Total:	___

PE Risk Interpretation:
0–1, Low risk
2–6, Intermediate risk
$\geq$ 7, High risk

Urine Toxicology Screening

Urine toxicology screening offers important information when illicit drug use may be a potential cause of chest pain. Substance use is prolific in the United States; in 2021, 21.9% of persons 12 years and older in the United States used some form of illegal substance in the past year.[9] The use of stimulants such as prescription medications, methamphetamines, and cocaine increase the risk of cardiac complications, including arrhythmia, vasospasm, and MI[10] The use of intravenous substances, such as heroin and fentanyl, increases the risk of embolism and endocarditis.[11]

Stable Chest Pain Diagnostics

Patients presenting with stable or nonspecific chest pain may undergo additional testing to determine the need for invention (**Fig. 3**). The choice of diagnostic testing is based on a patient's risk factors, ambulatory ability, and previous history of CAD as well as regional availability (**Table 4**). Contraindications for testing must be considered prior to referral.

Coronary Artery Calcium Scoring

Because nearly half all CV deaths are asymptomatic,[12] coronary artery calcium (CAC) scoring is a nonemergent means of using CT to measure the amount of plaque within the coronary arteries and assess cardiovascular disease (CVD) and risk of MI. Information gathered from CAC can be beneficial for medication management (eg, aspirin, HMG-CoA Reductase Inhibitors, etc.) and determining need for further intervention.

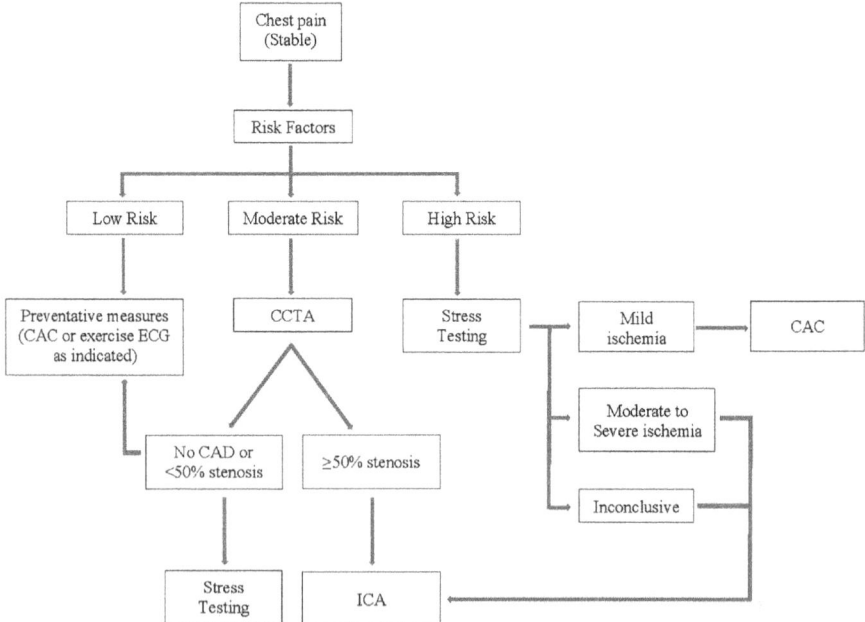

Fig. 3. Clinical pathway for stable chest pain diagnostic evaluation. (*Data from* Gulati M, Levy PD, Mukherjee D, et al. 2021 AHA/ACC/ASE/CHEST/SAEM/SCMR guideline for the evaluation and diagnosis of chest pain: a report of the American College of Cardiology/American Heart Association Joint Committee on clinical practice guidelines. J Am Coll Cardiol 2021;78(22);e187–e285.)

Table 4
Comparison of non-acute cardiac diagnostic testing

Test	Indication	Advantage	Disadvantage	Cost
CAC	Asymptomatic CAD screening for at risk patients	Evaluates plaque severity for determining CAD risk noninvasive low radiation noncontrast	Cannot identify noncalcium plaques less effective in older populations	$
CCTA	Potential symptoms of cardiac ischemia	Noninvasive high accuracy to rule out CAD noninvasive screening of coronary artery anatomy and obstruction	Requires further testing to determine significant of positive findings requires contrast	$
Exercise ECG	No known CAD Normal resting ECG	No radiation Readily available	Poor specificity and sensitivity can't localize	5
Stress Echo	Abnormal baseline ECG potential structural abnormality	No radiation high specificity and sensitivity detects structural issues	Accuracy technician dependent must be ambulatory	$$
Stress CMR	Known CAD Previous vascularization	high specificity and sensitivity May be non-ambulatory	less available expensive	$$$$
Stress SPECT	Known CAD	high specificity and sensitivity must be ambulatory	Decreased radiotracer uptake may lead to underestimation of CAD Radiation use	$$$
Stress PET	Known CAD potential microvascular disease	High specificity and sensitivity may be nonambulatory	Less available expensive radiation use	$$$$
ICA	Significant stenosis on CCTA or stress test ischemia	Contradictions to stress testing older patients or those who are not able complete stress testing (ie, dementia, mobility issues)	Invasive requires procedural sedation emboli/bleeding risk	$$$$

Coronary Computed Tomography Angiography

CCTA is a noninvasive diagnostic test using intravenous dye and CT to assess coronary artery anatomy and obstruction. It can be used to rule out atherosclerosis and coronary flow irregularities necessitating intervention. CCTA is a beneficial and cost-efficient test for patients unable to undergo in exercise testing.

Stress Testing

Stress testing offers a means of evaluating cardiac ischemia and function during exertion or the administration of pharmacologic agents. There are several types of stress tests available with some using radiation to achieve results.

A stress ECG test is a common, cost-effective means of determining exertional ischemia through the evaluation of electrical conduction. Ambulatory patients presenting with intermittent chest pain or pressure provoked by activity and relieved by rest benefit from exercise testing. While readily available, stress ECGs are the least accurate in locating specific coronary obstruction.

A stress echocardiogram examines for perfusion defects at rest and under exertion when myocardial ischemia is suspected. Testing may employ physical activity, medication utilization, or external pacing to achieve evaluation of wall motion and EF. Although more costly, stress echocardiogram is superior to exercise ECG, offering increased prognostic value.[13]

Nuclear Testing: Stress PET, Stress Single Photon Emission Computed Tomography

Nuclear testing uses the intravenous injection of a radioactive tracer to evaluate coronary artery flow. There are several types of cardiac nuclear testing: Cardiac PET and cardiac stress single photon emission computed tomography (SPECT), both of which offer better stress results, particularly in nonambulatory patients. Of the 2, stress PET is superior to stress SPECT, offering better image quality when obstructive coronary ischemia is considered.[14]

Stress Cardiac Magnetic Resonance

Stress cardiac magnetic resonance (CMR) myocardial perfusion imaging evaluates cardiac ischemia and function using contrast MRI. It is a highly sensitive and specific test, yet an expensive diagnostic.

Invasive Coronary Angiography

A coronary angiogram is a procedure in which an arterial catheter is introduced and migrated to the heart of a patient under sedation. Contrast dye is administered to evaluate for coronary artery obstruction. Indications for an invasive coronary angiography (ICA) are based on the suspected severity of coronary obstructions found using diagnostic testing.

SUMMARY

Chest pain complaints require the simultaneous evaluation of multiple key factors to determine the cause. PAs must ensure effective subjective and objective assessment to identify high-risk differentials that contribute to rapid instability. This method is the foundation for the development of sound clinical judgment and to establish a plan of care appropriate and specific to each patient presenting with chest pain.

CLINICS CARE POINTS

- There is no definitive tool to rule out acute coronary syndrome.
- Socioeconomic factors requiires evaluation when considering risk factors.
- Chest pain evaluation requires evaluation of signs, symptoms, and risk factors to determine cardiac cause.
- Initial chest pain evaluations must focus on findings consistent with risk of rapid deterioration.
- Diagnostics add to the assessment when symptom cause is unclear.
- Outpatient testing aids in assessing patients with stable chest pain to rule vascular or structural causes.

DISCLOSURE

The author has no disclosures or potential conflicts of interest, financial or otherwise.

REFERENCES

1. Harskamp RE, Laeven SC, Himmelreich JC, et al. Chest pain in general practice: a systematic review of prediction rules. BMJ Open 2019;9(2):e027081.
2. National Center for Health Statistics. Multiple cause of death 2018–2021 on CDC WONDER database. Available at: https://wonder.cdc.gov/mcd.html. Accessed February 2, 2023.
3. Tsao CW, Aday AW, Almarzooq ZI, et al. Heart disease and stroke statistics— 2023 update: a report from the American Heart Association. Circulation 2023; 147:e93–621.
4. Havranek EP, Mujahid MS, Barr DA, et al. Social determinants of risk and outcomes for cardiovascular disease: a scientific statement from the American Heart Association. Circulation 2015;132(9):873–98.
5. Homan TD, Bordes SJ, Cichowski E. Physiology, pulse pressure. In: StatPearls. 2024. Available at: https://www.ncbi.nlm.nih.gov/books/NBK482408/.
6. Fernando SM, Tran A, Cheng W, et al. Prognostic accuracy of the HEART score for prediction of major adverse cardiac events in patients presenting with chest pain: a systematic review and meta-analysis. Acad Emerg Med 2019;26: 140–51.
7. Thygesen K, Alpert JS, Jaffe AS, et al. Third universal definition of myocardial infarction. Circulation 2012;126(16):2020–35.
8. Gulati M, Levy P, Mukherjee D, et al. AHA/ACC/ASE/CHEST/SAEM/SCCT/SCMR guideline for the evaluation and diagnosis of chest pain: a report of the American college of cardiology/American heart association joint committee on clinical practice guidelines. J Am Coll Cardiol 2021;78(22):e187–285.
9. SAMHSA.gov. National survey on drug use and health: annual national report. 2021. Available at: https://www.samhsa.gov/data/release/2021-national-survey-drug-use-and-health-nsduh-releases#annual-national-report. Accessed June 14, 2024.
10. Pacor JM, Do A, Yeunjung K. Impact of drug abuse in acute coronary syndrome: analysis of the national inpatient sample 2012-2015. J Am Coll Cardiol 2019; 73:163.
11. Nishimura M, Bhatia H, Ma J, et al. The impact of substance abuse on heart failure hospitalizations. Am J Med 2020;133(2):207–13.e1.
12. Greenland P, Alpert JS, Beller GA, et al, American College of Cardiology Foundation; American Heart Association. 2010 ACCF/AHA guideline for assessment of

cardiovascular risk in asymptomatic adults: a report of the American college of cardiology foundation/American heart association task force on practice guidelines. J Am Coll Cardiol 2010;56(25):e50–103.

13. Mahenthiran J, Bangalore S, Yao SS, et al. Comparison of prognostic value of stress echocardiography versus stress electrocardiography in patients with suspected coronary artery disease. Am J Cardiol 2005;96(5):628–34.

14. Parker MW, Iskandar A, Limone B, et al. Diagnostic accuracy of cardiac positron emission tomography versus single photon emission computed tomography for coronary artery disease: a bivariate meta-analysis. Circulation: Cardiovascular Imaging 2012;5:700–7.

Management of Acute Coronary Chest Pain

Jennifer L. Barnett, DMSc, PA-C, DFAAPA[a,b,*]

KEYWORDS

- Acute coronary syndrome • Angina • Chest pain • Heart disease
- High sensitivity troponin • Unstable angina • Cardiac chest pain • STEMI

KEY POINTS

- Rapid evaluation identifying symptoms, history, and risk factors is important to guide treatment decisions. Obtaining an electrocardiogram and troponin tests is vital to target management.
- Primary percutaneous coronary intervention is preferred for ST-elevation myocardial infarction patients, while NSTE-ACS management may involve either early invasive strategies or ischemia-guided approaches based on risk assessment.
- Initial treatment for non-ST elevation acute coronary syndrome (NSTE-ACS) involves antiplatelet therapy (aspirin), anticoagulation, beta-blockers, and nitrates for pain relief, while oxygen is reserved for patients with low oxygen saturation.
- Post-ACS management includes medications like angiotensin-converting enzyme inhibitors and statins, along with lifestyle modifications to reduce the risk of future cardiovascular events.

INTRODUCTION

Acute Coronary Syndrome (ACS) is a spectrum of conditions caused by the sudden blocking of blood flow in the heart's blood vessels. It is noted in over 625,000 patients annually.[1] ACS includes ST elevation myocardial infarction (STEMI), Unstable Angina, and non-ST elevation myocardial infarction (NSTEMI). The term *non-ST Elevation Acute Coronary Syndromes* (NSTE-ACS) is used for both unstable angina and NSTEMI as the patients present similarly.[1] They are addressed together in the clinical practice guidelines.

DEFINITION

Chest pain or discomfort is common and can be described in various ways. Patients can describe the discomfort as pressure, tightness, squeezing, or other discomfort,

[a] Department of Hospital Medicine, MedStar Medical Group, MedStar Franklin Square Medical Center, 9000 Franklin Square Drive, Baltimore, MD 21237, USA; [b] Department of Graduate Studies, University of Maryland, Baltimore, MD, USA
* Corresponding author.
E-mail address: jennifer.l.barnett@medstar.net

Physician Assist Clin 10 (2025) 261–272
https://doi.org/10.1016/j.cpha.2024.11.004
physicianassistant.theclinics.com

Abbreviations	
ACE	angiotensin-converting enzyme
ACS	acute coronary syndrome
BMS	bare metal stents
CABG	coronary artery bypass grafting
CAD	coronary artery disease
CCB	calcium channel blockers
cTn	cardiac troponins
DAPT	dual antiplatelet therapy
DES	drug-eluting stents
ECG	electrocardiogram
GRACE	global registry of acute coronary events
IABP	intra-aortic balloon pump
IV	Intravenous
LAD	left anterior descending
LBBB	left bundle branch block
LV	left ventricular
MI	myocardial infarction
NSTE-ACS	non-ST elevation acute coronary syndrome
NSTEMI	non-ST elevation myocardial infarction
PCI	percutaneous coronary intervention
STEMI	ST elevation myocardial infarction
TIMI	thrombolysis in myocardial infarction
UFH	unfractionated heparin

which can be located in the chest, neck, arms, back, epigastric area, and jaw. It is important to note that although chest pain is often a presenting symptom of ACS, patients may also present with shortness of breath, exertional dyspnea, nausea, and fatigue. Specifically, women may present with nausea and shortness of breath and are typically more symptomatic than men.[2] Symptoms located on the left or right side of the chest that are stabbing, sharp, or in the throat or abdomen are more likely seen in diabetic women patients, or those who are elderly.[3]

Racial and ethnic disparities lead to poorer outcomes for Black, Hispanic, and South Asian individuals, among other groups.[3] Cultural competency training is advised, and considering race and ethnicity when approaching these patients is essential.[3]

Acute chest pain is noted when it is new, or the nature of the pain has changed in some way, such as frequency, length, or type of discomfort.[3] Chest pains are defined as *stable* if they are chronic, ongoing, and caused by stress.[3]

MOST COMMON SYMPTOMS

Although chest discomfort can present in a variety of ways, if a patient reports the following symptoms, their discomfort is more likely to be *cardiac or caused by ACS*[3]:

- Described as heaviness, tightness, pressure, constriction, or squeezing
- Retrostèrnal
- Gradually builds in intensity over a few minutes
- Precipitated by exercise or emotional stress, but can also occur at rest or with minimal exertion
- Radiates to left arm, neck, or jaw
- Associated with dyspnea, palpitations, diaphoresis, lightheadedness, presyncope or syncope, epigastric pain, heartburn unrelated to meals, nausea, or vomiting.

It is recommended that anyone with suspected ACS be rapidly categorized based on risk to determine the likelihood of ACS and adverse outcomes.[1] Key information that helps determine the risk includes history and physical examination, electrocardiogram (ECG), and blood tests, including cardiac troponins (cTn).[1] Evidenced-based risk assessments include thrombolysis in myocardial infarction (TIMI) risk score (42), the platelet glycoprotein iib/iiia in unstable angina: receptor suppression using integrilin therapy risk score (43), the global registry of acute coronary events (GRACE) risk score (44), and the National Cardiovascular Data Registry-Acute Coronary Treatment and Intervention Outcomes Network registry.[3,4]

RISK FACTORS SUGGESTING HIGHER PROBABILITY OF CORONARY CHEST PAIN

When obtaining a patient's history, the following factors increase the probability of NSTE-ACS[3,4]:

- Older age
- Male sex
- Positive family history of coronary artery disease (CAD)
- Presence of peripheral arterial disease
- Diabetes
- Renal insufficiency
- Prior myocardial infarction (MI)
- Prior Coronary Revascularization

During a physical examination, a clinician may hear an S4, paradoxic splitting of S2, or a new murmur of mitral regurgitation, but these are not pathognomonic of NSTE-ACS. Chest discomfort is less likely to be reproducible on examination. A pericardial friction rub would indicate acute pericarditis and pulsus paradoxus would indicate cardiac tamponade. A pleural friction rub may indicate pneumonitis or pleuritis. Often, the examination may be benign.

INITIAL APPROACH

The first step in managing acute coronary chest pain is to obtain an ECG. If symptom onset is within 12 hours, and if ST segment elevation is noted, coronary angiography should be immediately pursued to determine if reperfusion therapy should be performed.[4] ST elevation is defined as *new ST elevation at the J point in at least 2 contiguous leads of greater than 2 mm in men or 1.5 mm in women in leads v2-v3 and/or of greater than or equal to 1 mm in other contiguous chest or limb leads*[4] New or a presumed new left bundle branch block (LBBB) has been considered ST elevation equivalent in the past, but the 2013 guidelines state that LBBB should not be considered diagnostic of acute MI on its own.[4] The European Society of Cardiology/ACCF/AHA/World Heart Federation Task Force has defined Myocardial Infarction as new ST elevation at the J point in *at least 2 contiguous leads of ≥ 2 mm (0.2 mV) in men or ≥ 1.5 mm (0.15 mV) in women in leads V2–V3 and/or of ≥ 1 mm (0.1 mV) in other contiguous chest leads or the limb leads.*"[4] On rare occasions, hyperacute T wave changes are noted before ST elevation is present.[4] A right-sided ECG (V_3R to V_4R) can be performed when inferior STEMI is present, as it can show evidence of right ventricular infarction.[4]

Patients with NSTE-ACS may have a variety of changes on ECG, including ST depression, transient ST elevation, or new T wave changes. Sometimes, the ECG can be normal, noted in 1% to 6% of patients, or changes can develop over time.[1] If the ECG is normal in the beginning, repeating the ECG in 15 to 30 minutes over the first hour or more can be valuable.[1] Normal ECG can also suggest left circumflex or right coronary artery occlusions, and a posterior ECG to obtain leads V7- V9 can be useful.[1] A Wellens sign on ECG (deeply inverted or biphasic T waves) in leads V2 and V3 is highly specific for critical proximal stenosis of the left anterior descending (LAD) artery. Left ventricular hypertrophy, bundle branch blocks with repolarization, and ventricular pacing rhythms may hide signs of ischemia on ECG. The accuracy of the clinician for determining ECG changes is variable and harder to recognize with more minor degrees of ST-segment changes.[5,6] The ECGs should be compared to ECGs taken previously for comparison.[2]

ST ELEVATION MYOCARDIAL INFARCTION

STEMI is noted to be about 25%- 40 % of all Myocardial Infarction (MI) presentations with approximately 30% of patients with STEMI being women.[4] Risk of death has improved but remains 5% to 6% in hospital and 7% to 18% at 1-year post-event.[4]

PRIMARY PERCUTANEOUS CORONARY ANGIOGRAPHY

- Primary percutaneous coronary intervention (PCI) is the best method of reperfusion when it can be performed promptly and by experienced operators.[4]
- If there are no contraindications, fibrinolytic therapy should be given if the patient has an STEMI, is located at a non-PCI-capable hospital, or if the transportation to a PCI-capable hospital exceeds 120 minutes.[4]
- If fibrinolytic therapy is chosen as the method of reperfusion, it should be administered within 30 minutes of arrival at the hospital.[4]
- Primary PCI should be performed for patients with STEMI and ischemic symptoms of less than 12 hours duration who have contraindications to fibrinolytics.[4]
- Primary PCI is reasonable in patients with STEMI if there is clinical or ECG evidence of ongoing ischemia less than 24 hours after symptoms onset.[4]

During PCI, manual aspiration of the thrombus is reasonable.[4] Coronary stenting is often used at the time of primary PCI. Bare metal stents (BMS) are used in patients with high bleeding risk, inability to comply with 1 year of dual antiplatelet therapy (DAPT), or who will likely need invasive surgery in the next year.[4] Drug-eluting stents (DES) can prevent restenosis and maintain arteries but should not be used in patients who cannot tolerate a prolonged course of DAPT due to the risk of stent thrombosis if DAPT is prematurely discontinued.[4]

Medications recommended for managing coronary artery disease (CAD) after percutaneous coronary intervention (PCI) include aspirin, purinergic receptor type Y, subtype 12 $P2Y_{12}$ inhibitors, heparin or unfractionated heparin (UFH), and GP IIb/IIIa receptor antagonists. See **Box 1** for the guidelines for PCI medication management. Aspirin is loaded and then given daily. It is often administered prehospital and does not need to be repeated until the next day. $P2Y_{12}$ inhibitors are also loaded but are sometimes held until after PCI in case there is a multivessel disease that would indicate a need for coronary artery bypass grafting (CABG), and $P2Y_{12}$ inhibitors should be held before cardiac surgery. Administration of Glycoprotein IIb/IIa (GP IIb/IIIa) receptor antagonists such as eptifibatide or tirofiban can be considered for large thrombus burden or inadequate P2Y12 receptor antagonist loading, and the interventional cardiologist may best make this decision.

Box 1
Guidelines post percutaneous coronary intervention medication management (2013)

Antiplatelet Therapy

Aspirin
- 162 to 325 mg load before the procedure
- 81 to 325 mg daily maintenance dose (indefinite)
- 81 mg daily is the preferred maintenance dose

P2Y$_{12}$inhibitors

Loading Doses
- Clopidogrel 600 mg as early as possible or at the time of PCI
- Prasugrel 60 mg as early as possible or at the time of PCI
- Ticagrelor 180 mg as early as possible or at the time of PCI

Maintenance Doses and Duration
  If either DES or BMS is placed:
    One year of therapy
    - Clopidogrel 75 mg daily
    - Prasugrel 10 mg daily
    - Ticagrelor 90 mg two times a day
  After 1 year
    - Above can be continued beyond 1 year
    - Note: if STEMI and prior stroke or transient iscemic attack (TIA)- Prasugrel can cause harm

Heparin
- UFH can be considered through PCI with additional IV boluses as needed based on activated clotting time (ACT).
- Lovenox can continue through PCI
- Fondaparinux is noted to cause harm as the sole anticoagulant for PCI

Source O'Gara P, Kushner F, Ascheim D, et al. 2013 ACCF/AHA Guideline for the Management of ST-Elevation Myocardial Infarction: A Report of the American College of Cardiology Foundation/American Heart Association Task Force on Practice Guidelines. JACC 2013;61(4):e78–e140. https://doi.org/10.1016/j.jacc.2012.11.019.

FIBRINOLYTIC

If primary PCI is unavailable within a reasonable time from symptom onset, fibrinolytics should be considered and administered within 30 minutes of hospital arrival. Four options for fibrinolytics are Tenecteplase, Reteplase, Alteplase, and Streptokinase. The dosing and timing of administration are best discussed with a cardiologist or cardiologist specialist with pharmacy support and are not the purview of this discussion. **Box 2** lists the contraindications and cautions for fibrinolytics in STEMI.

Fibrinolytic therapy aims to restore flow to the arteries as indicated by improvement or resolution of chest discomfort, resolution of ST elevation, or the presence of reperfusion arrhythmias.[4] Complete or near complete ST-segment resolution 60 to 90 minutes after fibrinolytic suggests a patent culprit artery.[4] For patients who received thrombolytics, the following conditions indicate a need for additional interventional coronary angiography:[4]

- Cardiogenic shock or severe acute heart failure, regardless of the time of MI onset
- Failed perfusion or reocclusion
- As part of an invasive strategy in stable patients with PCI between 3 and 24 hours after successful fibrinolysis

---

Box 2
Contraindications and cautions for fibrinolytics in ST elevation myocardial infarction[4]

Absolute Contraindications
- Any prior intracranial hemorrhage (ICH)
- Known structural cerebral vascular lesion (eg, arteriovenous malformation)
- Known malignant intracranial neoplasm (primary or metastatic)
- Ischemia s troke within 3 months (except acute ischemic stroke within 4.5 h)
- Suspected aortic dissection
- Active bleeding or bleeding diathesis
- Significant close head or facial trauma within 3 months
- Intracranial or intraspinal surgery within 2 months
- Severe uncontrolled hypertension (unresponsive to emergency therapy)
- For streptokinase, prior treatment within 6 months

Relative Contraindications
- History of chronic, severe, poorly controlled hypertension
- Significant hypertension on presentation (SBP greater than 180 mm Hg or DBP >110 mm Hg)
- Dementia
- Known intracranial pathology not covered by the above
- Traumatic or prolonged cardiopulmonary resuscitation (CPR) (more than 10 min)
- Major surgery (less than 3 weeks)
- Recent (within 2–4 weeks) internal bleeding
- Non compressible vascular procedures
- Pregnancy
- Active peptic ulcer
- Oral anticoagulant therapy

Source O'Gara P, Kushner F, Ascheim D, et al. 2013 ACCF/AHA Guideline for the Management of ST-Elevation Myocardial Infarction: A Report of the American College of Cardiology Foundation/American Heart Association Task Force on Practice Guidelines. JACC 2013;61(4):e78–e140. https://doi.org/10.1016/j.jacc.2012.11.019.

NON-ST ELEVATION ACUTE CORONARY SYNDROME

ACS develops suddenly when there is a disruption of the fibrous cap of the fibrofatty deposits within heart arteries, stimulating thrombogenesis.[1] Thrombus formation and possible coronary vasospasm reduce arterial flow, causing chest pain due to ischemia.[1] Decrease blood flow to the coronary arteries can be complete or partial. ACS is typically caused by a blood vessel obstruction causing a mismatch between oxygen consumption (MVO_2) and demand, but can also include excessive myocardial oxygen demand due to a stable flow-limiting lesion, acute coronary insufficiency due to other causes (vasospastic angina), coronary embolism, and coronary arteritis.[1] There are times when demand mismatch can have causes not related to obstructed coronaries, including hypotension, severe anemia, tachycardia, hypertension, and severe aortic stenosis, among others.[1] Other causes of this mismatch can be stress (Takotsubo), cardiomyopathy, pulmonary embolus, severe heart failure, and sepsis.[1]

STRATEGY FOR MANAGEMENT

Patients with NSTE-ACS should receive optimal anti-ischemic and antithrombotic medical therapy and then can be treated with either an invasive strategy or initial ischemia-guided management.[1] An invasive strategy recommends coronary angiography within 24 hours of admission and possible PCI early, as clinically appropriate, and is generally better. Indications for early invasive strategy would be new or presumed new ST changes, elevation of troponin (cTn), or a GRACE score of more than 140. With ischemic guided management, the patient's condition may stabilize and not require coronary intervention. There is no benefit for the early invasive strategy for people with extensive comorbidities that likely outweigh the benefit and for those with acute chest pain and low likelihood of ACS and whose troponins are negative. Shared decision-making with clinically stable and lower-risk patients is recommended to determine the appropriate approach. Ischemia-guided management patients should be considered for invasive evaluation if, after 25 to 72 hours, they.

1. Fail medical therapy, noting persistent angina or angina at rest or minimal exertion despite maximal medical treatment.
2. Have objective evidence of ischemia noted on noninvasive stress test (ECG changes or myocardial perfusion defect)
3. Have clinical indicators of high prognostic risk by high TIMI or GRACE scores.

TESTING

cTn are the hallmark of cardiac testing specific for NSTE-ACS as they are the most sensitive and specific. A cTn concentration of over 99 percentile upper reference limit (assay dependent) indicates myocardial injury. Elevations of cTn are specific to the heart, but not the specific condition, as many ischemic, noncoronary cardiac, and noncardiac conditions can cause elevations in cTn. High Sensitivity cTn is preferred if available as they have an even higher negative predictive value, reaching over 99%.

Serial cTn testing should be performed 3 and 6 hours after symptom onset and trended until peak troponin level is obtained. If the exact timing of symptom onset is unclear, clinicians should consider the presentation time as symptom onset. Troponin elevations and trends have been helpful in prognostication, and it is reasonable to consider remeasuring on day 3 or 4 as an index of infarct size and dynamics of necrosis. Creatine kinase- MB (Ck-MB) testing is no longer indicated for diagnosis of ACS. Measurement of B-type natriuretic peptide or N-terminal proB type natriuretic peptide can be considered to assess risk with suspected ACS.

Assessment of the left ventricular (LV) function is recommended typically via echocardiogram, as a depressed LV function will influence medication management. If the LV function is significantly depressed, it may suggest the presence of more extensive CAD and lead to revascularization consideration versus CABG.

STRESS TESTING

Noninvasive stress testing is recommended for patients with a low or intermediate risk of CAD when the patient has been free of ischemia at rest or with low-level activity for a minimum of 12 to 24 hours (Level B evidence). Treadmill testing is helpful for patients who can tolerate it and whose ECG is free of resting ST changes. Stress testing with imaging is recommended for patients with ST changes and can add prognostic information. Pharmacologic stress testing with imaging is recommended for those with physical limitations precluding adequate stress tests.

MONITORING

All patients with acute cardiac chest pain should be placed on heart rhythm monitoring. Patients with recurrent symptoms, positive cTn, or ECG changes benefit from inpatient management.[1] Those patients with continuing angina, hemodynamic instability, large MI, and/or uncontrolled arrhythmias would benefit from a coronary care unit or similar unit that can provide a frequent assessment of vitals and mental status in addition to rapid cardioversion and defibrillation if needed for the first

24 hours.[1] Initial goals for treatment include immediate relief of ischemia and prevention of MI and death.[1] Consideration of ischemia-guided therapy and early invasive strategy are options. The medical management of patients with NSTE-ACS is multimodal, including antianginal, antiplatelet, and anticoagulant therapies.[1]

IMMEDIATE MEDICAL MANAGEMENT

Medications should be promptly administered and reassessed often (ie, every 5 minutes) for ongoing management in the first minutes to an hour of acute cardiac chest pain.

Antiplatelet Therapy

All patients presenting with chest pain due to NSTE-ACS and without contraindication should be given nonenteric coated chewable aspirin at a dose of 162 mg to 325 mg, then continued on a maintenance dose of 81 mg daily aspirin indefinitely.[1] If a patient cannot take aspirin due to allergy or gastrointestinal concerns, a loading dose of clopidogrel at 600 mg should be administered, followed by a daily dose of 75 mg. Dosing of P2Y12 inhibitors is the same for post-PCI medication management and can be found in **Box 1**. For medical management, Ticagrelor can be preferred over clopidogrel as a P2Y12 inhibitor for those with ischemia-guided and early invasive strategies.

Anticoagulation

For ALL patients with chest pain due to NSTE-ACS, anticoagulation should be administered and continued for hospitalization or until PCI is performed. Evidenced-based options include.[1]

- Enoxaparin 1 mg/kg subcutaneously every 12 hours, or renally dose as appropriate, as recurrent ischemic events and invasive procedures, were significantly reduced short term and at 1 year.
- Fondaparinux 2.5 mg subcutaneously daily. If PCI is performed, an additional anticoagulant with anti-IIa activity (UFH or bivalirudin) should be given due to the risk of catheter thrombosis.
- UFH with an initial loading dose of 60 IU/kg (max 4000 IU) and infusion of 12 IU/kg/hr (max 1000 IU) adjusted per activated partial thromboplastin time to maintain therapeutic anticoagulation according to hospital protocol, continued for 48 hours or until PCI performed.
- Argatroban is a direct thrombin inhibitor that can be used in patients with Heparin-induced thrombocytopenia and renal insufficiency. The usual dose is 2mcg/kg per minute continuous infusion followed by activated partial thromboplastin time of 1.5 to 3 times baseline.
- Bivalirudin 0.75 mg/kg/dose loading one time then 1.75 mg/kg/hr IV for procedure duration, then 0.25 mg/kg can be started for patients with early invasive management and continued until diagnostic angiography or PCI if the patient is also treated with dual antiplatelet therapy (DAPT). Bivalirudin is a direct thrombin inhibitor and was inferior when given alone.

Although patients with STEMI are indicated for thrombolytics if Primary PCI is not available in a reasonable amount of time, in NSTE-ACS patients, fibrinolytics should not be used as they cause an increased risk of intracranial hemorrhage and fatal/non-fatal MI.

Beta-Adrenergic Blockers

Oral beta-blockers should be given within the first 24 hours unless there are signs of heart failure, evidence of a low output state, increased risk of cardiogenic shock, or contraindications to beta-blockade.[1] Contraindications to beta-blockers include increased PR interval, second-degree or third-degree block, active asthma, or significant reactive airway disease. Patients should be reevaluated after 24 hours if beta-blockers were previously contraindicated to determine if the patient is now eligible.[1] For patients with NTSE-ACS and reduced systolic function but stabilized heart failure, one of the 3 medications to reduce mortality in heart failure should be used, including metoprolol succinate, carvedilol, or bisoprolol. It is also reasonable to continue beta-blocker therapy in patients with normal LV function. Intravenous (IV) beta-blockers can be harmful in patients with NSTE-ACS who have risk factors for shock. Risk factors for shock include age over 70 years, heart rate over 110 bpm, systolic blood pressure less than 120 mm Hg, and late presentation.

Beta-blockers decrease heart rate, blood pressure, and contractility, which help with oxygen demand. They decrease ischemia and reinfarction, decrease ventricular arrhythmia, and, most importantly, improve long-term survival.[1] Beta-blockers are recommended for patients with an ejection fraction less than 40% with or without pulmonary congestion before discharge. Patients with chronic obstructive lung disease or asthma can have beta-blockers if they do not have active bronchospasm, and beta one selective beta-blockers are preferred, starting at the lowest dose.[1]

Nitrates

For patients with ischemic pain, nitroglycerin should be administered sublingually every 5 minutes for up to 3 doses unless contraindicated.[1] Contraindications include low systolic blood pressure and use of phosphodiesterase inhibitor within 24 hours of sildenafil or vardenafil or within 48 hours of tadalafil.[1] Nitrates dilate the cardiac and peripheral blood vessels.[1] This dilation decreases preload and reduces ventricular wall tension.[1] There are effects of nitrates on afterload reduction and decreased oxygen consumption.[1] A mild increase in heart rate and contractility can counteract the reduction in oxygen consumption unless a beta-blocker is administered with nitrates.[1] Nitrates may also inhibit platelet aggregation.[1]

Nitrate use in NSTE-ACS is based on pathophysiological principles and extensive observations, as randomized clinical trials have not been shown to reduce major adverse cardiac events. Priority should be given to beta-blockers as they have mortality-reducing evidence in multiple randomized controlled trials. IV nitroglycerin should be administered for patients with persistent ischemia, heart failure, or hypertension unless contraindicated and may need periodic increases to maintain efficacy. If there is an ongoing need for IV nitroglycerin, it suggests the need for prompt coronary angiography and possible revascularization.[1]

Topical and oral nitrates can be used if available. Nitroglycerin's side effects include headache and hypotension. Patients may complain of headaches with nitrates, as blood vessels in the brain are also dilated. Hypotension is a side effect of nitroglycerin, and blood pressure should be assessed every 5 minutes before administering or changing the dose.

Analgesics

Morphine is reasonable to administer intravenously if there is continued ischemic chest pain despite treatment with maximally tolerated anti-ischemic medication. Morphine 1 - 5 mg IV can be repeated every 5 to 30 minutes to improve comfort and help symptoms.[1] However, some observational studies show increased adverse events in patients with ACS and acute decompensated heart failure with morphine. Similar to nitrates, no randomized controlled trials have assessed the use of morphine or reviewed specific dosing of morphine.[1] Hypotension and respiratory depression are the most severe complications of morphine, and naloxone can be used if a morphine overdose is suspected. NSAIDs, except aspirin, should not be given and should be discontinued during hospitalization as they are associated with an increased risk of adverse cardiac events.[1]

Oxygen

Oxygen, once applied to every patient with chest pain, is now recommended only for cyanotic patients with oxygen saturations less than 90%, in respiratory distress, or other high risk of hypoxemia. Applying oxygen to all patients with chest pain can cause increased coronary vascular resistance, reduced coronary blood flow, and increased risk of mortality.[1]

Calcium Channel Blockers

Non-dihydropyridine calcium channel blockers (CCB) such as verapamil or diltiazem should be used for NSTE-ACS patients with continued or frequent recurring ischemia and contraindications to beta-blockers if their LV function is normal and who are not at increased risk for shock and who do not have second-degree or third-degree heart block without a pacemaker or if the PR is less than 0.24 seconds. Non-dihydropyridine CCBs have significant negative inotropic, chronotropic, and dromotropic effects. They can help ischemia by decreasing heart rate and blood pressure and have been shown to decrease reinfarction in patients without LV dysfunction in some studies. Verapamil can help reduce long-term events after acute myocardial infarction (AMI) in hypertensive patients with normal LV function and patients with heart failure and MI when used with an ACE (angiotensin-converting enzyme) inhibitor.

If not contraindicated, oral non-dihydropyridine CCBs can be used as an additional agent after treating a patient with beta-blockers and nitrates. Short-acting dihydropyridine CCB should not be used as they increase mortality in patients with ACS. Coronary artery spasm is best treated with long-acting CCBs and nitrates.

Renin-Angiotensin-Aldosterone System Inhibitors

Angiotensin-converting enzyme inhibitors

ACE inhibitors reduce death from MI, particularly those with an left ventricular ejection fraction (LV EF) of less than 40%. For people with normal LV function, ACEs reduce mortality and major adverse cardiac events, particularly in patients with diabetes, hypertension, and stable chronic kidney disease. Data supports starting ACEs in the hospital before discharge with NSTE-ACS but should be used with caution in the first 24 hours after an MI due to the risk of hypotension or renal dysfunction. It is reasonable to use an angiotensin receptor blocker (ARB) instead of an ACE for patients who are ACE intolerant.

Aldosterone blockade medication such as eplerenone or spironolactone is recommended in patients after MI who have creatinine less than 2.5 mg/dL in men, and 2.0 mg/dL in women, and potassium is less than 5 mEq/L if they are also already on an ACE and beta-blocker and have an EF less than 40%, diabetes, or heart failure.

Cholesterol management

If not contraindicated, cholesterol management with a high-intensity statin should be continued or started in all patients with NSTE-ACS. Statins reduce the rate of recurrent MI, death from coronary artery disease, the need for revascularization, and stroke. Higher-risk patients benefit from a high-intensity statin such as atorvastatin rather than moderate or low-intensity statins such as pravastatin. Fasting lipid panels are reasonable to be assessed within 24 hours of the event.

Other Anti-ischemic Interventions

Ranolazine

Ranolazine is an antianginal medication used for chronic angina, but it has been shown useful in myocardial ischemia, particularly in women, and has shown a 29% reduction in recurrent ischemia. The starting dose of Ranolazine is 500 mg two times a day, and it can be increased to 1000 mg twice daily. The side effects are constipation, nausea, dizziness, and headache. Note that QTc interval can increase while taking Ranolazine, particularly at higher doses.

Intra-aortic balloon pump

Intra-aortic balloon Pump (IABP) counterpulsation has been a modality used for decades on patients with severe persistent or recurrent ischemia, particularly those waiting for angiography. It works by increasing diastolic blood pressure and augmenting coronary blood flow. In randomized controlled trials, IABP failed to reduce major adverse cardiac events, decrease infarct size, or diminish early mortality in patients with cardiogenic shock. The current recommendations are that intra-aortic balloon pump counterpulsation can be useful for patients with cardiogenic shock after STEMI who do not quickly stabilize with pharmacologic therapy, with additional research needed.

CLINICS CARE POINTS

- Acute Coronary Syndrome (ACS) is a life-threatening disease and should be evaluated urgently with an electrocardiogram, troponins, and physical examination.
- Patients with an acute ST elevation myocardial infarction (STEMI) should be treated with primary percutaneous coronary intervention, when available.
- A new or presumed new left bundle branch block is not considered an STEMI.
- Non-ST elevation ACS (NSTE-ACS) patients can be treated with early invasive treatment or medical management.
- Aspirin and anticoagulation should be given to all patients with NSTE-ACS unless contraindicated.
- Oxygen, once applied to every patient with chest pain, is now recommended only for cyanotic patients with oxygen saturations less than 90%, in respiratory distress, or other high risk of hypoxemia.
- Beta-blockers and ACE inhibitors have been shown to improve outcomes. They should be given unless contraindicated and prioritized over other less evidence-based approaches, including morphine, calcium channel blockers, and Ranolazine.
- If initially contraindicated, patients should be reevaluated daily while hospitalized to see if they are candidates for beta-blockers or ACE inhibitors.

DISCLOSURES

The author has nothing to disclose.

REFERENCES

1. Amsterdam EA, Wenger NK, Brindis RG, et al. 2014 AHA/ACC guideline for the management of patients with non–ST-elevation acute coronary syndromes. J Am Coll Cardiol 2014;64(24):e139–228.

2. Reynolds HR, Shaw LJ, Min JK, et al. Association of sex with severity of coronary artery disease, ischemia, and symptom burden in patients with moderate or severe ischemia: secondary analysis of the ISCHEMIA randomized clinical trial. JAMA Cardiol 2020;5:1–14.
3. Gulati M, Levy PD, Mukherjee D, et al. AHA/ACC/ASE/CHEST/SAEM/SCCT/SCMR guideline for the evaluation and diagnosis of chest pain: a report of the American College of Cardiology/American heart association joint committee on clinical practice guidelines. Circulation 2021;144(22).
4.. O'Gara P, Kushner F, Ascheim D, et al. 2013 ACCF/AHA guideline for the management of ST-elevation myocardial infarction: a report of the American College of Cardiology foundation/American Heart Association Task Force on practice guidelines. JACC (J Am Coll Cardiol) 2013;61(4):e78–140.
5. Lawton JS, Tamis-Holland JE, Bangalore S, et al. 2021 ACC/AHA/SCAI guideline for coronary artery revascularization: executive summary. J Am Coll Cardiol 2022;79(2):197–215.
6. Kontos MC, de Lemos JA, Deitelzweig SB, et al. ACC expert consensus decision pathway on the evaluation and disposition of acute chest pain in the emergency department: a report of the American College of Cardiology Solution Set Oversight Committee. J Am Coll Cardiol 2022;80:1925–60.

Heart Failure with Reduced and Preserved Ejection Fraction: Birds of a Different Feather

Lauren S. Eyadiel, MMS, MS, PA-C, SLP[a,b,c],*

KEYWORDS

- Heart failure • HFrEF • HFpEF • Guideline-directed medical therapy
- Heart failure device therapy • Atrial fibrillation • Iron deficiency

KEY POINTS

- Heart failure affects patients in primary care and all subspecialties where physician assistants practice.
- Heart failure is a clinical diagnosis that is confirmed by diagnostic testing.
- Patients with heart failure with reduced ejection fraction should be on all 4 pillars of guideline-directed medical therapy unless there are explicit contraindications.
- Patients with heart failure with preserved ejection fraction should have aggressive management of comorbidities, participate in supervised exercise training, and decongestive therapy.
- Patients with heart failure can and do get better with aggressive management.

INTRODUCTION

Heart failure is a complex, systemic syndrome where there is inadequate oxygen supply or blood flow from the heart to meet the metabolic demands of the tissue. This supply and demand mismatch is a result of any structural or functional impairment of ventricular filling or ejection of blood.[1] This leads to clinical symptoms of congestion or a low cardiac output state. Symptoms of heart failure are shown in **Table 1**. Heart failure is classified using left ventricular ejection fraction (LVEF) as this helps to differentiate prognosis and evidence-based treatment of the disease process. Heart failure with reduced ejection fraction (HFrEF) is defined as an LVEF of less than or equal to

[a] Department of PA Studies, Wake Forest University School of Medicine; [b] Division of Cardiovascular Medicine, Department of Internal Medicine, Advanced Heart Failure, Heart Transplant, and Mechanical Circulatory Support; [c] Atrium Health Wake Forest Baptist, Winston Salem, NC, USA
* Wake Forest University School of Medicine, Department of PA Studies, Atrium Health Wake Forest Baptist, Advanced Heart Failure, Heart Transplant, and Mechanical Circulatory Support, Medical Center Boulevard, Winston-Salem, NC 27157.
E-mail address: lesykes@wakehealth.edu
Twitter: @leyadiel (L.S.E.)

Physician Assist Clin 10 (2025) 273–285
https://doi.org/10.1016/j.cpha.2024.11.002
physicianassistant.theclinics.com
2405-7991/25/© 2024 Elsevier Inc. All rights reserved, including those for text and data mining, AI training, and similar technologies.

Table 1	
Symptoms of heart failure[1]	
Symptoms of Congestion	**Symptoms of Low Cardiac Output**
Shortness of breath	Altered mental status
Lower extremity edema	Cardiac cachexia
Abdominal bloating	Renal dysfunction
Orthopnea	Fatigue
Paroxysmal nocturnal dyspnea	

40%, heart failure with preserved ejection fraction (HFpEF) as an LVEF of greater than or equal to 50%, heart failure with mildly reduced ejection fraction (HFmrEF) as an LVEF of 41% to 49%, and heart failure with improved ejection fraction (HFimpEF) as a previous LVEF less than or equal to 40% and a follow-up measurement of greater than 40%.[1] Symptoms of both congestion and a low cardiac output state are common in HFrEF, while symptoms of congestion are more prevalent in patients with HFpEF.

The New York Heart Association (NYHA) functional classification is often used to describe the functional capacity of a patient with symptomatic heart failure.[2]

The NYHA functional class has been an independent predictor of mortality and can be trended over the continuum of care for patients with heart failure. NYHA Classification is summarized in **Table 2**.

Currently, about 6.7 million Americans are living with heart failure, with a lifetime risk of 1 in 4 persons to develop heart failure, which is expected to continue to increase over the next decade.[3] Therefore, no matter what specialty of medical practice, the clinically practicing physician assistant (PA) will care either directly or indirectly for patients with heart failure.

DIAGNOSTIC EVALUATION FOR PATIENTS WITH HEART FAILURE

Heart failure is a clinical diagnosis based on history and physical examination, which is confirmed by diagnostic testing. A thorough history and physical examination are essential as this allows the PA to not only identify patients with overt signs and symptoms of heart failure but also ascertain history, which can identify patients at risk for the disease. When taking a history for patients for whom the PA has concerns for heart failure, there should be attention to a family history of sudden cardiac death, heart failure, and conditions associated with the causes of cardiomyopathy in addition to the common signs and symptoms of heart failure.[1] These causes are discussed in more detail later based on the classification of heart failure type by ejection fraction. While there are various causes of shortness of breath and fatigue, both of which are common in patients with heart failure, the most specific signs are orthopnea and paroxysmal

Table 2	
New York Heart Association functional classification[2]	
Class	**Patient Symptoms**
I	No limitation in physical activity.
II	Slight limitation of physical activity, comfortable at rest.
III	Marked limitation of physical activity including with basic activities of daily living, comfortable at rest.
IV	Symptoms of heart failure at rest.

nocturnal dyspnea.[4] Physical examination should include vital signs, a comprehensive cardiovascular examination to include inspection of the chest, palpation to identify the site of the patient's point of maximal impulse and location, careful auscultation for murmurs as well as additional heart sounds, evaluation of jugular venous distention, peripheral pulses, pulmonary auscultation, and evaluation for lower extremity edema.[4] Additional physical examination should be chosen based on the suspected underlying cause of heart failure.

Following a comprehensive history and physical examination, additional diagnostic testing should be ordered to confirm the diagnosis and classify heart failure based on ejection fraction to guide management. Initial laboratory and diagnostic testing should include:

1. Electrocardiogram to evaluate for underlying arrhythmias.
2. Complete blood count and iron profile should be obtained to evaluate for anemia, a common comorbidity of heart failure.
3. Basic metabolic panel and magnesium levels to check renal function and electrolytes, which may be affected by treatments for heart failure.
4. N-terminal (NT)-pro brain natriuretic peptide (BNP) or BNP, which is a nonspecific but a sensitive way to indirectly measure volume overload.
5. Transthoracic echocardiogram to evaluate the LVEF, right ventricular function, and valvular function.[1]

The LVEF on transthoracic echocardiogram allows for the classification of LVEF, which in turn guides the treatment of heart failure. If the patient is diagnosed with HFrEF, an ischemic evaluation should be completed, as this is the most common cause of HFrEF.[1] Additional laboratory and diagnostic testing should be completed based on the suspected underlying cause to determine the etiology. A summary of the recommended diagnostic approach for patients with suspected heart failure is summarized in **Fig. 1**.

HEART FAILURE WITH REDUCED EJECTION FRACTION
Pathophysiology

HFrEF is a complex neurohormonal process that involves the activation of compensatory mechanisms, which, when sustained, result in systolic dysfunction and reduced cardiac output.[5] These compensatory mechanisms include the activation of sympathetic nervous system, renin angiotensin aldosterone system (RAAS), and cytokine system. These compensatory mechanisms are initially protective but, when sustained, lead to adverse cardiac remodeling. The sympathetic nervous system is activated by a reduction of cardiac output, which results in increased peripheral vasoconstriction, increased heart rate, and increased myocardial contractility. A decrease in cardiac output also leads to a reduction in renal blood flow activating RAAS, which triggers sodium and increases circulating volume and preload. The increase in preload leads to increased myocardial contractility based on the Frank-Starling mechanism, which states that cardiac fiber length increases contractile strength.[6] Left unchecked, these mechanisms result in adverse cardiac remodeling. **Fig. 2** provides an overview of the basic pathophysiology of HFrEF.

Etiology

Causes of HFrEF are divided into 2 broad categories: ischemic and nonischemic causes. In the United States and Europe, the most common cause of HFrEF is ischemic heart disease whereas a nonischemic cause is more common in the

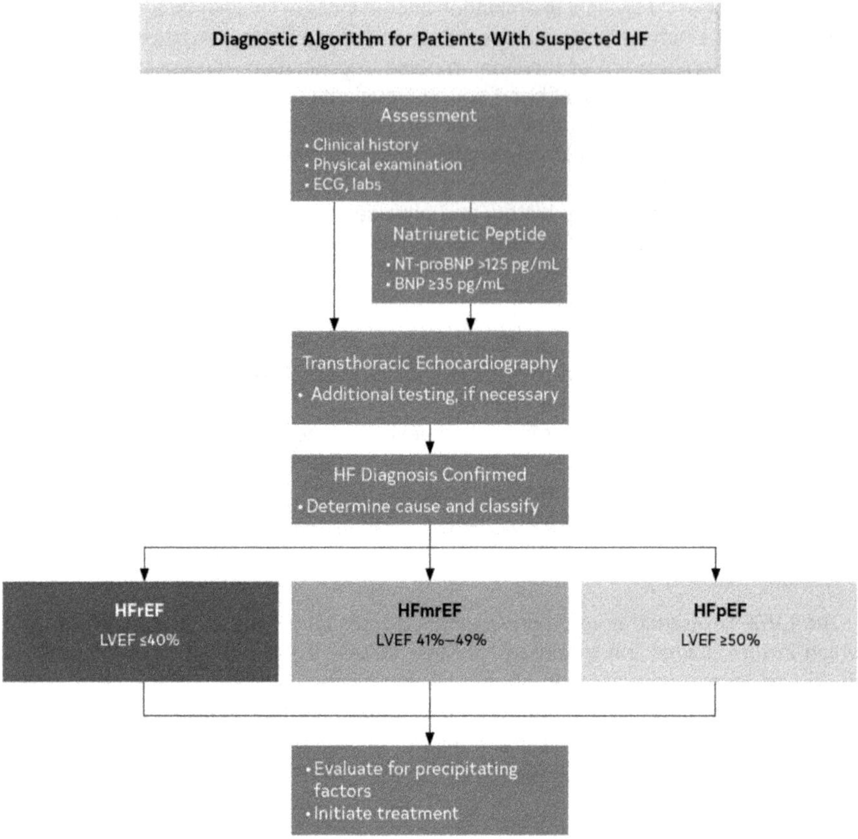

Fig. 1. Recommended diagnostic approach for patients with suspected heart failure. (*Adapted from* the ACC/AHA/HFSA 2022 Guidelines for the Management of Heart Failure.[1])

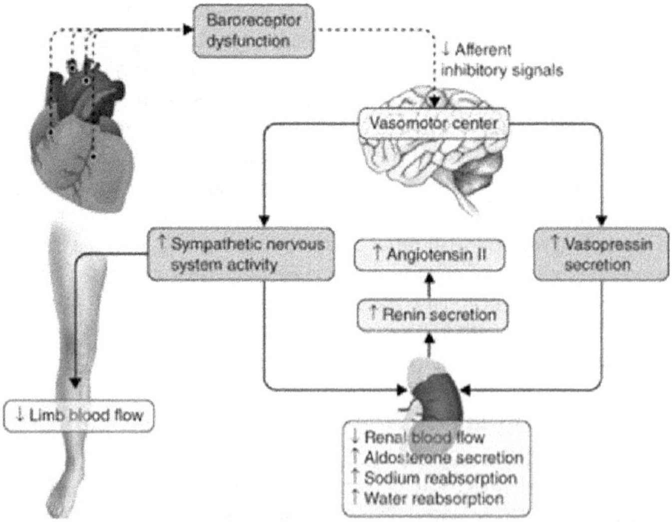

Fig. 2. Pathophysiology of HFrEF. (*Adapted from* Harrison's Principles of Internal Medicine.[7])

Caribbean, sub-Saharan Africa, and Latin America.[3] In the United States, there are about 115 million people with hypertension, 100 million with obesity, 92 million with prediabetes, 26 million with diabetes, and 125 million with atherosclerotic cardiovascular disease, which predisposes them to a risk for ischemic disease.[1] With advances in intervention and management for ischemic disease, the prevalence of HFrEF is increasing.[3]

Nonischemic causes of HFrEF include hypertensive disease, arrhythmias, valvular disease, and cardiomyopathy.[1,5,7] While hypertension alone is a risk factor for the development of ischemic heart disease, this also represents an independent risk factor for the development of HFrEF. Arrhythmia-mediated causes include atrial arrhythmias (eg, atrial flutter and atrial fibrillation), ventricular arrhythmias (eg, ventricular tachycardia and ventricular fibrillation), frequent premature ventricular contractions, and right ventricular pacing. Valvular heart disease, particularly mitral and aortic valve disease, disrupts the normal intracardiac filling pressures, creating an inciting event that results in adverse cardiac remodeling, as detailed earlier. Lastly, cardiomyopathy is a category of a broad range of diseases where the heart muscle structure or function is abnormal in the absence of coronary artery disease, valvular heart disease, or congenital defects.[1,7] This category includes restrictive, dilated, hypertrophic, stress, and arrhythmogenic right ventricular cardiomyopathy. A broad overview of common causes of HFrEF is shown in **Table 3**.

Treatment

Medical therapy
The cornerstone of treatment for HFrEF is pharmacologic management with the 4 pillars of guideline-directed medical therapy (GDMT): beta blockers (BBs), angiotensin

Table 3
Common causes of heart failure with reduced ejection fraction

Causes of HFrEF				
Ischemic	Nonischemic			
	Hypertensive	Arrhythmia mediated	Valvular	Cardiomyopathy Restrictive • Amyloidosis • Sarcoidosis • Hemochromatosis Dilated • Familial/Genetic • Peripartum • Myocarditis • Autoimmune • Toxin mediated (chemotherapy, medications, alcohol, cocaine, methamphetamine) • Thyroid disease Hypertrophic Stress cardiomyopathy
				Arrhythmic right ventricular cardiomyopathy

Adapted from the 2022 ACC/AHA/HFSA Guideline for the Management of Heart Failure.[1]

receptor neprilysin inhibitors (ARNi), mineralocorticoid receptor antagonists (MRAs), and SGLT2 inhibitors (SGLT2i).[1] While historically, GDMT was implemented in a step-wise manner, the data support rapid simultaneous initiation of 4-drug therapy followed by dose escalation.[8] The rapid initiation of 4 drug therapy has been proven to improve the outcomes for patients with HFrEF, including both morbidity and mortality.[8] If an ARNi cannot be tolerated due to symptomatic hypotension or there are barriers with affordability, an angiotensin converting enzyme inhibitor (ACEi) or angiotensin receptor blocker (ARB) should be considered.[1]

In addition to the pillars of GDMT, there are agents shown to improve outcomes other than morbidity in patients with heart failure. These agents include ivabradine, vericiguat, digoxin, hydralazine and nitrates, and diuretic therapies. Ivabradine, a sino-atrial node modulator, reduces the heart rate in patients with heart failure. This medication was shown to reduce the risk of heart failure hospitalization and cardiovascular death in patients with symptomatic heart failure with a heart rate greater than or equal to 70 beats per minute on maximally tolerated BB.[9] Of note, ivabradine cannot be used in patients with a history of atrial fibrillation or atrial flutter. Vericiguat is a sodium gua-nylate cyclase inhibitor that was shown to reduce cardiovascular death or heart failure hospitalization in patients with worsening heart failure and can be considered as an additional agent in patients with recent decompensated heart failure.[10] Digoxin causes an increase in intracellular sodium, driving an influx of calcium that results in increased contractility.[11] This drug was first created as an antiarrhythmic but has since been used for its inotropic properties for patients with HFrEF. Digoxin has been shown to improve exercise tolerance but not reduce mortality in patients with late-stage HFrEF, and drug levels should be monitored given significant known toxicities.[11] A combination of vasodilation and afterload reduction using hydralazine and nitrates in combination has been shown to reduce morbidity and mortality in patients who self-identify as African Americans.[12,13] This drug combination has an additional indica-tion for use in all patients with HFrEF who are unable to tolerate ACEi, ARB, or ARNi due to underlying renal dysfunction.[1]

Diuretics have historically been the mainstay of treatment for congestion in heart failure. That said, they have never been shown to improve mortality in patients with heart failure but do improve symptoms associated with congestion, such as shortness of breath, orthopnea, paroxysmal nocturnal dyspnea, and lower extremity edema.[14] The addition of a SGLT2i has changed the approach to the overall management of congestion in heart failure, but diuretics continue to be used as the first-line manage-ment. Loop diuretics are used as the initial diuretic of choice in patients with heart fail-ure. It is best to dose these medications in the morning due to frequent urination because of their mechanism of action. Oral furosemide is typically used initially due to cost but has poor oral bioavailability. If diuretic resistance is present, an alternative loop diuretic such as torsemide or bumetanide can be considered. If loop diuretics alone are insufficient to manage congestion, a thiazide diuretic can be added for augmentation. When considering equivalent diuretic dosing, 40 mg of oral furose-mide = 20 mg of oral torsemide = 1 mg of oral bumetanide = 20 mg of IV furosemide.

A summary of common medications used in the treatment of HFrEF is shown below in **Table 4**.

Device therapy
About 50% of patients with HFrEF have ventricular arrhythmias that result in sudden car-diac death. Therefore, implantable cardiac defibrillators (ICDs) are recommended for pa-tients with an LVEF of less than or equal to 35% on an optimized regimen of GDMT for 3 months with a life expectancy of greater than 1 year.[1] ICDs do not provide any benefit

Table 4
Summary of common medications used in heart failure with reduced ejection fraction

4 Pillars of GDMT			
BB	*ARNi*	*MRA*	*SGLT2i*
Bisoprolol	Sacubitril/Valsartan	Spironolactone	Dapagliflozin
Carvedilol		Eplerenone	Empagliflozin
Metoprolol succinate			
Additional HFrEF Medical Therapies			
Ivabradine	Vericiguat	Digoxin	Hydralazine/Nitrates
Diuretic Therapy			
Loop diuretics		*Thiazide diuretics*	
Furosemide		Metolazone	
Torsemide		Hydrochlorothiazide	
Bumetanide			

in reverse remodeling or symptomatic improvement in patients with HFrEF, but instead solely prevent sudden cardiac death. That said, cardiac resynchronization therapy (CRT) is a different device strategy for selected patients that leads to reverse remodeling and can prevent sudden cardiac death if a defibrillator lead is added (cardiac resynchronization therapy with defibrilator [CRT-D]). CRT is indicated in patients with an LVEF of less than or equal to 35% on an optimized regimen of GDMT for 3 months with a left bundle branch block with a QRS of greater than or equal to 150 milliseconds and a New York Heart Association functional class of II–IV.[1] The New York Heart Association functional class scale is described in **Table 2**.

ADVANCED HEART FAILURE THERAPIES

If patients do not have improvement in functional status or LVEF with implementation of GDMT and/or CRT therapy when indicated, a referral to an advanced heart failure specialist should be considered. There are many high-risk features for progression to advanced heart failure, which include recurrent ICD shocks, need for a reduction of GDMT, worsening end organ function, high heart rate with low blood pressures, and/or recurrent heart failure hospitalizations.[1] Advanced heart failure therapies include left ventricular assist devices and cardiac transplantation. Each of these therapies has certain criteria for consideration and requires management by an advanced heart failure cardiology team.

HEART FAILURE WITH PRESERVED EJECTION FRACTION
Pathophysiology

HFpEF is a systemic disease that involves primary and secondary myocardial injury resulting in a cascade of events resulting in adverse cardiac remodeling, pulmonary hypertension, and renal dysfunction with volume overload and shortness of breath with exertion.[7,15] Primary myocardial diseases, such as cardiac amyloidosis, hypertrophic cardiomyopathy, chest radiation, and cardiotoxicity result in direct adverse cardiac remodeling.[7] Secondary myocardial injury occurs in the setting of comorbidities such as obesity, hypertension, diabetes mellitus, chronic kidney disease, coronary artery disease, atrial fibrillation, and obstructive sleep apnea. These comorbidities result in systemic inflammation and endothelial dysfunction, leading to secondary myocardial injury and resultant adverse cardiac remodeling.[7] Whether the cause is primary or secondary myocardial injury, the final common pathway is concentric left ventricular remodeling and hypertrophy, which subsequently leads to remodeling of the left atria and right ventricular dysfunction. The patient will then experience pulmonary and systemic vascular congestion symptoms, which manifests as shortness of breath, orthopnea, paroxysmal nocturnal dyspnea, and fatigue. Interestingly, systemic inflammation and endothelial dysfunction also result in changes to the skeletal muscle composition, leading to dysfunction and worsening exercise tolerance.[5,7,15] The pathophysiology of HFpEF is summarized in **Fig. 3**.

Treatment

Treatment for HFpEF focuses on a 3-fold treatment strategy.

1. Medical management of congestion,
2. Management of comorbidities that contribute to the disease, and
3. Exercise training.[7,15]

Medical management has focused primarily on decongestion and, thus, prevention of heart failure hospitalizations. While many agents have been studied, at present, only SGLT2 inhibitors have been shown to reduce the risk for cardiovascular mortality in patients with HFpEF, which is driven by a reduction in heart failure hospitalization.[16,17] In addition to SGLT2 inhibitors, loop diuretics play a key role in decongestion but have not demonstrated a mortality benefit. Both ARNis and MRAs have also been studied to determine their role in patients with HFpEF and have shown promising results in select patients.[18–21] While multiple agents may play a role in decongestion, none of these medical therapies have improved exercise intolerance.

Aggressive management of comorbidities resulting in secondary myocardial injury is imperative in HFpEF as the disease is systemic and not solely a cardiac disease. The semaglutide in patients with heart failure with preserved ejection fraction and obesity (STEP-HFpEF) trial (2023) identified the first pharmacologic agent, semaglutide, to demonstrate a statistically significant benefit in exercise intolerance in patients' with HFpEF and obesity.[22] However, the endpoint for reduction in heart failure hospitalization was not met and mortality was not studied. In addition to the use of semaglutide, weight loss and exercise should be targeted for patients with obesity. Obstructive sleep apnea, atrial fibrillation, coronary artery disease, chronic kidney disease, hypertension, and diabetes mellitus should all be managed aggressively based on current guidelines for these conditions in the treatment of concomitant HFpEF.

At present, the most effective treatment for disease modification with an impact on exertional fatigue, exercise intolerance, and dyspnea in HFpEF is supervised exercise training, such as cardiac rehabilitation.[23] This has been shown to improve exercise tolerance by improving cardiac output, reverse remodeling of peripheral vasculature, and improving skeletal muscle dysfunction by increasing oxidative muscle fibers and reducing muscle wasting.[15]

MANAGEMENT OF COMMON COMORBIDITIES

The 2022 ACC/AHA/HFSA Guidelines on the Management of Heart Failure identify common comorbidities that require management in patients with both HFrEF and HFpEF. These include iron deficiency, hypertension, sleep disorders, and atrial fibrillation.[1] Recommendations for these comorbidities are summarized in **Table 5**.

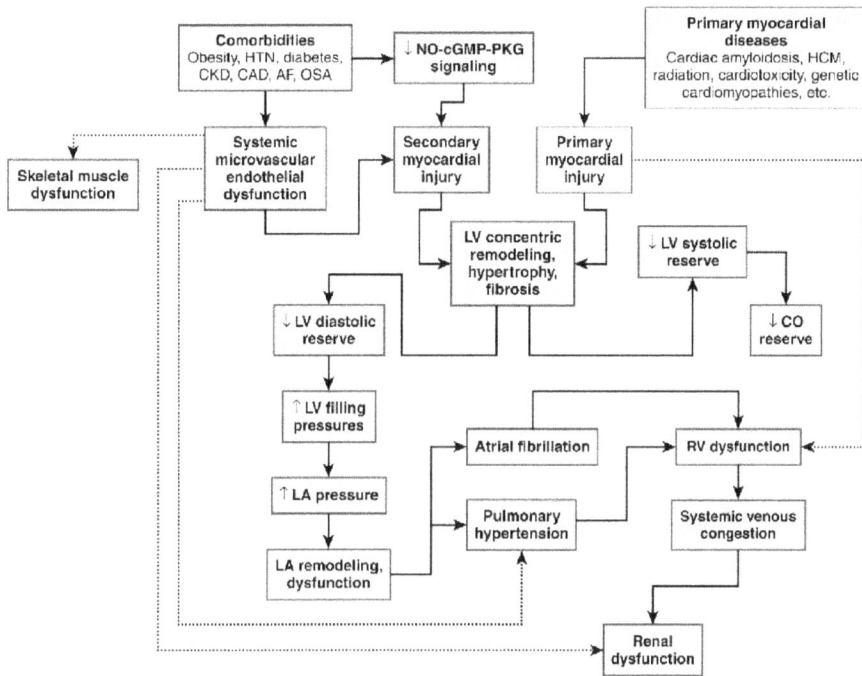

Fig. 3. Summary of pathophysiology of HFpEF. (*Adapted from* Braunwald's Heart Disease: A Textbook of Cardiovascular Medicine.[7])

Iron Deficiency and Anemia

Iron deficiency is common in patients with heart failure and associated with increased symptoms compared with patients with heart failure without iron deficiency with or without anemia.[24] The use of intravenous iron in patients with iron deficiency has been shown to improve exercise tolerance and quality of life in patients with heart failure.[1,25] However, the same improvement has not been seen with oral iron repletion and improvement in cardiovascular mortality remains unclear.[26]

Hypertension

There are currently no clinical trials that evaluate optimal blood pressure targets in patients with HFrEF or HFpEF. That said, it is well established that blood pressure should be optimized to the lowest blood pressure tolerated, without orthostasis, with the highest GDMT doses, as the evidence clearly demonstrates that "more is better" when it comes to GDMT.[1] For patients with HFpEF, guidelines for the management of hypertension are recommended to be followed. Nondihydropyridine calcium channel blockers are not recommended.[1]

Sleep Disorders

There is a strong association between central and obstructive sleep apnea with deleterious outcomes in patients with heart failure. The presence of these disorders ultimately leads to increased afterload, which can contribute to hypertension, development of atrial fibrillation, and fluid retention.[1] Continuous positive airway pressure is the recommended treatment to prevent these outcomes and worsened heart failure.

Table 5
Summary of recommendations for the treatment of heart failure and selected comorbidities

Comorbidity	Recommendation	Criteria
Iron deficiency	IV iron replacement	Ferritin <100 mcg/L Ferritin 100–200 mcg/L if transferrin saturation <20%
Hypertension	*HFrEF:* GDMT *HFpEF:* ARB or ARNi	*HFrEF:* blood pressure (BP) as low as patient can tolerate without symptoms. *HFpEF:* BP <140/90
Sleep disorders	Continuous positive airway pressure	Presence of obstructive sleep apnea on polysomnography.
Atrial fibrillation	Anticoagulation	Determine eligibility based on $CHADS_2VASC$ score
	Atrial fibrillation ablation	Patient with heart failure symptoms attributed to atrial fibrillation.
	AV nodal ablation with CRT placement	Patients with atrial fibrillation and LVEF ≤50% if rhythm control strategy fails with persistent rapid ventricular rates.

Adapted from 2022 ACC/AHA/HFSA Guidelines for Management of Heart Failure.[1]

Atrial Fibrillation

Heart failure and atrial fibrillation have many shared risk factors, and either can predispose a patient to the other. There is a higher prevalence of atrial fibrillation in patients with HFpEF versus HFrEF.[27] In patients with HFrEF and atrial fibrillation, an aggressive rhythm control strategy is recommended.[27] Catheter ablation should be favored in patients who are felt to benefit from this in terms of quality of life, procedural tolerance, with less left atrial remodeling. In patients who are not felt to benefit from catheter ablation, cardioversion plus or minus antiarrhythmic drug therapies should be considered. Early rhythm control in patients with HFpEF is less well understood. However, there is data suggestive of a benefit for rhythm control in these patients and, in the event that is not feasible, a rate control strategy should be implemented.[27] If persistent atrial fibrillation with rapid ventricular response is present in patients who have failed both rate and rhythm control, atrioventricular node ablation with CRT placement can be considered.

SUMMARY

Heart failure is a common condition with significant morbidity and mortality that affects patients that PAs care for, regardless of where they practice. For patients with HFrEF, the goal is rapid titration of the 4 pillars of GDMT: BBs, ARNi, MRA, and SGLT2 inhibitors. If LVEF fails to improve with GDMT, device and advanced heart failure therapies should be considered. Conversely, the treatment for HFpEF targets the systemic disease process and includes exercise therapy, aggressive management of comorbidities (iron deficiency, arrhythmias, hypertension, obesity, and sleep disorders), decongestion with SGLT2 inhibitors and loop diuretics, plus or minus use of MRAs.

CLINICS CARE POINTS

Heart failure with reduced ejection fraction (HFrEF):
- Start with the 4 pillars of guideline-directed medical therapy (GDMT)—beta blockers, angiotensin receptor neprilysin inhibitors, sodium glucose co-transporter 2 (SGLT2) inhibitors, and mineralocorticoid receptor antagonists.
  - There is a need for speed! Aim to have patients on 4 drugs within 4 weeks and rapidly titrate!
- Consider device-based therapy if patients have a left ventricular ejection fraction less than or equal to 35% on maximally tolerated GDMT for 3 months with a life expectancy of greater than a year.
  - Think implantable cardiac defibrillator in patients without a wide left bundle branch block. These save your patients' life if they have a ventricular arrhythmia but do not treat the HFrEF itself.
  - Think CRT-D in patients with a wide left bundle branch block. This device does have the potential to improve exercise tolerance and reverse remodeling.
- You have lots of other tools in your toolkit from a medical therapy perspective, consider your patient and choose based on their phenotypic presentation.
- If your patient is not improving with any of these therapies, consider referral to advanced heart failure cardiology.

Heart failure with preserved ejection fraction (HFpEF):
- Decongest, exercise, and aggressively treat comorbidities.
- SGLT2 inhibitors are the only mortality reducing agent in treatment of HFpEF.
- In obesity and HFpEF, semaglutide is the only pharmacologic agent that improves exercise tolerance.
- Supervised exercise training is good for all comers with HFpEF and improves exercise tolerance while treating the underlying cause of the disease.

DISCLOSURE

The author has nothing to disclose.

REFERENCES

1. Heidenreich PA, Bozkurt B, Aguilar D, et al. 2022 AHA/ACC/HFSA guideline for the management of heart failure: executive summary: a report of the American college of cardiology/American heart association joint committee on clinical practice guidelines. Circulation 2022;145(18):e876–94.
2. Caraballo C, Desai NR, Mulder H, et al. Clinical implications of the New York heart association classification. J Am Heart Assoc 2019;8(23):e014240.
3. Bozkurt B, Ahmad T, Alexander KM, et al. Heart failure epidemiology and outcomes statistics: a report of the heart failure society of America. J Card Fail 2023;29(10):1412–51.
4. Thibodeau JT, Drazner MH. The role of the clinical examination in patients with heart failure. JACC Heart Fail 2018;6(7):543–51.
5. Schwinger RHG. Pathophysiology of heart failure. Cardiovasc Diagn Ther 2021;11(1):263–76.
6. Kosta S, Dauby PC. Frank-Starling mechanism, fluid responsiveness, and length-dependent activation: unravelling the multiscale behaviors with an in silico analysis. PLoS Comput Biol 2021;17(10):e1009469.
7.. Mann DL, Zipes DP, Libby P, et al. Braunwald's heart disease: a textbook of cardiovascular medicine. 10th edition. Philadelphia, PA: Elsevier/Saunders; 2015.

8. Mebazaa A, Davison B, Chioncel O, et al. Safety, tolerability and efficacy of up-titration of guideline-directed medical therapies for acute heart failure (STRONG-HF): a multinational, open-label, randomised, trial. Lancet 2022; 400(10367):1938–52.

9. Swedberg K, Komajda M, Böhm M, et al. Ivabradine and outcomes in chronic heart failure (SHIFT): a randomised placebo-controlled study. Lancet 2010; 376(9744):875–85.

10. Armstrong PW, Pieske B, Anstrom KJ, et al. Vericiguat in patients with heart failure and reduced ejection fraction. N Engl J Med 2020;382(20):1883–93.

11. The effect of digoxin on mortality and morbidity in patients with heart failure. N Engl J Med 1997;336(8):525–33.

12. Ziaeian B, Fonarow GC, Heidenreich PA. Clinical effectiveness of hydralazine-isosorbide dinitrate in african-American patients with heart failure. JACC Heart Fail 2017;5(9):632–9.

13. Cohn JN, Archibald DG, Ziesche S, et al. Effect of vasodilator therapy on mortality in chronic congestive heart failure. Results of a Veterans Administration Cooperative Study. N Engl J Med 1986;314(24):1547–52.

14. Ellison DH, Felker GM. Diuretic treatment in heart failure. N Engl J Med 2017; 377(20):1964–75.

15. Sachdev V, Sharma K, Keteyian SJ, et al. Supervised exercise training for chronic heart failure with preserved ejection fraction: a scientific statement from the American heart association and American college of cardiology. Circulation 2023; 147(16):e699–715.

16. Packer M, Butler J, Zannad F, et al. Effect of empagliflozin on worsening heart failure events in patients with heart failure and preserved ejection fraction: EMPEROR-preserved trial. Circulation 2021;144(16):1284–94.

17. Peikert A, Martinez FA, Vaduganathan M, et al. Efficacy and safety of dapagliflozin in heart failure with mildly reduced or preserved ejection fraction according to age: the DELIVER trial. Circ Heart Fail 2022;15(10):e010080.

18. Chandra A, Polanczyk CA, Claggett BL, et al. Health-related quality of life outcomes in PARAGON-HF. Eur J Heart Fail 2022;24(12):2264–74.

19. Tridetti J, Nguyen Trung ML, Ancion A, et al. [The PARAGON-HF trial]. Rev Med Liege 2020;75(2):130–5. L'étude clinique du mois. PARAGON-HF : sacubitril/valsartan (Entresto®) dans l'insuffisance cardiaque à fraction d'éjection préservée (HFpEF).

20. Vaduganathan M, Mentz RJ, Claggett BL, et al. Sacubitril/valsartan in heart failure with mildly reduced or preserved ejection fraction: a pre-specified participant-level pooled analysis of PARAGLIDE-HF and PARAGON-HF. Eur Heart J 2023;44(31):2982–93.

21. Pitt B, Pfeffer MA, Assmann SF, et al. Spironolactone for heart failure with preserved ejection fraction. N Engl J Med 2014;370(15):1383–92.

22. Kosiborod MN, Abildstrøm SZ, Borlaug BA, et al. Semaglutide in patients with heart failure with preserved ejection fraction and obesity. N Engl J Med 2023; 389(12):1069–84.

23. Sachdev V, Sharma K, Keteyian SJ, et al. Supervised exercise training for chronic heart failure with preserved ejection fraction: a scientific statement from the American heart association and American college of cardiology. J Am Coll Cardiol 2023;81(15):1524–42.

24. Ponikowski P, Kirwan BA, Anker SD, et al. Ferric carboxymaltose for iron deficiency at discharge after acute heart failure: a multicentre, double-blind, randomised, controlled trial. Lancet 2020;396(10266):1895–904.

25. Anker SD, Comin Colet J, Filippatos G, et al. Ferric carboxymaltose in patients with heart failure and iron deficiency. N Engl J Med 2009;361(25):2436–48.

26. Lewis GD, Malhotra R, Hernandez AF, et al. Effect of oral iron repletion on exercise capacity in patients with heart failure with reduced ejection fraction and iron deficiency: the IRONOUT HF randomized clinical trial. JAMA 2017;317(19):1958–66.
27. Joglar JA, Chung MK, Armbruster AL, et al. 2023 ACC/AHA/ACCP/HRS guideline for the diagnosis and management of atrial fibrillation: a report of the American college of cardiology/American heart association joint committee on clinical practice guidelines. Circulation 2024;149(1):e1–156.

Atrial Fibrillation

Review and Update of the Most Common Arrhythmia

David J. Bunnell, MSHS, PA-C, DFAAPA*

KEYWORDS

- Atrial fibrillation • Review • Diagnosis • Treatment • Management

KEY POINTS

- Rate vs. rhythm control: In atrial fibrillation treatment, rhythm control may improve symptoms and long-term outcomes in select patients compared to rate control.
- Catheter ablation: Early electrophysiology referral for symptomatic AF can optimize rhythm control, reduce recurrence, and improve outcomes through strategies like catheter ablation.
- Anticoagulation therapy: Use the CHA2DS2-VASc score to assess stroke risk in AF patients and consider non-vitamin K anticoagulants for safer, convenient alternatives to warfarin.
- Comorbidities and lifestyle: Manage hypertension, diabetes, and lifestyle factors (OSA, weight, smoking). Incorporate patient preferences to reduce AF risk and improve outcomes.
- Multidisciplinary care: Utilize a team-based approach, collaborating with cardiologists, dietitians, and specialists to deliver comprehensive, patient-centered management for atrial fibrillation.

INTRODUCTION

Atrial fibrillation (AF), the most common cardiac arrhythmia, presents a complex health care challenge.[1] This condition not only elevates the risk for critical complications like stroke, heart failure (HF), and thromboembolism but also markedly contributes to the global burden of cardiovascular-related mortality.[2] For physician associates/assistants (PAs) across diverse specialties, encounters with AF are not just probable, but inevitable. As the population ages and the prevalence of obesity and hypertension continues to rise, the incidence of AF is increasing, underscoring the urgent need for a skilled and comprehensive approach to management.[3,4] PAs play a critical

University of Maryland School of Graduate Studies, Doctor of Medical Science Progam, 620 W. Lexington Street, Baltimore, MD 21201, USA
* Corresponding author.
E-mail address: dbunnell@umaryland.edu

Physician Assist Clin 10 (2025) 287–296
https://doi.org/10.1016/j.cpha.2024.11.005   physicianassistant.theclinics.com
2405-7991/25/© 2024 Elsevier Inc. All rights are reserved, including for text and data mining, AI training, and similar technologies.

Abbreviations	
AF	atrial fibrillation
ECG	electrocardiogram
HF	heart failure
HFpEF	preserved ejection HF
HFrEF	reduced ejection fraction HF
OSA	obstructive sleep apnea
PA	physician associate/assistant
POAF	postoperative atrial fibrillation
TTE	transthoracic echocardiography
USPSTF	US Preventive Services Task Force

role in the early detection and management of AF, as well as in coordinating comprehensive care for these patients. Their expertise and involvement are key to optimizing patient outcomes across various health care settings. This underscores the necessity for a comprehensive understanding of its pathophysiology, evolving diagnostic modalities, and effective therapeutic strategies.

This review provides PAs with essential knowledge for effective AF management. It aligns with the most recent AF guidelines established by leading cardiology societies.[5] Additionally, the review emphasizes the value of adopting a patient-centered approach in AF treatment, combining evidence-based methods with an awareness of each patient's unique needs. Through this approach, PAs can enhance patient well-being, helping people to achieve better health outcomes and improved quality of life.

EPIDEMIOLOGY

Epidemiologic studies have extensively examined AF trends. The Framingham Heart Study, a longitudinal research project conducted over 50 years from 1958 to 2007, analyzed more than 202,000 person-years of data.[3] This study identified significant increases in both the prevalence and incidence rates of AF, while simultaneously observing improvements in associated outcomes.[3] Additionally, a cohort study involving 500,684 patients from a rural Pennsylvania health care system noted a 3% annual increase in AF incidence from 2006 to 2018.[4] Remarkably, 74% of the diagnosed cases in this study were secondary, indicating that AF commonly occurs as a comorbidity. Older individuals in the Pennsylvania study, particularly those aged above 85 years, exhibited the steepest rise in AF incidence over the study period.[4] Both the Framingham and Pennsylvania studies also reported an upward trend in body mass index and hypertension over the years under investigation.[3,4] It has been suggested that expanded health care screening capabilities could also be a contributing factor to increased AF detection.[4]

PATHOPHYSIOLOGY

AF is marked by rapid, chaotic atrial electrical activity due to changes in the electrical properties of atrial tissue, affecting impulse conduction and formation. The arrhythmia manifests in various forms: paroxysmal, persistent, and permanent.[6] Although most AF cases originate in the pulmonary veins, other atrial sites can also be involved, often indicating more advanced disease stages.[7] This variability in origin points to the complexity and heterogeneity of AF as a cardiac condition.

In chronic AF, structural remodeling of the atria occurs, which includes both dilation and fibrosis.[7] This remodeling further exacerbates the arrhythmic environment, as the dilated and fibrotic atrial tissue alters normal electrical pathways and tissue responsiveness. Fibrosis leads to increased tissue stiffness and disrupts electrical connectivity, which can sustain and propagate irregular rhythms. This structural alteration not only perpetuates AF but also presents challenges in treatment, as it can reduce the effectiveness of both pharmacologic and interventional strategies, necessitating a more nuanced approach to managing chronic AF cases.[7]

COMORBID CONDITIONS AND ATRIAL FIBRILLATION

Comorbid conditions like hypertension, HF, and diabetes contribute to AF development. Additionally, behaviors such as alcohol consumption and exercise also contribute to AF. Lifestyle modifications, including moderation of alcohol intake and tailored exercise programs, are integral to reducing AF risk and enhancing patient outcomes.

Hypertension

Chronic hypertension is a well-established risk factor for AF, primarily due to its role in causing structural and electrophysiological alterations in the atria.[8] Hypertension leads to left ventricular hypertrophy and subsequent diastolic dysfunction, increasing left atrial pressure and size.[9] This atrial stretch can induce fibrotic remodeling, which disrupts normal electrical conduction pathways and predisposes to AF.[9] Hypertension can also lead to alterations in ion channel expression and function, contributing to atrial electrical remodeling and increasing the vulnerability to AF.[9]

Heart Failure

The relationship between HF and AF is complex and bidirectional.[8] HF can lead to AF by inducing atrial structural and electrical remodeling. This remodeling includes atrial enlargement, fibrosis, and changes in the expression of various ion channels and gap junction proteins.[10] Conversely, AF can exacerbate or even precipitate HF by impairing atrial contractility and leading to a loss of atrioventricular synchrony, which reduces cardiac output.[8] The interplay between HF and AF is pronounced in both reduced ejection fraction HF (HFrEF) and preserved ejection HF (HFpEF), each influencing the other's progression and management.[10]

Valvular Heart Disease

Valvular heart disease, particularly mitral valve disorders, impacts atrial structure and function, thereby promoting AF. Mitral valve regurgitation and stenosis increase left atrial pressure and volume, leading to atrial stretch and hypertrophy.[8] These changes predispose to fibrosis and electrical remodeling, which disrupt normal atrial conduction and increase the risk of AF. Management of valvular heart disease is thus crucial in preventing the onset or progression of AF.

Diabetes Mellitus

Diabetes mellitus contributes to AF development through various mechanisms.[11] Hyperglycemia and insulin resistance, hallmark features of diabetes, are associated with increased atrial size and fibrosis, oxidative stress, and inflammation, all of which contribute to atrial remodeling. Additionally, diabetes can exacerbate other AF risk factors like hypertension and obesity, further increasing the risk of AF.[12] The management of diabetes and its associated metabolic derangements is, therefore, vital in reducing AF risk.

Obstructive Sleep Apnea

Obstructive sleep apnea (OSA) contributes to AF development through intermittent hypoxia and intrathoracic pressure changes.[8] The repetitive upper airway obstructions in OSA lead to fluctuations in intrathoracic pressure, hypoxemia, and sympathetic activation. These events can cause electrical instability in the atria and promote structural remodeling, including atrial enlargement and fibrosis. The management of OSA is an essential component in the prevention and treatment of AF.

Cardiac Surgery

Patients undergoing cardiac surgery face a significant risk of developing postoperative atrial fibrillation (POAF). A meta-analysis reported a prevalence of 23.7%, highlighting the substantial burden of this complication.[13] POAF typically manifests within 4 to 6 weeks after surgery and may serve as a predictor of future episodes.[13,14] Factors believed to contribute to the development of POAF include inflammatory processes, oxidative stress, and electrolyte imbalances.[15] Additionally, increasing age and various pre-existing medical conditions are associated with a heightened risk. Notably, traditional cardiovascular risk factors such as a history of AF, hypertension, and HF, alongside noncardiovascular comorbidities like pulmonary, thyroid, kidney diseases, and obesity, all contribute to the increased likelihood of POAF.[15]

Alcohol Consumption

Alcohol consumption, particularly in excessive amounts, is associated with an increased risk of AF.[16] The relationship between alcohol intake and AF is dose-dependent, with higher consumption leading to a greater risk.[16] Alcohol can lead to atrial enlargement and fibrosis, alter ion channel function, and induce oxidative stress and inflammation, all of which contribute to the development of AF.[17] Binge drinking is associated with a higher risk of AF episodes, known as "holiday heart syndrome."[17]

Smoking

Smoking is a significant risk factor for AF. It contributes to the development of AF through mechanisms such as oxidative stress, systemic inflammation, and endothelial dysfunction.[18] These processes can lead to atrial structural and electrical remodeling, increasing the susceptibility to AF.[18] Smoking cessation is, thus, a crucial component in reducing AF risk and improving overall cardiovascular health.

Obesity

Obesity, and particularly central adiposity, is a critical risk factor for AF.[5] Obesity leads to an increase in atrial size and fibrosis, partly due to the secretion of proinflammatory adipokines and the development of systemic inflammation.[19] Additionally, obesity often coexists with other AF risk factors such as hypertension, diabetes, and sleep apnea, exacerbating the risk. Weight management and lifestyle modifications to reduce obesity are essential strategies in preventing AF.[5] Targeted interventions aimed at reducing obesity could decrease the incidence of atrial fibrillation and improve overall cardiovascular health.

Exercise

While moderate exercise has a protective effect against cardiovascular diseases, including AF, excessive high-intensity exercise may increase the risk of AF, especially in men.[5] High-intensity endurance training can lead to atrial enlargement and alterations in autonomic tone, all of which can predispose to AF.[20] It is important to strike a balance in exercise intensity and duration to maximize cardiovascular benefits while minimizing AF risk.

Genetics

Genetic factors can predispose individuals to AF.[5] Understanding these genetic links can aid in risk assessment and personalized treatment approaches. The Framingham Heart Study discovered that individuals with a family history of AF had a 40% increased chance of developing the arrhythmia.[21] The Framingham Heart Study's findings emphasize the importance of familial history in assessing AF risk, particularly noting the significance of premature onset AF as a strong indicator. Building on this, research has uncovered genetic factors, including specific mutations that impact ion channel functions, which influence AF development.[22] Genetic research has also discovered loci in individuals of Japanese and Korean descent that contribute to developing AF.[22] These insights suggest a future shift toward personalized AF management, with consideration for tailored interventions based on a combination of genetic insights and familial patterns. Further research is necessary to improve patient AF outcomes through more precise and individualized treatment strategies, acknowledging the complex interplay of genetic factors in AF pathophysiology.

Social Determinants

AF's complexity is further compounded by the influence of various social determinants, including race and ethnicity, economic status, access to health care, geographic location, and educational level.[23] These elements affect the disease's incidence, the efficacy of its management, and patient outcomes, highlighting critical disparities in health care access and treatment effectiveness across different population segments. While it has been found that White patients have increased incidence of AF compared to people who are Black, Hispanic, or Asian, worse health outcomes have been observed in these groups.[24] Despite the acknowledged impact of these social determinants, there remains a substantial gap in the literature concerning their comprehensive evaluation and integration into AF management strategies.[23] Future research is needed to explore the intersectionality of these determinants and their collective impact on AF, with a focus on identifying effective interventions to address these disparities. Such studies are essential for developing tailored, equitable health care approaches that consider the multifaceted influences on AF treatment outcomes, aiming to improve care for diverse patient populations.

CLINICAL PRESENTATION

The clinical presentation of AF varies among individuals, with some experiencing "silent AF," where the condition presents without symptoms.[5] Among those who do experience symptoms, fatigue and shortness of breath are the most common, alongside palpitations, chest discomfort, and dizziness. These symptoms can impact daily life, causing exercise intolerance and psychological distress, which may reduce quality of life. A German observational study with 1857 participants found that psychological factors, diabetes, and coronary artery disease to be associated with symptoms associated with decreased quality of life.[25] The manifestation of symptoms also varies across demographic groups, with differences observed in symptom severity and type between genders, age groups, and racial or ethnic backgrounds, highlighting the need for further research to understand these disparities and improve AF management strategies.[26]

DIAGNOSIS

AF requires a careful diagnostic and management approach. Initial clinical assessment is pivotal in confirming the diagnosis and identifying key clinical determinants influencing treatment strategies. This process includes a detailed history and physical examination, to be revisited periodically due to the dynamic risk of thromboembolism and therapeutic symptom response.[5] To enhance diagnostic precision, subsequent evaluations often incorporate advanced imaging and laboratory tests that further evaluate the structural and functional cardiac status.

Initial Confirmation with Electrocardiography

The 12-lead electrocardiogram (ECG) stands as the foundational diagnostic tool for AF, scrutinizing electrical irregularities, including Wolff–Parkinson–White syndrome, concurrent atrial arrhythmias, and other anomalies impacting pharmacologic choices, such as bradycardia and QT interval variations.[5] The ECG typically reveals missing discrete P waves and a variable ventricular rate.[27] Detailed ECG analysis assists clinicians in distinguishing AF from other supraventricular tachycardias, crucial for tailoring appropriate therapeutic interventions.

Comprehensive Evaluation for Underlying Conditions

Laboratory and clinical investigations play a significant role in unearthing disorders critical to management decisions, especially regarding stroke and hemorrhage risks. Transthoracic echocardiography (TTE) is indispensable for assessing chamber dimensions, functionality, valvular integrity, and right ventricular pressure. The left ventricular ejection fraction influences the choice of antiarrhythmic drugs and rhythm control interventions, such as catheter ablation.[5] Additionally, laboratory tests may identify AF-related conditions, including chronic kidney disease, liver anomalies, and thyroid dysfunction, thus guiding therapeutic approaches.[5]

Further Diagnostic Testing

Continuous ambulatory ECG monitoring and advanced imaging techniques have a role following initial assessments, enabling ongoing observation of heart rhythms over extended periods and facilitating the detection of intermittent atrial fibrillation that may not be captured during a standard ECG. Importantly, the presence of AF does not inherently raise the risk for myocardial ischemia, acute coronary syndromes, or pulmonary embolism, rendering routine testing for these conditions unnecessary in the absence of indicative symptoms.[5] This understanding helps streamline the diagnostic process and focus health care resources on managing the primary condition effectively, without the distraction of unwarranted investigations.

Left Atrium

Assessing the left atrium is pivotal in managing AF, as its size and function influence the arrhythmia's pathophysiology, treatment decisions, and prognostication.[5,27] TTE is instrumental in evaluating left atrial enlargement—a marker of AF risk and therapeutic outcomes. Furthermore, cardiology specialists may consider advanced imaging modalities like cardiac MRI to provide insights into atrial anatomy and fibrosis, which are essential for planning effective ablation strategies.[5] Left atrial appendage evaluation, particularly for thrombus detection via transesophageal echocardiography, plays a crucial role in stroke risk assessment and anticoagulation management in patients with AF.[5]

Screening

The 2023 guidelines underscore the importance of comprehensive risk factor screening as a critical component of AF diagnosis and management.[5] This process is guided by the mnemonic HEAD 2 TOES, designed to aid health care providers in remembering and assessing the major risk factors associated with AF.[5] These include HF, which often exacerbates or triggers AF episodes; exercise habits, which can influence cardiovascular health; arterial hypertension, a key contributor to cardiac stress; diabetes, which complicates cardiac function; tobacco use, a significant risk enhancer for cardiovascular diseases; obesity, which impacts heart structure and function; ethanol (alcohol) consumption; and sleep disorders, such as sleep apnea, which disrupt normal cardiac rhythms.[5] By systematically identifying and addressing these factors, clinicians can more effectively tailor interventions to mitigate the individual risk profiles of their patients, ultimately aiming to improve outcomes and reduce the incidence of AF.

Screening for AF primarily targets high-risk individuals aged over 65 years and employs methods ranging from one-time to continuous ECG recordings. Research suggests that intermittent or continuous recordings are more effective at detecting AF, especially in those at higher risk.[5] Population-level screenings with smartwatch apps rarely yield new AF diagnoses.[5] Screening efficacy, cost-effectiveness, and their impact on clinical outcomes, such as reducing stroke rates and improving survival, remain to be proven.[5] Cardiac monitoring is recommended for patients with AF to detect recurrences, screening, or monitor therapy responses.[5] As consumer-based wearable heart monitors are becoming more common, their accuracy and best-use practices, particularly in AF screening, require further validation.[5]

The US Preventive Services Task Force (USPSTF) has found insufficient evidence to support routine AF screening in asymptomatic adults aged over 50 years.[28] Although AF is a significant risk factor for ischemic stroke, the USPSTF found that the potential benefits and harms of screening asymptomatic individuals remain uncertain. Consequently, the task force does not recommend screening asymptomatic patients for AF, emphasizing the need for additional research to determine if such screening could effectively lower stroke risk without causing unnecessary harm.

MANAGEMENT

AF management requires a sophisticated, multidisciplinary approach to address this prevalent and complex arrhythmia. Innovations and research advancements have broadened the therapeutic landscape, offering clinicians a variety of tools to tailor treatment to individual patient needs. This overview explores the nuances of AF management strategies in greater detail.

Rate Versus Rhythm Control

Understanding the balance between rate control and rhythm control is fundamental to managing AF. Rate control strategies aim to manage the patient's heart rate within a normal range, focusing on alleviating symptoms and preventing the deleterious effects of sustained tachycardia on cardiac function. This approach often employs beta-blockers, calcium channel blockers, and sometimes digoxin, tailored according to patient-specific factors such as age, comorbidities, and medication tolerance.[27]

Rhythm control, conversely, seeks to restore the heart's normal sinus rhythm, which can improve symptoms, exercise tolerance, and quality of life. This strategy may utilize antiarrhythmic drugs, electrical cardioversion, or catheter ablation. The choice between rate and rhythm control is influenced by several factors, including the patient's symptom burden, AF duration, and the presence of HF. Notably, recent studies suggest that an early initiation of rhythm control may offer benefits in select patient populations, challenging the traditional reliance on rate control as the initial strategy.[5]

Anticoagulation Therapy

Anticoagulation remains a cornerstone of AF management, crucial for the prevention of AF-related stroke and systemic embolism. The choice of anticoagulant therapy is increasingly leaning toward non-vitamin K oral anticoagulants due to their predictable pharmacokinetic profiles, fewer dietary interactions, and reduced need for monitoring, compared to warfarin.[5] Decision-making about anticoagulation incorporates assessment of stroke risk using tools such as the CHA2DS2-VASc (congestive heart failure, hypertension, age $\geq$75 (doubled), diabetes, stroke (doubled), vascular disease, age 65 to 74, sex category) score and balancing it against the risk of bleeding using the HAS-BLED (Hypertension, Abnormal renal/liver function, Stroke, Bleeding history or predisposition, Labile INR, Elderly, Drugs/alcohol) score.[5,27]

Catheter Ablation

Catheter ablation, especially pulmonary vein isolation, has gained prominence as a rhythm control strategy for AF. Indicated for patients with symptomatic AF refractory to at least one antiarrhythmic drug, catheter ablation can also be considered as a first-line treatment in specific scenarios. Ablation is associated with reduced mortality and hospitalization for patients with HF, underscoring its integral role in AF management.[5]

Management in Heart Failure

HF and AF frequently coexist, each exacerbating the other's progression and complicating management. The integration of rhythm control strategies, including catheter ablation, has been shown to provide significant benefits in patients with HF, potentially reversing some of the adverse effects of AF on cardiac function. These interventions require careful patient selection and consideration of the underlying type of HF, with a growing body of evidence supporting their use in both HFrEF and HFpEF.[5]

FUTURE DIRECTIONS

The future of AF management is poised for significant advancements, with ongoing research into novel therapeutic agents, ablation technologies, and personalized medicine approaches. The development of more precise risk stratification models and the integration of wearables and digital health tools for remote monitoring and management of AF promise to enhance patient outcomes and quality of life further. These innovations aim to allow for an earlier detection and a more effective management of AF, reducing the burden of this condition on patients and health care systems alike.

SUMMARY

AF is a growing public health concern due to its increasing prevalence and association with significant complications like stroke and HF. Effective management of AF requires a comprehensive understanding of its pathophysiology, risk factors, and diverse treatment modalities. This review provided PAs with a foundation in AF management, emphasizing the importance of a patient-centered approach that considers individual needs and preferences.

CLINICS CARE POINTS

- *Early detection and intervention*: Prioritize an early detection of AF through regular screening based on symptoms and other clinical indications for obtaining an ECG, especially in high-risk populations. Routine screening for asymptomatic patients is not currently recommended.

- *Risk factor management*: Actively manage modifiable risk factors in your patients, including controlling blood pressure, managing obesity, and treating sleep apnea, to help prevent the onset or progression of AF.

- *Developing individualized treatment plans:* For patients experiencing symptomatic AF, consider early referral to electrophysiology to explore rhythm control options, such as catheter ablation, as part of a personalized treatment plan that takes into account family history, genetic factors, and patient preferences.

- *Collaborative multidisciplinary care:* Engage in multidisciplinary collaboration, working with cardiologists, primary care providers, and other health care professionals to create and implement a cohesive management plan for patients with AF.

- *Patient education and lifestyle counseling:* Educate patients on the importance of lifestyle changes, including diet, exercise, and smoking cessation, as part of a comprehensive strategy to manage AF and improve their quality of life.

By understanding the complexities of AF and remaining updated on evolving treatment strategies, PAs can contribute to improving the well-being of patients living with this condition.

ACKNOWLEDGMENTS

The author acknowledges the assistance of OpenAI's ChatGPT 4.0, which was instrumental in enhancing the readability and coherence of this article.

DISCLOSURE

The author has no commercial or financial conflicts of interest related to this topic.

REFERENCES

1. Jame S, Barnes G. Stroke and thromboembolism prevention in atrial fibrillation. Heart Br Card Soc 2020;106(1):10–7.
2. Roth GA, Johnson C, Abajobir A, et al. Global, regional, and national burden of cardiovascular diseases for 10 causes, 1990 to 2015. J Am Coll Cardiol 2017; 70(1):1–25.
3. Schnabel RB, Yin X, Gona P, et al. 50 year trends in atrial fibrillation prevalence, incidence, risk factors, and mortality in the Framingham Heart Study: a cohort study. Lancet 2015;386(9989):154–62.
4. Williams BA, Chamberlain AM, Blankenship JC, et al. Trends in atrial fibrillation incidence rates within an integrated health care delivery system, 2006 to 2018. JAMA Netw Open 2020;3(8):e2014874.
5. Joglar JA, Chung MK, Armbruster AL, et al. 2023 ACC/AHA/ACCP/HRS guideline for the diagnosis and management of atrial fibrillation: a report of the American college of cardiology/American heart association joint committee on clinical practice guidelines. Circulation 2024;149(1):e1–156.
6. Wijesurendra RS, Casadei B. Mechanisms of atrial fibrillation. Heart Br Card Soc 2019;105(24):1860–7.
7. Iwasaki Y, Nishida K, Kato T, et al. Atrial fibrillation pathophysiology. Circulation 2011;124(20):2264–74.

8. Heijman J, Linz D, Schotten U. Dynamics of atrial fibrillation mechanisms and co-morbidities. Annu Rev Physiol 2021;83:83–106.

9. Verdecchia P, Angeli F, Reboldi G. Hypertension and atrial fibrillation. Circ Res 2018;122(2):352–68.

10. Carlisle MA, Fudim M, DeVore AD, et al. Heart failure and atrial fibrillation, like fire and fury. JACC Heart Fail 2019;7(6):447–56.

11. Gherasim L. Association of atrial fibrillation with diabetes Mellitus, high risk co-morbidities. Maedica 2022;17(1):143–52.

12. Bavishi A, Patel R. Addressing comorbidities in heart failure: hypertension, atrial fibrillation, and diabetes. Heart Fail Clin 2020;16(4):441–56.

13. Eikelboom R, Sanjanwala R, Le ML, et al. Postoperative atrial fibrillation after cardiac surgery: a systematic review and meta-analysis. Ann Thorac Surg 2021;111(2):544–54.

14. Lee SH, Kang DR, Uhm JS, et al. New-onset atrial fibrillation predicts long-term newly developed atrial fibrillation after coronary artery bypass graft. Am Heart J 2014;167(4):593–600.e1.

15. Greenberg JW, Lancaster TS, Schuessler RB, et al. Postoperative atrial fibrillation following cardiac surgery: a persistent complication. Eur J Cardio Thorac Surg 2017;52(4):665–72.

16. Kim YG, Han KD, Choi JI, et al. Frequent drinking is a more important risk factor for new-onset atrial fibrillation than binge drinking: a nationwide population-based study. Europace 2020;22(2):216–24.

17. Surma S, Lip GYH. Alcohol and atrial fibrillation. Rev Cardiovasc Med 2023;24(3):73.

18. Elliott AD, Middeldorp ME, Van Gelder IC, et al. Epidemiology and modifiable risk factors for atrial fibrillation. Nat Rev Cardiol 2023;20(6):404–17.

19. Wong CX, Sun MT, Odutayo A, et al. Associations of epicardial, abdominal, and over-all adiposity with atrial fibrillation. Circ Arrhythm Electrophysiol 2016;9(12):e004378.

20. Abdulla J, Nielsen JR. Is the risk of atrial fibrillation higher in athletes than in the general population? A systematic review and meta-analysis. Europace 2009;11(9):1156–9.

21. Lubitz SA, Yin X, Fontes JD, et al. Association between familial atrial fibrillation and risk of new-onset atrial fibrillation. JAMA 2010;304(20):2263–9.

22. Sagris M, Vardas EP, Theofilis P, et al. Atrial fibrillation: pathogenesis, predisposing factors, and genetics. Int J Mol Sci 2021;23(1):6.

23. Essien UR, Kornej J, Johnson AE, et al. Social determinants of atrial fibrillation. Nat Rev Cardiol 2021;18(11):763–73.

24. Ugowe FE, Jackson LR, Thomas KL. Racial and ethnic differences in the preva-lence, management, and outcomes in patients with atrial fibrillation: a systematic review. Heart Rhythm 2018;15(9):1337–45.

25. Sadlonova M, Senges J, Nagel J, et al. Symptom severity and health-related quality of life in patients with atrial fibrillation: findings from the observational ARENA study. J Clin Med 2022;11(4):1140.

26. Streur M. Atrial fibrillation symptom perception. J Nurse Pract JNP 2019;15(1):60–4.

27. Rosenthal L, McManus D, Sardana M. Atrial fibrillation: practice essentials, back-ground, pathophysiology. Medscape 2019. Available at: https://emedicine.medscape.com/article/151066-overview. Accessed March 16, 2024.

28. Davidson KW, Barry MJ, Mangione CM, et al. US Preventive Services Task Force. Screening for atrial fibrillation: US preventive Services Task Force recommenda-tion statement. JAMA 2022;327(4):360.

Evaluation and Management of Ventricular Arrhythmias from Diagnosis to Treatment

Navigating the Complexities of Ventricular Arrhythmias

Kimberly A. Berggren, DMSc, PA-C[a],*, Robert Hill, DMSc, PA-C[b,1]

KEYWORDS

- Ventricular tachycardia • Ventricular arrhythmia • Sudden cardiac death
- Catheter ablation • Device therapy

KEY POINTS

- Ventricular arrhythmias (VAs) are significant causes of sudden cardiac death, often linked to structural heart disease and inherited disorders.
- Diagnostic tools such as electrocardiograms, echocardiography, and cardiac MRI are crucial for assessing VAs and guiding treatment decisions.
- Treatment options range from pharmacologic interventions to advanced methods such as device therapy and catheter ablation, targeting the underlying conditions of arrhythmias.
- Proper diagnosis and timely management of ventricular arrhythmias can greatly reduce the risk of sudden cardiac death and improve overall cardiovascular health.

INTRODUCTION TO VENTRICULAR ARRHYTHMIAS (DIAGNOSIS AND EVALUATION)

Normal cardiac electrical conduction begins with a pacemaker impulse generated in the sinoatrial node, passing through the atrioventricular (AV) node, the bundle of His, bundle branches, and the Purkinje fibers of the ventricles. An arrhythmia occurs when there is any deviation from this normal electrical conduction pathway. Ventricular arrhythmias (VAs) originate in the ventricle and can occur in both structurally normal and abnormal hearts.[1]

VAs are a significant cause of sudden cardiac death (SCD) in the United States, with an annual incidence of 60 per 100,000 people in the United States.[1] Ventricular

[a] Florida State University College of Medicine, School of Physician Assistant Practice, Tallahassee, FL, USA; [b] Bradley University, Department of Physician Assistant Practice, Peoria, IL, USA
[1] Present address: PO Box 1724, Glen Allen, VA 23060.
* Corresponding author. 1115 West Call Street, Tallahassee, FL 32306-4300.
E-mail address: kimberly.berggren@med.fsu.edu

Physician Assist Clin 10 (2025) 297–305
https://doi.org/10.1016/j.cpha.2024.11.006
2405-7991/25/Published by Elsevier Inc.
physicianassistant.theclinics.com

Abbreviations	
ARVC	arrhythmic right ventricular cardiomyopathy
AV	atrioventricular
CMR	cardiac magnetic resonance
CRT	cardiac resynchronization therapy
EKG	electrocardiogram
EP	electrophysiology
HF	heart failure
ICD	implantable cardioverter-defibrillator
LGE	late gadolinium enhancement
LVEF	left ventricular ejection fraction
MI	myocardial infarction
PVCs	premature ventricular contractions
SCD	sudden cardiac death
VA	ventricular arrhythmia
VF	ventricular fibrillation
VT	ventricular tachycardia

arrhythmias include isolated premature ventricular contractions (PVCs), nonsustained and sustained ventricular tachycardia (VT), and ventricular fibrillation (VF). Underlying structural heart disease is present in most SCD cases, with VT or VF in patients with heart failure accounting for 50% of cardiovascular deaths.[2]

VT is defined as 3 consecutive ventricular beats at a rate greater than 100 beats per minute and a QRS duration exceeding 120 milliseconds.[1] Nonsustained VT, lasting under 30 seconds, does not usually cause hemodynamic instability. On the other hand, sustained VT, which lasts 30 seconds or more, can significantly decrease cardiac output, particularly in the presence of coronary artery disease, reduced left ventricular ejection fraction (LVEF), and other comorbidities.[3,4]

Wide-complex tachycardia on an electrocardiogram (EKG) is diagnosed as VT about 80% of the time.[5] Other potential causes include supraventricular tachycardias with bundle branch block or accessory pathways, atrial flutter or fibrillation with aberrancy, and QRS widening from drugs or electrolyte derangements.[1] The diagnosis requires careful patient history and EKG comparison. Because of the significant mortality associated with ventricular tachycardia, a wide complex tachycardia should be treated as VT until proven otherwise.[6]

Most sustained monomorphic VTs arise from reentry due to slow conduction in diseased myocardium caused by ischemia, inflammation, infiltrative cardiomyopathy, or scar tissue. Structurally normal hearts may experience VT due to ion channel defects or calcium cycling issues such as idiopathic ventricular outflow tract tachycardia and long QT syndromes. VT from enhanced automaticity, although rare, can occur in conditions like catecholaminergic VT, transient inflammation, excess digoxin levels, electrolyte imbalance, and following myocardial reperfusion.[7]

OUTPATIENT EVALUATION OF VENTRICULAR ARRHYTHMIA

Ventricular arrhythmias can manifest in various ways, ranging from subtle signs like an irregular pulse during a physical examination to more severe presentations such as cardiac arrest. Common symptoms include palpitations, dizziness, syncope, shortness of breath, and chest pain. These arrhythmias may signify underlying structural heart disease; thus, the onset of frequent PVCs or VT necessitates a thorough diagnostic evaluation.[2]

The evaluation encompasses a comprehensive medical history and physical examination. Identifying conditions such as coronary artery disease, left ventricular systolic dysfunction, or other structural heart disease is crucial. A thorough history helps determine the etiology of arrhythmia and assesses the patient's risk of systemic hypotension, coronary and cerebral hypoperfusion, syncope, and SCD. In cases of a structurally normal heart, syncope and cardiac arrest are less common, with symptoms typically emerging during physical exertion or emotional stress.[6]

A detailed family history is critical, especially when VT is suspected. Current guidelines recommend obtaining a 3-generation family history to search for premature SCD, dilated cardiomyopathy, or another inherited cause of VT. VT related to inherited conditions can initially manifest as syncope, cardiac arrest, or SCD, typically affecting individuals between 20 and 40 years. Genetic testing should be considered for people with a family history of dilated cardiomyopathy or premature SCD. Furthermore, genetic testing is recommended for asymptomatic first-degree relatives of patients diagnosed with genetically linked VT.[2]

Diagnostic testing, including an EKG during sinus rhythm and, when possible, during arrhythmic events, plays a pivotal role in diagnosing and localizing ventricular arrhythmias. The findings on an EKG can guide risk stratification and influence therapeutic strategies. An EKG can also detect underlying issues like myocardial ischemia, long QT syndrome, hypertrophic cardiomyopathy, Brugada syndrome, and arrhythmogenic right ventricular cardiomyopathy. For people with symptoms triggered by exertion, exercise stress testing is also recommended.[6] Additionally, coronary angiography with computed tomography or left heart catheterization may be used to ascertain the presence of coronary artery abnormalities and coronary artery disease.[6]

For ongoing symptom monitoring, particularly in patients with histories of syncope, presyncope, or palpitations where arrhythmias remain undetected by standard EKG or telemetry, ambulatory EKG monitoring is helpful. These monitors allow for the continuous recording of heart rhythms, linking symptoms with arrhythmic events, and assessing the frequency of arrhythmias. In cases where symptoms are infrequent, or syncope remains unexplained, implantable loop recorders can be used.[2]

ECHOCARDIOGRAM

In patients with VAs, a transthoracic echocardiogram evaluates cardiac structure and function. It helps diagnose conditions such as hypertrophic cardiomyopathy, dilated cardiomyopathy, valvular heart disease, and other structural heart diseases. Serial echocardiograms are used to monitor disease progression and assess the effectiveness of therapeutic interventions.[2]

CARDIAC MAGNETIC RESONANCE

Cardiac magnetic resonance (CMR) offers excellent soft-tissue characterization and provides detailed cardiac morphology and function assessments.[7] CMR is beneficial for patients suspected of having conditions like sarcoidosis or arrhythmogenic right ventricular cardiomyopathy, and it plays a role in risk stratification for various cardiomyopathies. Late gadolinium enhancement CMR (LGE-CMR) can detect and localize myocardial injury, inflammation, fibrotic remodeling, and edema. It helps elucidate the etiology of nonischemic cardiomyopathies or concealed structural disease by identifying distinct patterns of regional distribution of LGE. This imaging technique can also pinpoint areas of fibrotic remodeling that may serve as substrates for arrhythmias, aiding electrophysiologists in planning targeted VT ablation procedures. It is important to perform CMR before implanting cardiac devices, as cardiac devices can delay the timing of CMR imaging or cause artifacts.[2]

CARDIAC ELECTROPHYSIOLOGY TESTING

An electrophysiology (EP) study is a detailed analysis of the heart's conduction system to identify mechanisms and specific origins of an arrhythmia. Cardiac mapping during an EP study identifies the exact distribution of myocardial tissue responsible for arrhythmias, enabling electrophysiologists to locate and target the abnormal tissue for radiofrequency ablation. This study is particularly beneficial for patients with underlying heart disease and recurrent syncope when other cardiac evaluations do not reveal a clear cause. Additionally, an EP study is valuable for assessing the risk of SCD in patients where the necessity for an implantable cardioverter-defibrillator (ICD) is unclear[1]

CAUSES OF VENTRICULAR TACHYCARDIA
Ischemic Heart Disease

Ischemic heart disease is the most common cause of VT in older persons. VT and VF can develop within minutes to hours following a myocardial infarction (MI) and are responsible for a significant proportion of out-of-hospital SCD.[2] The risk of SCD is highest in the first month post MI, although VT may occur up to 20 years later. Nonsustained VT occurs in up to 80% of patients with dilated ischemic cardiomyopathy.[1,8]

Hypertrophic Cardiomyopathy

Hypertrophic cardiomyopathy is a well-known cause of VT and SCD, particularly among young people and athletes, accounting for over one-third of SCD cases in these groups. It is characterized by the unexplained thickening of the ventricular walls, predominantly the interventricular septum. Assessing the risk of SCD involves a history of syncope, documented nonsustained VT, septal thickness greater than 3 cm, and a paradoxic drop in blood pressure during exercise. LGE-CMR is proving useful as a predictor of serious VA in these patients.[9]

Long QT-Syndrome

Caused by mutations that prolong the QT interval, congenital long QT syndrome increases the risk of Torsade de Pointes (TdP), a type of polymorphic VT.[9] Episodes of TdP tend to resolve spontaneously but can evolve into sustained VF. A QTc greater than 500 ms is a predictor for life-threatening arrhythmias.[10] Acquired long QT is caused by medications that prolong the QT interval. The list of these medications is extensive and includes antiarrhythmic drugs (particularly dofetilide, ibutilide, and sotalol), antipsychotics, antidepressants, antibiotics, antimalarials, gastrointestinal medications, and anesthetic agents. Medications that can prolong the QT interval should be identified and managed carefully to reduce VT risk.[2,9]

The first-line therapy for preventing TdP in patients with congenital long QT syndrome is ß-blockers: however, patients should be monitored for bradycardia exacerbations. Despite full-dose ß-blocker therapy, about 25% of patients continue to experience VA and may require an ICD. In the acute setting with frequently recurrent TdP, intravenous magnesium sulfate is useful. Both bradycardia and pauses increase the risk of TdP in predisposed patients. Temporary pacing may also be considered in excessive bradycardia or prolonged pauses seen on telemetry, and discontinuing medications that cause bradycardia may be beneficial.

Idiopathic Outflow Tract Tachycardias

Idiopathic VT is uncommon and typically presents in adults aged 20 to 40 years and occurs in structurally normal hearts, seldom progressing to VF. Significant arrhythmia burden may lead to a reversible form of LV systolic dysfunction. Symptoms such as palpitations and presyncope are usually triggered by exertion or stress. Catheter ablation of the outflow tract is highly effective, with a success rate exceeding 90%, and should be considered the first-line treatment. β-Blockers or calcium channel blockers may be used temporarily or if ablation is not an option.[11]

Brugada Syndrome

Brugada syndrome is a rare genetic disorder that predisposes individuals to VT and SCD in an otherwise structurally normal heart. It is identifiable on an EKG by a specific right bundle branch block pattern with ST-segment elevations.[9] Increased clinical awareness and genetic screening have led to more asymptomatic diagnoses. An ICD is the primary preventive treatment for high-risk patients, with EP studies and genetic testing helping to clarify treatment decisions.[10,12]

Inflammatory and Infiltrative Disease

Infiltrative and inflammatory heart diseases such as cardiac sarcoidosis, cardiac amyloidosis, hemochromatosis, systemic lupus erythematosus, and rheumatoid arthritis can have significant cardiac implications. Among patients with sarcoidosis, about 40% to 50% exhibit cardiac involvement, which may initially manifest as progressive AV block, VT, or both. Arrhythmogenic right ventricular cardiomyopathy (ARVC) is a congenital cardiomyopathy characterized by arrhythmogenic fibrofatty infiltration of the ventricular myocardium, typically presenting as sustained VT and SCD in individuals aged 20 to 40 years. Exercise can trigger VT in ARVC and exacerbate the progression of cardiomyopathy and the incidence of VT. Treatment involves moderating exercise, implanting an ICD, and using antiarrhythmic drugs to manage VT and prevent ICD shocks. VT ablation can be considered in infiltrative diseases, although its success is often limited due to the multifocal nature of the substrate and the progressive course of these conditions.[13,14]

EVALUATION OF UNSTABLE VENTRICULAR TACHYCARDIA

Patients with acute VT require immediate, evidence-based interventions, particularly in the emergency setting or following cardiac arrest. For hemodynamically unstable patients with sustained VT, prompt defibrillation and advanced cardiac life support are crucial. Hemodynamically stable patients may undergo pharmacologic cardioversion using intravenous amiodarone, lidocaine, or procainamide. Intravenous calcium-channel blockers should be avoided unless the exact cause of the arrhythmia is known and the patient has no structural heart disease.[2]

Identifying and addressing any factors that provoke VT is essential for preventing recurrence. Evaluations should consider myocardial ischemia, acute heart failure (HF), electrolyte imbalances, metabolic acidosis, and arrhythmia-inducing medications. Prompt revascularization and treatment of electrolyte imbalance are critical. An EKG is necessary to assess cardiac structure and function, while medication reconciliation helps identify any drugs that might prolong the QT interval or cause electrolyte imbalances. Intravenous amiodarone is the primary antiarrhythmic drug used to reduce VT recurrence.[2,12]

An electrical storm—3 or more episodes of VT or VF within 24 hours—rarely occurs in a structurally normal heart. The initial drug of choice is typically intravenous amiodarone, although procainamide, lidocaine, and quinidine are alternatives. Managing ischemic heart disease to relieve ischemia is vital. Device interrogation can confirm appropriate ICD shocks and allow reprogramming of the device to optimize antitachycardic pacing and minimize unnecessary shocks. In refractory cases, sedation and intravenous ß-blockers may be used to break the cycle by reducing sympathetic drive. Urgent catheter ablation is indicated if VT does not respond to medical interventions.[2]

PREMATURE VENTRICULAR CONTRACTIONS

For patients experiencing symptomatic PVCs, ß-blockers are considered safe and effective first-line therapy. In cases of heart failure with reduced ejection fraction (HFrEF), more aggressive interventions such as early cardiac ablation are recommended to prevent the progression of cardiomyopathy. Additionally, frequent PVCs may diminish the effectiveness of cardiac resynchronization therapy (CRT). Reducing the burden of PVCs with antarrhythmic drugs or through cardiac ablation can improve LVEF and alleviate symptoms.[2]

DEVICE THERAPY

Device therapy with an ICD is the most effective method to prevent SCD. An ICD terminates VA using antitachycardia pacing (ATP) and, if necessary, direct current shocks. While ICDs can be lifesaving, they do not prevent the occurrence of VAs and may decrease the quality of life due to inappropriate or frequent shocks. Other risks include device-related infections and lead fractures.[1,2,15]

Indications for an ICD include patients who have experienced sustained VT or VF without a reversible cause, regardless of LVEF. For primary prevention, an ICD should be considered for patients with HF symptoms and an LVEF of ≤35%. Asymptomatic patients with ischemic cardiomyopathy and an LVEF ≤30% are recommended to have an ICD. Patients with HFrEF must receive maximally tolerated guideline-directed medical therapy for HF for 3 months, and ICD implantation should be delayed for 40 days post acute MI or revascularization to confirm nonimprovement of LVEF. People with a life expectancy of less than 1 year are generally not considered candidates for an ICD.[1,2,6,15]

There are several types of ICDs as follows:

- Single-Chamber ICD: Contains a single lead in the right ventricle to deliver shocks or ATP, suitable for patients without the need for cardiac pacing or atrial arrhythmia detection.
- Dual-Chamber ICD: Contains a lead in both the right atrium and right ventricle, enabling arrhythmia detection and ventricular pacing, and is useful in patients who require a pacemaker or monitoring for atrial arrhythmias such as atrial fibrillation.
- ICD with CRT (CRT-D): Enhances both symptoms and survival by improving ventricular function, reducing VA burden, and decreasing the frequency of ICD-delivered therapies. Candidates for CRT include people with an LVEF ≤35%, HF symptoms, and a left bundle branch block or QRS duration ≥ 150 ms of any morphology.
- Subcutaneous ICD (S-ICD): An alternative for patients at high risk for infections or young patients who might face complications from long-term transvenous leads. The S-ICD does not offer pacing, ATP, or CRT capabilities.[2]

The appropriate device and configuration should be tailored based on individual patient needs and underlying medical conditions.

CATHETER ABLATION

Catheter ablation has significantly reduced the frequency of recurrent VT and ICD discharges. The VANISH trial showed that patients with ischemic cardiomyopathy experiencing recurrent VT despite antiarrhythmic drugs saw a 28% reduction in mortality, VT storms, or ICD shocks following catheter ablation. Risks associated with cardiac ablation are rare but include vascular access complications, cardiac perforation, and induction of arrhythmias.[1,2,7]

Despite the proven benefits of early catheter ablation in reducing VT recurrence, referrals for this procedure often occur late in a patient's clinical course. Candidates for catheter ablation include patients with ischemic or nonischemic cardiomyopathy who have symptomatic VT; those experiencing frequent PVCs, nonsustained, or sustained VT in the context of HFrEF; patients with symptomatic VT originating from the right ventricular outflow tract; and people with bundle branch reentrant VT. Catheter ablation is also advantageous for patients with recurrent sustained VT and VF that are refractory to antiarrhythmic drugs or who prefer to avoid these drugs due to side effects or concerns for long-term toxicity.[1,2,7]

ANTIARRHYTHMIC MEDICATIONS

Several antiarrhythmic drugs are used to manage ventricular arrhythmias and reduce their recurrence. Although ICDs and advances in catheter ablation have taken precedence in preventing SCD, antiarrhythmic drugs remain crucial for controlling VAs, especially in patients who continue to receive ICD therapies despite cardiac ablation or in those who either failed cardiac ablation or are not candidates for the procedure.[12]

- *Amiodarone* is commonly prescribed for VAs due to its efficacy but it has significant long-term side effects including thyroid dysfunction, pulmonary fibrosis, hepatic toxicity, photosensitivity, corneal deposits, and polyneuropathy. Monitoring laboratory and diagnostic studies for the liver, thyroid, and pulmonary function are essential with long-term use.[12]
- *Beta-blockers* are widely used for their antiarrhythmic effects resulting from sympathetic blockade and membrane stabilization. They are particularly effective in treating HFrEF, and ß-blockers offer antiischemic benefits, decrease myocardial oxygen demand, slow the heart rate, and are recommended as first-line therapy for preventing VAs in congenital heart disease.[2,12]
- *Sotalol*, a nonselective ß-blocker with antiarrhythmic properties, is used as a second-line medication for managing VT, particularly in patients who cannot tolerate amiodarone. Its dosing requires careful adjustments based on QTc interval and renal function, and it requires regular monitoring.[12]
- *Lidocaine and Mexiletine* are often used as an adjunct to other antiarrhythmic agents like amiodarone and sotalol to enhance their effectiveness.[12]
- *Nondihydropyridine calcium channel blockers* such as verapamil and diltiazem are generally contraindicated in most cases of VAs due to risks of severe hemodynamic collapse and death. However, they can be useful in structurally normal hearts to manage outflow tract PVCs and terminate fascicular VT.[12]
- *Flecainide and Propafenone* are suitable for suppressing PVCs in patients with structurally normal hearts and no history of MI or HF. These drugs are also effective for right ventricular outflow tract PVCs and exercise-induced VAs but must be used cautiously due to their potential to provoke serious arrhythmias, especially in patients with coronary artery disease, reduced LVEF, or Brugada syndrome. Alcohol can increase propafenone levels, raising the risk of proarrhythmic effects.[12]

SUMMARY

Managing ventricular arrhythmias requires a deep understanding of the underlying pathophysiology and the array of treatment options available. Clinicians must balance the immediate need for arrhythmia control with long-term management strategies, including lifestyle modifications, device function optimization, and medication regimens. Appropriate and comprehensive diagnostic evaluations with EKGs, echocardiography, appropriate use of ischemic evaluations, and CMR are crucial to evaluate the patient with ventricular arrhythmia. Additionally, careful patient selection, consultation with cardiology and electrophysiology specialists, and patient-specific treatment plans can significantly improve clinical outcomes. As medical technology and knowledge of cardiac electrophysiology continue to evolve, ongoing research and clinical vigilance remain imperative to advancing treatment protocols and enhancing preventive measures for patients with ventricular arrhythmias.

CLINICS CARE POINTS

Pearls
- The workup for ventricular arrhythmia includes a complete medical history of the patient, a complete and accurate medication reconciliation, a comprehensive review of previous EKGs, other previous diagnostic studies (eg, echocardiograms, cardiac angiography, cardiac MRI, and device data), and previous cardiovascular procedures.
- An appropriate workup includes a physical examination, EKG, and echocardiogram. Ischemic evaluation, CMR, and EP study should be obtained when indicated.
- A 12-lead EKG capturing ventricular arrhythmia helps determine etiology and guide the management plan.
- Younger patients (ages 20–40 years) also develop VT and SCD—a family history and workup are needed in the setting of syncope or palpitations.
- Consider ablation as the primary treatment for PVCs and VT, particularly ischemic VT, idiopathic outlet tract VT, and recurrent VT/Shocks refractory to medical therapy. Early referral to electrophysiology (EP) is crucial.

Pitfalls
- Do not overlook PVCs; frequent PVCs at a rate of 10 to 20 per hour or any occurrence of VT should prompt further evaluation.
- Failure to ensure a complete and accurate medication reconciliation during transitions in care, ensuring medications for VT are not inappropriately held or discontinued without clear guidance from cardiology and accurate documentation.
- Not recognizing that a history of MI, particularly in patients with reduced LVEF, significantly elevates the risk of VT and SCD.
- Failure to monitor patients on common antiarrhythmic drugs, such as amiodarone, sotalol, flecainide, and propafenone, for potential adverse effects or drug interactions.

DISCLOSURE

The authors have nothing to disclose.

REFERENCES

1. Guandalini GS, Liang JJ, Marchlinski FE. Ventricular tachycardia ablation: past, present, and future perspectives. JACC Clin Electrophysiol 2019;5(12):1363–83.
2. Vazquez-Calvo S, Roca-Luque I, Althoff TF. Management of ventricular arrhythmias in heart failure. Curr Heart Fail Rep 2023;20(4):237–53.
3. Janse MJ, Rosen MR. History of arrhythmias. Handb Exp Pharmacol 2006;(171):1–39.

4. Al-Khatib SM, Stevenson WG, Ackerman MJ, et al. 2017 AHA/ACC/HRS guideline for management of patients with ventricular arrhythmias and the prevention of sudden cardiac death: executive summary: a report of the American college of cardiology/American heart association task force on clinical practice guidelines and the heart rhythm society. J Am Coll Cardiol 2018;72(14):1677–749.
5. Kashou AH, Evenson CM, Noseworthy PA, et al. Differentiating wide complex tachycardias: a historical perspective. Indian Heart J 2021;73(1):7–13.
6. Whitaker J, Wright MJ, Tedrow U. Diagnosis and management of ventricular tachycardia. Clin Med 2023;23(5):442–8.
7. Lopez EM, Malhotra R. Ventricular tachycardia in structural heart disease. J Innov Card Rhythm Manag 2019;10(8):3762–73.
8. Koplan BA, Stevenson WG. Ventricular tachycardia and sudden cardiac death. Mayo Clin Proc 2009;84(3):289–97.
9. Locati ET, Bagliani G, Cecchi F, et al. Arrhythmias due to inherited and acquired abnormalities of ventricular repolarization. Card Electrophysiol Clin 2019;11(2):345–62.
10. Singh M, Morin DP, Link MS. Sudden cardiac death in long QT syndrome (LQTS), Brugada syndrome, and catecholaminergic polymorphic ventricular tachycardia (CPVT). Prog Cardiovasc Dis 2019;62(3):227–34.
11. Nan J, Sugrue A, Ladas TP, et al. Anatomic considerations relevant to atrial and ventricular arrhythmias. Card Electrophysiol Clin 2019;11(3):421–32.
12. Apte N, Kalra DK. Pharmacotherapy in ventricular arrhythmias. Cardiology 2023;148(2):119–30.
13. Krahn AD, Wilde AAM, Calkins H, et al. Arrhythmogenic right ventricular cardiomyopathy. JACC Clin Electrophysiol 2022;8(4):533–53.
14. Tan JL, Fong HK, Birati EY, et al. Cardiac sarcoidosis. Am J Cardiol 2019;123(3):513–22.
15. Jaiswal V, Taha AM, Joshi A, et al. Implantable cardioverter defibrillators for primary prevention in patients with ischemic and non-ischemic cardiomyopathy: a meta-analysis. Curr Probl Cardiol 2024;49(2):102198.

Valvular Heart Disease
Classic Presentations and Contemporary Treatment

Check for updates

Amy E. Simone, PA-C, FACC

KEYWORDS

- Valve • Valvular • Heart • Disease

KEY POINTS

- Recognize valvular heart disease (VHD) and outline currently available treatment options.
- Acknowledge that VHD is prevalent, deadly, and treatable, however, is underdiagnosed and undertreated.
- Demonstrate how the Multidisciplinary Heart Team supports patients suffering from VHD across the care continuum.
- Highlight rapidly evolving surgical and percutaneous treatment options.

INTRODUCTION

Valvular heart disease (VHD) refers to any deviation or departure from normal valve anatomy or function[1] and affects people of all ages across the globe. While the forthcoming discussion is technical in nature, there is a distinctly humanistic element of creativity and innovation that has propelled us to the current management and treatment of VHD. Valve disease includes conditions caused by genetic, environmental, or acquired pathologic processes that vary with geographic location and demography.[1] Left untreated, valve disease is associated with increased morbidity and mortality, diminished quality of life, increased rate of hospitalizations, and various cardiovascular sequelae including heart failure (HF). We live in an exciting era of rapidly evolving indications for the treatment and advances of percutaneous therapies to address VHD. The paradigm of care has shifted to a multidisciplinary approach that leverages the vast training, experience, and perspectives of the clinicians on the Heart Team and integrates the patient's goals, wishes, and voice across the continuum of care.

Clinical Affairs, Transcatheter Heart Valves, Edwards Lifesciences, 1 Edwards Way, Irvine, CA 92614, USA
E-mail address: AmyESimone@gmail.com
Twitter: @AmySimonePA (A.E.S.)

Physician Assist Clin 10 (2025) 307–332
https://doi.org/10.1016/j.cpha.2024.12.001
physicianassistant.theclinics.com
2405-7991/25/© 2024 Elsevier Inc. All rights reserved, including those for text and data mining, AI training, and similar technologies.

Abbreviations	
AF	atrial fibrillation
AR	aortic regurgitation
AS	aortic stenosis
AVC	aortic valve calcification
AVR	aortic valve replacement
BAV	bicuspid aortic valve
BMC	balloon mitral commissurotomy
CAD	coronary artery disease
CMR	cardiac magnetic resonance
CT	computed tomography
DSE	dobutamine stress echocardiography
EuroSCORE II	European System for Cardiac Operative Risk Evaluation
GDMT	goal-directed medical therapy
HF	heart failure
LFLG AS	low-flow, low-gradient aortic stenosis
LVEDP	LV end diastolic pressure
LVEF	left ventricular ejection fraction
MDHT	Multidisciplinary Heart Team
MR	mitral regurgitation
MS	mitral stenosis
MVA	mitral valve area
RCT	randomized clinical trial
RhD	rheumatic disease
SDM	shared decision making
STS-PROM	Society of Thoracic Surgeons' Predicted Risk of Mortality
TAVR	transcatheter aortic valve replacement
TEER	transcatheter edge-to-edge repair
TMVR	transcatheter mitral valve replacement
TR	tricuspid regurgitation
TS	tricuspid stenosis
TTE	transthoracic echocardiography
VHD	valvular heart disease
VWF	von Willebrand factor

INCIDENCE/PREVALENCE

Valve disease is a global problem estimated to affect 2.5% of the world's population.[1] The etiology of valve disease differs between industrially underdeveloped versus developed regions. Rheumatic disease (RhD) remains the most common cause of valve disease in underdeveloped countries[1]; in contrast, age-induced calcific aortic stenosis (AS) and secondary (or functional) mitral regurgitation (MR) are most common in developed countries.[1] In the United States, 13% of VHD is observed in patients older than 75 years of age.[1] As the life expectancy continues to increase in developed countries, clinicians will be faced with caring for more patients with VHD. Globally, VHD has many causes including infective endocarditis, systemic lupus erythematosus, carcinoid tumors, and iatrogenic causes such as radiation, chemotherapy, and degeneration of bioprosthetic devices. Unfortunately, VHD remains underdetected and undertreated globally because of the significant variations in access to health care.

THE ROLE OF THE MULTIDISCIPLINARY HEART TEAM

The 2020 ACC/AHA Guideline for the Management of Valvular Heart Disease formalized a Class I indication that "patients with severe VHD should be evaluated by a

Multidisciplinary Heart Valve Team when intervention is considered[2]" with equipoise by both cardiology and cardiac surgery. Importantly, treatment plans must consider surgical and percutaneous intervention, medical management, palliative care, and patient preference. Team-based care is essential when evaluating and treating patients with heart valve disease, and the Multidisciplinary Heart Team (MDHT) plays the central role. The high-functioning MDHT embodies a common understanding of goals and responsibilities,[3] placing the patient at the center of a team that supports them collectively across the care continuum[3] (**Fig. 1**). A paradigm of multidisciplinary care has become best-practice; ideally, every patient should be evaluated by both an interventional cardiologist and a cardiothoracic surgeon to establish the correct diagnosis, perform risk stratification, and discuss preferred treatment plans that optimize clinical outcomes. Although the interventional cardiologist and cardiothoracic surgeon are at the core of the MDHT, critical insight and expertise by the extended members including cardiac imagers, anesthesiologists, HF specialists, advanced practice providers, nurses, valve program coordinators, cardiac navigators, and more are essential. Each member of the MDHT draws from disparate training, experience, and scope of practice to add to the collaborative-care model for a holistic approach. This is a patient-centric model in which shared decision making (SDM) tools and decision aids ensure patient understanding of the disease process, treatment options, and the risk-benefit ratio.

SURGICAL RISK ASSESSMENT

Defining a patient's surgical risk is crucial in identifying potential treatment options. For example, patients of unacceptably elevated risk for traditional open-heart surgery may be better candidates for minimally invasive transcatheter interventions or clinical research trial options. Surgical risk considers an array of anatomic features, comorbidities, surgical history, life expectancy, functional, and cognitive assessments. The Society of Thoracic Surgeons' Predicted Risk of Mortality[4] (STS-PROM) and the

CENTRAL ILLUSTRATION: Conceptual Framework for the MDHT

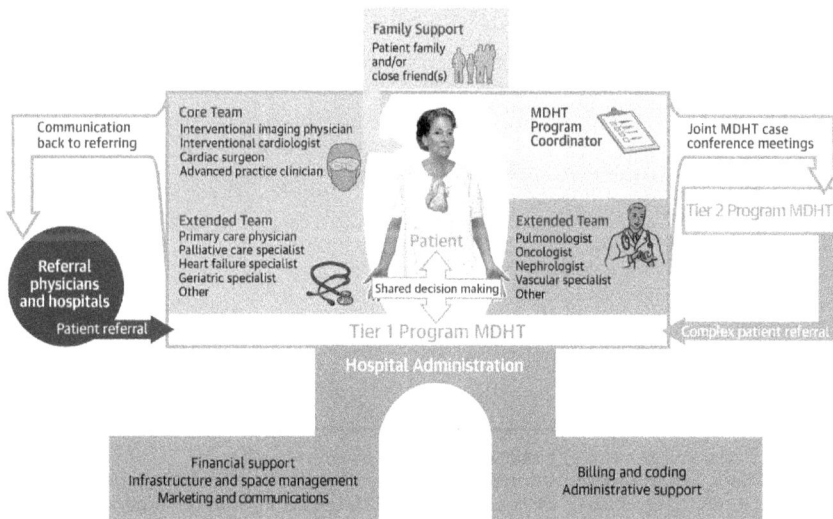

Fig. 1. The multidisciplinary heart team.[3]

European System for Cardiac Operative Risk Evaluation[5] (EuroSCORE II) are the most utilized risk assessment prediction models. It is important to note that these calculators are specifically designed to prospectively analyze patients undergoing traditional open-heart cardiac surgery. The calculated risk assessment score is a starting point for discussion as there are inherent limitations to the calculations. For example, the calculators consider many variables and discreet data fields; however, they do not include functional or cognitive assessments, frailty metrics (gait speed, grip strength, serum albumin, and activities of daily living), or a number of comorbidities that can negatively impact outcomes and elevate surgical risk[1] (**Table 1**). A methodical approach should assess a patient's surgical risk, including baseline clinical data, comorbidities, and STS score and followed by functional and cognitive assessments, resulting in the determination of overall procedure risk[1] (**Table 2**). Surgical risk is characterized as: low risk, intermediate risk, high risk, or prohibitive risk. After surgical risk has been determined, the MDHT, utilizing SDM, offers a personalized treatment plan.

THE AORTIC VALVE
Aortic Stenosis

Background
AS is characterized by the formation of calcium in and around the valve apparatus. The deposition of calcific material on the leaflets and in the annulus inhibits proper function of the valve by decreasing the effective orifice area (EOA), therefore, impeding blood flow. The most common causes of AS include age-related calcific aortic valve disease, congenital aortic valve disease, and RhD.[1] Less common etiologies of AS include

Table 1
Examples of procedure-specific risk factors for interventions not incorporated into existing risk scores[1]

SAVR	TAVI	Surgical Mitral Valve Repair or Replacement	TEER
Technical or anatomic			
Prior mediastinal radiation	Aorto-iliac occlusive disease precluding transfemoral approach	Prior sternotomy	Multivalve disease
Ascending aortic calcification (porcelain aorta may be prohibitive)	Aortic arch atherosclerosis (protuberant lesions)	Prior mediastinal radiation	Valve morphology (eg, thickening, perforations, clefts, calcification, and stenosis)
	Severe MR or TR	Ascending aortic calcification (porcelain aorta may be prohibitive)	Prior mitral valve surgery
	Low-lying coronary arteries		
	Basal septal hypertrophy		
	Valve morphology (eg, bicuspid or unicuspid valve)		
	Extensive LV outflow tract calcification		
Comorbidities			
Severe COPD or home oxygen therapy	Severe COPD or home oxygen therapy	Severe COPD or home oxygen therapy	Severe COPD or home oxygen therapy
Pulmonary hypertension	Pulmonary hypertension	Pulmonary hypertension	Pulmonary hypertension
Severe RV dysfunction	Severe RV dysfunction	Hepatic dysfunction	Hepatic dysfunction
Hepatic dysfunction	Hepatic dysfunction	Frailty[a]	Frailty[a]
Frailty[a]	Frailty[a]		
Futility			
STS score >15	STS score >15	STS score >15	STS score >15
Life expectancy <1 y	Life expectancy <1 y	Life expectancy <1 y	Life expectancy <1 y
Poor candidate for rehabilitation	Poor candidate for rehabilitation	Poor candidate for rehabilitation	Poor candidate for rehabilitation

[a]Validated frailty scores include the Katz activities of daily living score.[10]

Abbreviations: COPD, chronic obstructive pulmonary disease; MR, mitral regurgitation; RV, right ventricular; SAVR, surgical aortic valve replacement; STS, society of thoracic surgeons; TAVI, transcatheter aortic valve implantation; TEER, transcatheter edge-to-edge repair; TR, tricuspid regurgitation.

Table 2
Risk assessment combining clinical data, STS risk estimate, frailty, major organ system dysfunction, and procedure-specific impediments[1]

Step 1: Initial Assessment		
Valve related symptoms and severity	Symptoms	Intensity, acuity
	AS severity	Echocardiography and other imaging
Baseline clinical data	Cardiac history	Prior cardiac interventions
	Physical examination and laboratory results	Routine blood tests, pulmonary function tests
	Chest irradiation	Access issues other cardiac effects
	Dental evaluation	Treat dental issues before TAVR
	Allergies	Contrast, latex, medications
	Social support	Recovery, transportation, postdischarge planning
Major CV comorbidity	Coronary artery disease	Coronary angiography
	LV systolic dysfunction	LV ejection fraction
	Concurrent valve disease	Severe MR or MS
	Pulmonary hypertension	Assess pulmonary pressures
	Aortic disease	Porcelain aorta (CT scan)
	Chest or vascular access	Prohibitive reentry after previous open heart surgery (CT scan)
		Hostile chest
		Peripheral vascular disease
Major noncardiovascular comorbidity	Malignancy	Remote or active, life expectancy
	Gastrointestinal and liver disease, bleeding	IBD, cirrhosis, varices, GIB—ability to take antiplatelets/anticoagulation
	Kidney disease	eGFR < 30 mL/min/1.73 m² or dialysis
	Pulmonary disease	Oxygen requirement, FEV1 < 50% predicted or DLCO < 30% predicted
	Neurologic disorders	Movement disorders, dementia
Step 2: Functional Assessment		
Frailty and disability	Frailty assessment	Gait speed (>0.5 m/s or <0.83 m/s with disability/cognitive impairment)
	Nutritional risk/status	Frailty (not frail or frail by assessments)
		Nutritional risk status (BMI < 21 kg/m², albumin < 3.5 mg/dL, >10-lb weight loss in past year, or ≤11 on MNA)
Physical function	Physical function and endurance	6 min walk <50 m or unable to walk
	Independent living	Dependent in ≥1 activities
Cognitive function	Cognitive impairment	MMSE < 24 or dementia
	Depression	Depression history or positive screen
	Prior disabling stroke	
Futility	Life expectancy	<1 year of life expectancy
	Lag time to benefit	Survival with benefit of < 25% at 2 years
Step 3: Overall Procedural Risk		
Risk categories	Low risk	STS-PROM < 4% and
		No frailty and
		No comorbidity and
		No procedure-specific impediments
	Intermediate risk	STS-PROM 4%–8% or
		Mild frailty or
		1 major organ system compromise not to be improved postoperatively or
		A possible procedure-specific impediment
	High risk	STS-PROM > 8% or
		Moderate-severe frailty or
		>2 major organ system compromises not to be improved postoperatively or
		A possible procedure-specific impediment
	Prohibitive risk	PROM > 50% at 1 year or
		≥3 major organ system compromises not to be improved postoperatively or
		Severe frailty or
		Severe procedure specific impediments

Abbreviations: AS, aortic stenosis; DLCO, carbon dioxide diffusing capacity; eGFR, estimated glomerular filtration rate; FEV, forced expiratory volume; GIB, gastrointestinal bleeding; IBD, irritable bowel syndrome; MMSE, mini-mental status examination; MNA, mini nutritional assessment; MR, mitral regurgitation; MS, mitral stenosis; STS-PROM, Society of Thoracic Surgeons Predicted Risk of Mortality; TAVR, transcatheter aortic valve replacement.

Data from Otto CM, Kumbhani DJ, Alexander KP, et al. 2017 ACC expert consensus decision pathway for transcatheter aortic valve replacement in the management of adults with aortic stenosis: a report of the American College of Cardiology task force on Clinical Expert Consensus Documents. J Am Coll Cardiol 2017;69:1313-1346.

metabolic conditions, chest or mediastinal radiation, and subvalvular or supravalvular anatomic anomalies.[1] The aortic valve is typically comprises 3 leaflets; however, bicuspid aortic valve (BAV) disease is often associated with early onset AS. Calcific AS in trileaflet valves is rarely seen in patients prior to age 50 unless drug or radiation induced.

DIAGNOSIS AND CLASSIFICATION

Two-dimensional (2D) transthoracic echocardiography (TTE) is the gold-standard imaging modality and is recommended for initial assessment, ongoing valve surveillance, or the emergence of new symptoms or changes in physical examination in a patient with known AS.[1] Echocardiography visualizes the degree and distribution of valve calcification, which typically correlates to severity of the disease. Restricted opening of the aortic valve can be quantified by measuring the aortic valve area (AVA) and hemodynamic data including mean gradient and max velocity. The stages of AS range from "at risk" to "symptomatic severe AS" and are classified based on anatomy, hemodynamics, functionality of the left ventricle, and symptoms[2] (**Table 3**). Severe AS is classified as a mean gradient $\geq$ 40 mm Hg or maximum velocity (V_{max}) $\geq$ 4 m/s typically illustrating an AVA $\leq$ 1.0 cm^2. Low-flow, low-gradient aortic stenosis (LFLG AS) is observed in patients with a low stroke volume index of $\leq$35 mL/m^2 which results in a V_{max} less than 4.0 m/s but with an AVA less than 1.0 cm^2. The 2 main causes of LFLG AS are reduced left ventricular ejection fraction (LVEF) or a small left ventricular chamber.[1] LFLG AS in the setting of decreased LVEF can be further explored by low-dose dobutamine stress echocardiography (DSE). Paradoxic LFLG AS occurs with a discordance between gradients and valve area in the setting of preserved ejection fraction and is quite challenging to diagnose.[1] Computed tomography (CT) can be useful in quantification of aortic valve calcification (AVC) by applying the Agatston scoring method to assess disease severity when faced with low gradients by echocardiography. AVC values for severe AS are sex-specific: AVC greater than 1200 AU for women or greater than 2000 AU for men.[1] Artificial intelligence is an evolving tool to predict the rate of disease progression based on echocardiography and CT. Exercise stress testing can be useful to evaluate asymptomatic patients and is considered safe when supervised appropriately.[1] In a patient with known symptomatic, severe AS (stage D1) exercise stress testing is not recommended.[1] The diagnostic work-up for a patient with AS is guided by data collection and symptoms[1] (**Fig. 2**).

CLINICAL PRESENTATION

Symptoms attributed to AS tend to manifest once the degree of obstruction is significant, however, symptom onset is case dependent. The classic triad of symptoms includes dyspnea on exertion, angina, and syncope. Most commonly, the initial symptoms of decreased exercise tolerance and dyspnea on exertion are related to diastolic dysfunction and elevated left ventricular filling pressures.[1] The progression of AS is insidious, and at times elderly patients mistake diminished exercise tolerance, shortness of breath, and fatigue for normal signs of aging. A percentage of patients with severe AS are characterized as asymptomatic, however, 18% to 37% of this group of patients experience symptoms when performing exercise.[1] Obtaining an accurate history of functional changes over time is essential, and clinicians are urged to ask open-ended questions to illicit any symptoms of AS. Angina is the second most common symptom of patients with AS and typically stems from myocardial oxygen supply-demand mismatch.[1] Symptoms of angina must be explored to rule out concomitant coronary artery disease (CAD). Exertional dizziness or lightheadedness, near-syncope, or true syncope is the least common in the classic triad of symptoms. Syncope in patients with AS indicates significant valvular obstruction during increased demand resulting in reduced cardiac output. Other causes of near-syncopal symptoms in a patient with AS can include cardiac arrhythmias or a baroreceptor-mediated vasodilatory and bradycardic reflex during high LV wall stress.[1]

PHYSICAL EXAMINATION

Upon auscultation, a systolic ejection murmur secondary to turbulent flow across the narrowed aortic valve orifice is heard best at the right second intercostal space with

Table 3
Stages of aortic stenosis

Stage	Definition	Valve Anatomy	Valve Hemodynamics	Hemodynamic Consequences	Symptoms
A	At risk of AS	BAV (or other congenital valve anomaly) Aortic valve sclerosis	Aortic V_{max} <2 m/s with normal leaflet motion	None	None
B	Progressive AS	Mild to moderate leaflet calcification/fibrosis of a bicuspid or trileaflet valve with some reduction in systolic motion or Rheumatic valve changes with commissural fusion	Mild AS: aortic V_{max} 2.0–2.9 m/s or mean ΔP<20 mm Hg Moderate AS: aortic V_{max} 3.0–3.9 m/s or mean ΔP 20–39 mm Hg	Early LV diastolic dysfunction may be present Normal LVEF	None
C: Asymptomatic severe AS					
C1	Asymptomatic severe AS	Severe leaflet calcification/ fibrosis or congenital stenosis with severely reduced leaflet opening	Aortic V_{max} ≥4 m/s or mean ΔP≥40 mm Hg AVA typically is ≤1.0 cm² (or AVAi 0.6 cm²/m²) but not required to define severe AS Very severe AS is an aortic V_{max} ≥5 m/s or mean P ≥60 mm Hg	LV diastolic dysfunction Mild LV hypertrophy Normal LVEF	None Exercise testing is reasonable to confirm symptom status
C2	Asymptomatic severe AS with LV systolic dysfunction	Severe leaflet calcification/ fibrosis or congenital stenosis with severely reduced leaflet opening	Aortic V_{max} ≥4 m/s or mean ΔP≥40 mm Hg AVA typically ≤1.0 cm² (or AVAi 0.6 cm²/m²) but not required to define severe AS	LVEF <50%	None
D. Symptomatic severe AS					
D1	Symptomatic severe high-gradient AS	Severe leaflet calcification/ fibrosis or congenital stenosis with severely reduced leaflet opening	Aortic V_{max} ≥4 m/s or mean ΔP≥40 mm Hg AVA typically ≤1.0 cm² (or AVAi ≤0.6 cm²/m²) but may be larger with mixed AS/AR	LV diastolic dysfunction LV hypertrophy Pulmonary hypertension may be present	Exertional dyspnea, decreased exercise tolerance, or HF Exertional angina Exertional syncope or presyncope
D2	Symptomatic severe low-flow, low-gradient AS with reduced LVEF	Severe leaflet calcification/ fibrosis with severely reduced leaflet motion	AVA ≤1.0 cm² with resting aortic V_{max} <4 m/s or mean ΔP<40 mm Hg Dobutamine stress echocardiography shows AVA <1.0 cm² with V_{max} ≥4 m/s at any flow rate	LV diastolic dysfunction LV hypertrophy LVEF <50%	HF Angina Syncope or presyncope
D3	Symptomatic severe low-gradient AS with normal LVEF or paradoxical low-flow severe AS	Severe leaflet calcification/ fibrosis with severely reduced leaflet motion	AVA ≤1.0 cm² (indexed AVA ≤0.6 cm²/m²) with an aortic V_{max} <4 m/s or mean ΔP<40 mm Hg and Stroke volume index <35 mL/m² Measured when patient is normotensive (systolic blood pressure <140 mm Hg)	Increased LV relative wall thickness Small LV chamber with low stroke volume Restrictive diastolic filling LVEF ≥50%	HF Angina Syncope or presyncope

Abbreviations: ΔP, pressure gradient between the LV and aorta; AR, aortic regurgitation; AS, aortic stenosis; AVA, aortic valve area circulation; AVAi, AVA indexed to body surface area; BAV, bicuspid aortic valve; HF, heart failure; LV, left ventricular; LVEF, left ventricular ejection fraction; V_{max}, maximum velocity.

(Otto CM, Nishimura RA, Bonow RO, et al. 2020 ACC/AHA Guideline for the Management of Patients With Valvular Heart Disease: A Report of the American College of Cardiology/American Heart Association Joint Committee on Clinical Practice Guidelines. J Am Coll Cardiol 2021;77(4):e25-e197. https://doi.org/10.1016/j.jacc.2020.11.018. With permission from Elsevier Inc.)

radiation to the right clavicular area and carotid artery.[1] The volume of the murmur is not indicative of disease severity and varies based on body habitus.[1] The carotid arterial pulse is an important feature of the physical examination as the obstruction secondary to AS produces a weak and slowly rising carotid pulse (pulsus parvus et tardus).[1]

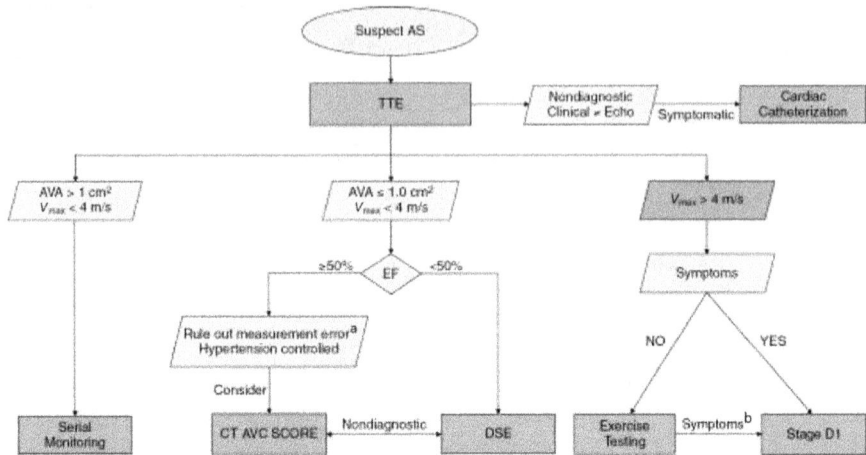

Fig. 2. Flowchart of the diagnostic workup for AS.[1] [b]Symptoms with exercise testing are defined as angina, syncope, and dyspnea.

CLINICAL COURSE

Patients can develop HF as a result of LV pressure overload and ensuing dysfunction. The LV ejection fraction tends to remain preserved until late in the disease process, however, the combination of diastolic dysfunction and elevated filling pressures can lead to symptoms of fatigue, shortness of breath, exertional dyspnea, and diminished exercise capacity.[1] Atrial fibrillation (AF) occurs commonly in patients with AS and appears more often as the disease progresses. Gastrointestinal bleeding (ie, Heyde syndrome) is observed in 1% to 3% of adults with AS.[1] This phenomenon is due to angiodysplastic vessels in the GI tract and promotes an acquired von Willebrand factor (VWF) deficiency.[1] Aortic valve replacement (AVR) restores VWF activity and typically improves clinical status. An asymptomatic patient with severe AS has a less than 1% risk of sudden death per year; however, once a patient develops symptoms the risk increases to nearly 2% per month.[1] The rates of sudden death without preceding symptoms is highest in patients with very severe AS ($V_{max} \geq 5.0$ m/s or mean gradient ≥ 60 mm Hg).[1] Sudden cardiac death in the setting of AS is potentially due to ventricular arrhythmia.[1]

TIMING OF INTERVENTION AND TREATMENT OPTIONS

It is a class I recommendation that patients with severe, symptomatic AS undergo AVR and management of comorbid conditions[2] (**Fig. 3**).[1] The timing of intervention depends on the classification of AS, symptoms, and impact on left ventricle[2] (**Fig. 4**). Surgical aortic valve replacement was the long-standing gold-standard treatment until the advent of transcatheter aortic valve replacement (TAVR). Through the course of the PARTNER randomized clinical trials (RCTs), the FDA in the United States has approved TAVR for patients of all-risk stratification who meet anatomic criteria for technical feasibility. TAVR is a fully percutaneous procedure in which a transcatheter valve is deployed into the diseased aortic valve with catheters, most commonly through a transfemoral approach. The diseased aortic valve is not removed during TAVR, but a new bioprosthetic valve is placed inside. TAVR is a minimally invasive therapy that does not require cardiopulmonary bypass. TAVR is not appropriate for

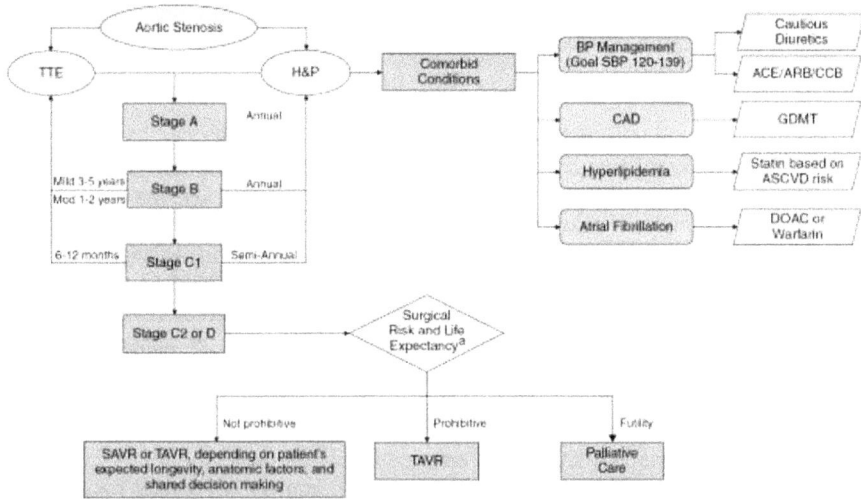

Fig. 3. Management of a patient with AS.[1] [a]Surgical risk includes an assessment which includes the Society of Thoracic Surgery (STS) predicted risk of mortality, frailty, anatomic considerations, and consideration of comorbidities. [b]Strength of recommendations in the AHA/ACC 2017 focused update of valvular guidelines.

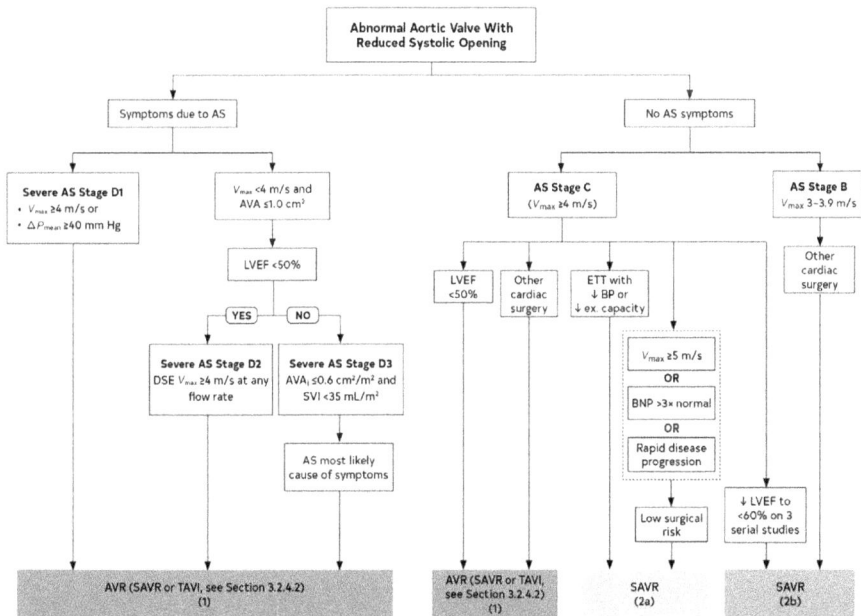

Fig. 4. Timing of intervention for AS. (Otto CM, Nishimura RA, Bonow RO, et al. 2020 ACC/AHA Guideline for the Management of Patients With Valvular Heart Disease: A Report of the American College of Cardiology/American Heart Association Joint Committee on Clinical Practice Guidelines. CirculationJ Am Coll Cardiol 2021;7 (4):e25-e197. https://doi.org/10.1016/j.jacc.2020.11.018. With permission from Elsevier Inc.)

patients with significant aortopathy, concomitant CAD or VHD, concerning calcium distribution in the aortic annulus, or futility.

AORTIC REGURGITATION
Background

Aortic regurgitation (AR), or aortic insufficiency, is the reflux of blood during diastole from the aorta back into the left ventricle. The prevalence of AR was estimated at 4.9% in the Framingham study and slightly more prevalent in men.[6] However, recent large-scale, community-based studies report 15% to 67.5% of adult patients 65 years of age or greater demonstrate $\geq$ mild AR and of these 1.6% to 15% are estimated to exhibit clinically significant AR (3+ or greater).[7] AR can be caused by congenital or acquired abnormalities of the aortic valve leaflets, aortic root, or ascending aorta[1] (**Table 4**). Abnormalities of the aortic valve causing AR most commonly include congenital bicuspid valve morphology, RhD, infective endocarditis, calcific degeneration, and myxomatous degeneration.[1] AR is most commonly due to chronic degenerative disease and almost 50% of these patients are found to have congenital abnormalities such as BAV,[7] which is the most common congenital heart defect observed globally.[8] There is a high correlation between BAV and associated aortopathy, which can result in aortic dilation and increased risk of aortic dissection alongside worsening AR.[6] Patients can exhibit a diseased and dilated aorta secondary to genetic disorders such as Marfan syndrome, idiopathic annuloaortic ectasia, or degenerative aneurysms.[1] During dilation of the ascending aorta and aortic root, the aortic annulus expands, which results in failure of aortic leaflet apposition and central AR.[6] In developed countries, congenital BAV and degenerative calcific AV leaflet are the most common causes of AR while in developing countries RhD remains the most common cause.[6] In RhD, fibrous tissue infiltrates the aortic cusps causing inleaflet retraction and inability for proper leaflet coaptation resulting in central AR.[6]

DIAGNOSIS AND CLASSIFICATION

AR can be classified as either acute or chronic. Severe, acute AR is often associated with dramatic hemodynamic compromise due to acute volume overload into a

---

Table 4
Causes of aortic regurgitation[1]

Leaflet abnormalities	Rheumatic disease
	Aortic valve sclerosis and calcification
	Congenital abnormalities (bicuspid, unicuspid, and quadricuspid valves; and aortic regurgitation associated with discrete subaortic stenosis and ventricular septal defect)
	Infective endocarditis
	Myxomatous valve disease
	Complicating balloon valvuloplasty and transcatheter aortic valve implantation
	Rare causes (drugs, leaflet fenestration, irradiation, nonbacterial endocarditis, trauma)
Aortic root abnormalities	Chronic hypertension
	Marfan syndrome
	Annulo-aortic ectasia
	Aortic dissection
	Ehlers-Danlos syndrome
	Osteogenesis imperfecta
	Atherosclerotic aneurysm
	Syphilitic aortitis
	Other systemic inflammatory disorders (giant cell aortitis, Takayasu disease, Reiter syndrome)
Combined valve and aortic root abnormalities	Bicuspid aortic valve
	Ankylosing spondylitis

Table 5
Severity grades of aortic regurgitation[1]

Parameters	Mild	Moderate	Severe
Qualitative			
Aortic valve morphology	Normal/abnormal	Normal/abnormal	Abnormal/flail/large coaptation defect
Color flow AR jet width[a]	Small in central jets	Intermediate	Large in central jet, varied eccentric jets
CW signal of AR jet	Incomplete/faint	Dense	Dense
Diastolic flow reversal in the descending aorta	Brief, protodiastolic flow reversal	Intermediate	Holodiastolic flow reversal (end-diastolic velocity >20 cm/s)
Diastolic flow reversal in the abdominal aorta	Absent	Absent	Present
Semiquantitative			
VC width (mm)	<3	Intermediate	≥6
Pressure half-time (ms)[b]	>500	Intermediate	<200
Quantitative			
EROA (mm²)	<10	10–19, 20–29[d]	≥30
RVol (mL)	<30	30–44, 45–59[d]	>60
+LV size[c]			

[a]At a Nyquist limit of 50–60 cm/s.
[b]Pressure half-time is shortened with increasing LV diastolic pressure, vasodilator therapy, and in patients with a dilated, compliant aorta or lengthened in chronic AR.
[c]Unless for other reasons, the LV size is usually normal in patients with mild AR. In acute severe AR, the LV size is often normal. Accepted cutoff values for nonsignificant LV enlargement: LV end-diastolic diameter < 56 mm, LV end-diastolic volume < 82 mL/m², LV end-systolic diameter < 40 mm, LV end-systolic volume < 30 mL/m².
[d]Grading of the severity of AR classifies regurgitation as mild, moderate, or severe and subclassifies the moderate regurgitations group as mild to moderate (EROA = 10–19 mm or an RVol of 20–44 mL) and moderate to severe (EROA = 20–29 mm² or an RVol of 45–59 mL).
Abbreviations: AR, aortic regurgitation; CW, continuous wave; EROA, effective regurgitant office area; LA, left atrium; LV, left ventricle; RVol, regurgitant volume; VC, vena contracta.
From Lancellotti P, Tribouilloy C, Hagendroff A, et al, Recommendations for the echocardiographic assessment of native valvular regurgitation; an executive summary from the European Association of cardiovascular imaging. Eur Heart J Cardiovasc Imaging 2013;14:611-644

noncompliant LV. In this situation, the LV end diastolic pressure (LVEDP) and filling pressures increase rapidly above the left atrial pressure, which results in premature closure of the mitral valve in diastole.[6] This cascade produces severe MR, an increase in pulmonary venous pressure, limited stroke volume, and decreased cardiac output, which presents as respiratory failure and cardiogenic shock.[6] Chronic AR is more common, and due to the slow progression of the disease, the LV remodels over time with increased wall tension, hypertrophy, and dilation.[6] Left untreated, the LV systolic function decreases, and irreversible remodeling occurs.

The imaging modality initially utilized to assess AR is TTE, which encompasses multiple methods to assess AR severity (**Table 5**). No single echocardiographic method is superior, and a combination of modalities for an integrated approach to imaging is recommended.[7] Cardiac magnetic resonance (CMR) is growing in clinical practice as an adjunct to echocardiography. The American College of Cardiology/American Heart Association and European Society of Cardiology/European Association of Cardio-Thoracic Surgery guidelines recommend conducting CMR when the degree of AR is indeterminate or to provide further insight into mechanism of failure, degree of regurgitant volume/fraction, aortic valve morphology, LV volume and systolic function.[2] CMR provides left ventricular volumetric assessment, which can reveal early LV dysfunction and remodeling not detected by echocardiography's longitudinal assessment.

CLINICAL PRESENTATION

Most commonly, patients initially complain of dyspnea on exertion in the setting of AR likely related to exercise-induced elevated LVEDP.[1] Chronic AR is insidious, and patients who experience a gradual reduction in exercise tolerance or capacity could attribute this to "normal signs of aging" or other comorbidities. Exercise testing may be useful in an asymptomatic patient to illicit symptoms and assess exercise capacity. Systolic HF may be the initial symptom in severe AR secondary to LV dilation and dysfunction. Patients may experience anginal symptoms even in the absence of CAD related to lower myocardial perfusion pressure, increased myocardial oxygen demand, and a decreased ratio of coronary artery size to myocardial mass.[1] Interestingly, patients may have an initial complaint of feeling their heart beat forcefully or palpitations, both of which can be related to increased pulse pressure.

PHYSICAL EXAMINATION

Patients with mild or moderate AR will likely present with a diastolic murmur on examination, which is high-frequency and begins immediately following S2 and continues to S1 while decreasing in intensity.[1] Unfortunately, the diastolic murmur has a high likelihood of going unnoticed on auscultation. For example, compared with Doppler echocardiography or aortic angiography, the sensitivity for detecting the diastolic AR murmur is 37% to 73%.[1] The loudness and duration of the murmur tends to correlate to some degree of AR severity.[1] During blood pressure measurement, there is a widened pulse pressure that can be observed in the setting of AR. One may also note a bounding carotid pulse, which manifests peripherally in a "water hammer pulse" or "Corrigan pulse"[1] (**Table 6**). In the case of LV dilation, the apex point of maximal impulse may be laterally displaced to palpation.

CLINICAL COURSE

The severity of AR and the patient's clinical course correlates to the degree of LV dilation.[7] For example, it is not uncommon for a patient to remain asymptomatic if the LVEF remains preserved. Medical management of these patients is recommended

Table 6 Peripheral signs of chronic severe aortic regurgitation[6]	
Physical signs	Description of physical findings
Becker sign	Arterial pulsations visible in the retinal arteries and pupils
de Musset sign	Head bob with each heartbeat
Duroziez sign	Systolic murmur over the femoral artery when compressed proximally and diastolic murmur when compressed distally
Müller sign	Systolic pulsation of the uvula
Quincke sign	Visible capillary pulsation detected at the tip of a fingernail
Traube sign	Pistol shot sounds heard over the femoral arteries in both systole and diastole
Water hammer or Corrigan pulse	Rapid upstroke followed by quick collapse of arterial pulse

Source Griffin B. Valvular heart disease. In: Griffin BP, Callahan TD, Menon V, editors. 4th edition. Manual of Cardiovascular Medicine, vol 1. Philadelphia, PA: Lippincott Williams & Wilkins; 2013. p. 238-355. Accessed 4.08.17.

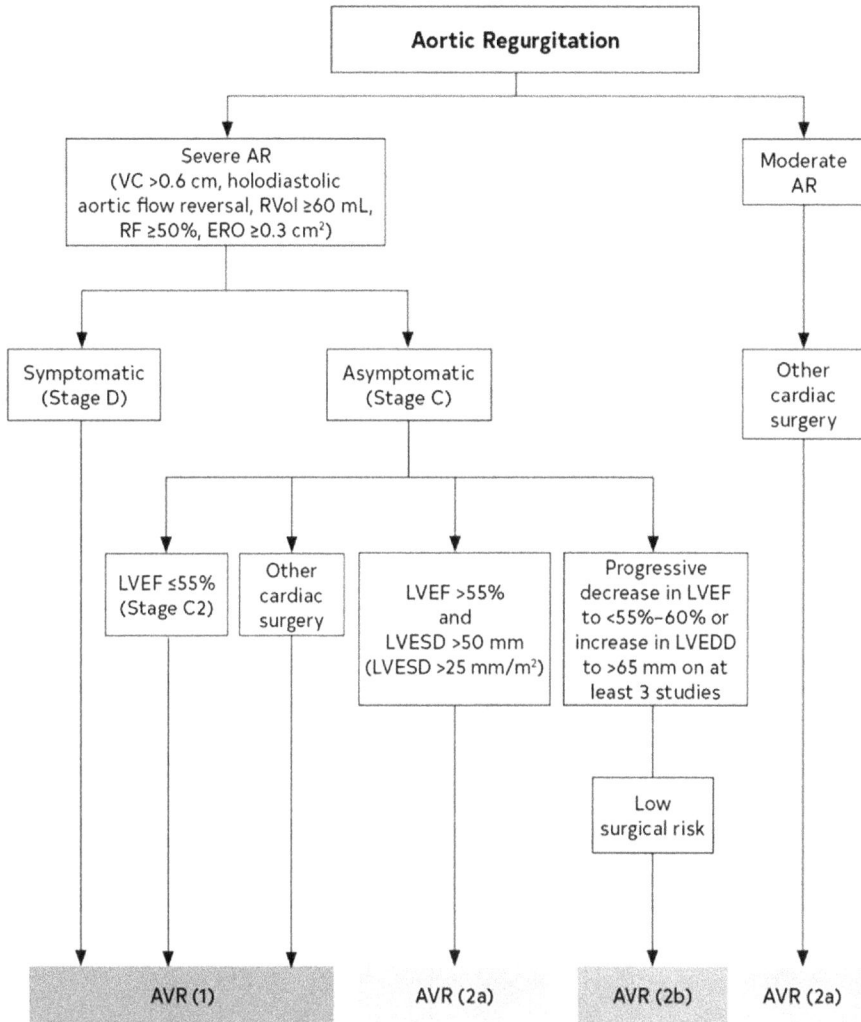

Fig. 5. Timing of intervention for AR. (Otto CM, Nishimura RA, Bonow RO, et al. 2020 ACC/ AHA Guideline for the Management of Patients With Valvular Heart Disease: A Report of the American College of Cardiology/American Heart Association Joint Committee on Clinical Practice Guidelines. CirculationJ Am Coll Cardiol 2021;7 (4):e25-e197. https://doi.org/10. 1016/j.jacc.2020.11.018. With permission from Elsevier Inc.)

with close monitoring of symptoms to identify the optimal timing for intervention to prevent LV remodeling. There is no evidence that vasodilating drugs reduce severity of AR, however, goal-directed medical therapy (GDMT) for hypertension and HF are beneficial for patients with AR even if asymptomatic.[2] As the LV dilates, patients begin to experience a decrease in exercise capacity and functional status.

TIMING OF INTERVENTION AND TREATMENT OPTIONS

Timing of intervention for AR depends on severity, symptoms, and the need for other types of cardiac surgery.[2] Once chronic AR is verified as severe, symptom onset is the indication for treatment.[1] An asymptomatic patient who demonstrates a struggling LVEF less than 50% and/or LV end-systolic diameter greater than 50 mm is recommended for treatment to avoid further LV damage and remodeling[2] (**Fig. 5**). Open heart surgery is the gold standard for treating AR. A technically conservative approach including valve-sparing operations and aortic cusp repair should be considered.[1] Surgical management of AR typically requires AVR, however, in surgical centers of excellence some patients may be candidates for aortic valve repair depending on anatomy and other factors.[1] In the United States, AR accounts for over 50% of AVRs.[6] Age, lifestyle, comorbidities, potential pregnancy, and aortopathy are a few considerations when discussing treatment options. Patients with AR and congenital BAV are often quite young, therefore, specific attention is paid to the lifelong management plan. Mechanical valves require only one intervention in a patient's lifetime, however, the patient must commit to lifelong oral anticoagulation with warfarin and strict INR monitoring. Bioprosthetic valves become degenerative over time and will require multiple interventions. Commercially available TAVR devices are currently not approved or appropriate to treat AR.[9] There is need for dedicated transcatheter devices to percutaneously treat AR, and presently there are a few TAVR devices at various stages of clinical research trials in this arena.

THE MITRAL VALVE
Mitral Regurgitation

Background
MR occurs when the mitral valve fails to close completely and allows blood to move backward into the left atrium. MR is the most common form of VHD and the incidence increases each decade to greater than 9% after 75 years of age.[1] MR is classified as either primary (degenerative) or secondary (functional) (**Fig. 6**). Primary MR is due to an abnormality within the mitral valve apparatus and might include the valve leaflets, subvalvular apparatus, chordae, or papillary muscles.[1] For example, mitral valve prolapse results from excessive systolic movement of a leaflet beyond

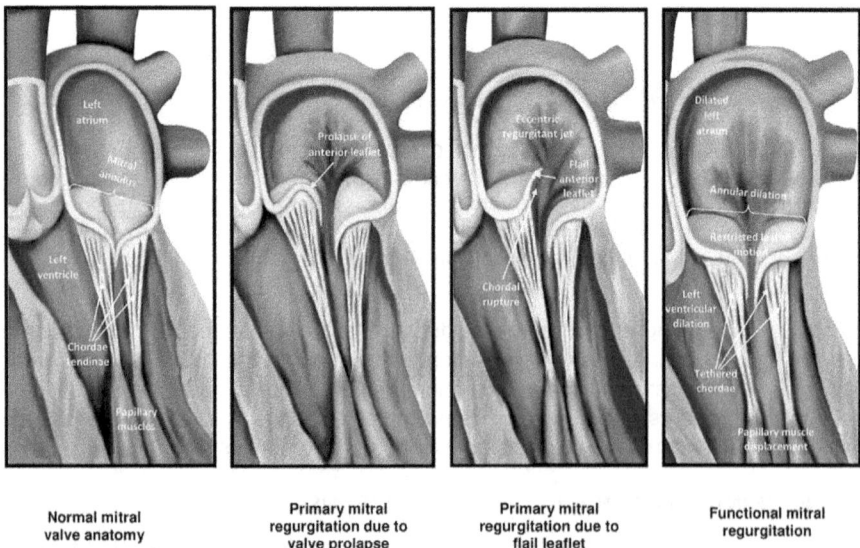

| Normal mitral valve anatomy | Primary mitral regurgitation due to valve prolapse | Primary mitral regurgitation due to flail leaflet | Functional mitral regurgitation |

Fig. 6. Mitral valve apparatus and etiologies for MR.[10]

the annulus due to an elongated chorda and/or leaflet.[1] Flail mitral valve leaflets are typically caused decision tree for distinguishing primary from secondary MR by rupture of the chordae with complete failure of leaflet coaptation due to abnormal movement of the leaflet tip into the left atrium.[1] Myxomatous disease of the mitral valve leaflets results in leaflet thickening and elongated chordae such as seen in Barlow's disease.[1] Secondary MR is due to left ventricular remodeling due to ischemic heart disease or dilated cardiomyopathy. Due to LV dilation, the mitral annulus expands, resulting in incomplete coaptation of the mitral leaflets. A new classification of *atrial functional MR* is applied to patients with isolated AF in the presence of normal mitral valve morphology and preserved LV anatomy/function.[10] Atrial functional MR is attributed to dilation of the left atrium, which in turn dilates the mitral annulus leading to mitral leaflet malcoaptation.[10] To distinguish between primary and secondary MR, the mitral valve morphology, LV size/function, and LA size must be investigated closely[11] (**Fig. 7**). Prevalence of significant primary MR is estimated to be 2.4% in the general population based on Framingham data, but prevalence of any degree of MR in the Oxvalve study from the United Kingdom was noted to be 20.1%.[1]

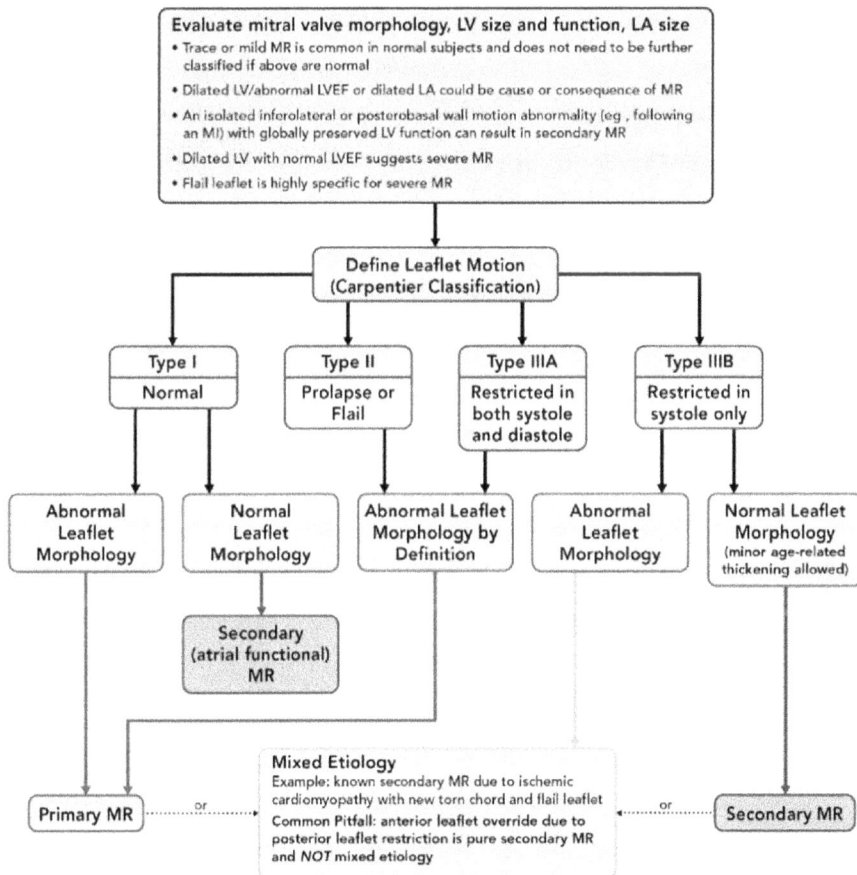

Fig. 7. Decision tree for distinguishing primary from secondary MR.[11] LA, left article; LV, left ventricle; LVEF, left ventricle ejection fraction; MR, mitral regurgitation.

DIAGNOSIS AND CLASSIFICATION

Acute MR refers to a sudden and severe backflow of blood through the mitral valve during systole. Etiology of acute MR includes myocardial infarction affecting the papillary muscles or chordae tendineae, infective endocarditis, or trauma.[1] Chronic MR refers to a long-standing abnormal backflow of blood from the left ventricle into the left atrium during systole due to a structural abnormality of the mitral valve apparatus or dysfunction of the left ventricle. Transthoracic and transesophageal echocardiography remains the cornerstones for diagnosing and quantifying MR. The stages of MR are defined by measuring valve hemodynamics and assessing patient symptoms and range from "at risk for MR" to "symptomatic severe MR" as illustrated in this table (Table 7). Classification of chronic MR considers the severity of regurgitation based on echocardiographic parameters such as regurgitant volume, effective regurgitant orifice area, and vena contracta width.

Table 7
Stages of mitral regurgitation in chronic primary and secondary mitral regurgitation[10]

Grade	Definition	Valve hemodynamics	Symptoms
A	At risk for MR	• No jet or small central jet area < 20% LA • VC < 0.3 cm	None
B	Progressive MR	• Central jet MR 20–40% LA or late systolic eccentric jet MR • VC < 0.7 cm • Rvol < 60 mL • RF < 50% • ERO < 0.4 cm^2 • Angiographic grade 1 to 2+	None
C	Asymptomatic severe MR	• Central jet MR >40% LA or holosystolic eccentric jet MR • VC ≥0.7 cm • Rvol ≥60 mL • RF ≥50% • ERO ≥0.4 cm^2 • Angiographic grade 3 to 4+	None
D	Symptomatic severe MR	• Central jet MR >40% LA or holosystolic eccentric jet MR • VC ≥0.7 cm • Rvol ≥60 mL • RF ≥50% • ERO ≥0.4 cm^2 • Angiographic grade 3 to 4+	Decreased exercise tolerance Exertional dyspnea

Abbreviations: ERO, effective orifice area; LA, left atrium; MR, mitral regurgitation; Rvol, regurgitant volume; RF, regurgitant fraction; VC, vena contracta.

CLINICAL PRESENTATION

Acute MR results in abrupt and significant left atrial and LV volume overload. Sudden increase of volume into a noncompliant left atrium results in the elevation of left atrial and pulmonary venous pressures, causing acute pulmonary edema.[10] In acute MR, patients may present with sudden onset dyspnea, chest pain, and hemodynamic instability. Chronic MR typically presents with symptoms such as dyspnea, fatigue, and palpitations, often exacerbated by physical activity. Patients may also report orthopnea, paroxysmal nocturnal dyspnea, and additional signs of HF such as peripheral edema and jugular venous distension.[1]

Physical Examination

A patient experiencing acute MR may display tachycardia, hypotension, and signs of poor organ perfusion. Auscultation of the heart may reveal a loud holosystolic murmur best heard at the apex, radiating to the axilla. In severe cases, a third heart sound (S3) indicative of rapid ventricular filling may also be present. Pulmonary auscultation may reveal crackles indicative of pulmonary congestion. Physical examination findings may vary depending on the severity and duration of MR. Auscultation typically reveals a pansystolic murmur at the apex, often radiating to the axilla. The murmur may be softer in chronic MR compared with acute MR. In both acute and chronic MR, signs of left-sided HF may be present. Additional findings may include hepatojugular reflux and pulsatile liver indicative of right-sided congestion in advanced stages.[1]

CLINICAL COURSE

Untreated severe MR, irrespective of etiology, carries a poor prognosis with decreased survival and diminished quality of life[10] (**Box 1**). Without intervention, primary MR can lead to complications such as AF, pulmonary hypertension, and left ventricular dysfunction.[1] Patients with severe functional MR who experience worse outcomes include symptoms of HF, new-onset AF, right ventricular dysfunction, severe tricuspid regurgitation (TR), and specific echocardiographic parameters.[10] The clinical course of secondary MR is often intertwined with the progression of the underlying cardiac condition. Both primary and secondary MRs require careful monitoring and management to mitigate symptoms, slow disease progression, and prevent complications. The clinical course for all patients with MR underscores the importance of timely diagnosis, risk stratification, and multidisciplinary management to optimize clinical outcomes and quality of life.

Box 1
Factors associated with worse outcomes with significant mitral regurgitation[10]

- Development of heart failure symptoms (Survival worse in NYHA functional class III/IV)
- New atrial fibrillation
- Right ventricular dysfunction[a]
- Severe tricuspid regurgitation[a]
- Functional etiology
- Echocardiographic parameters
  - Effective regurgitant orifice area $\geq$40 mm^2 (primary MR)
  - Effective regurgitant orifice area $\geq$20 mm^2 (secondary MR)
  - LV ejection fraction <60% (LV systolic dysfunction)

[a]When studied with functional mitral regurgitation.

TIMING OF INTERVENTION AND TREATMENT OPTIONS

Prompt surgery is recommended for all patients who present with acute, severe, symptomatic MR. Vasodilator therapies and percutaneous hemodynamic support devices (ie, intra-aortic balloon pump or Impella left-ventricular assist device) can be used to augment cardiac output to support and stabilize the patient awaiting intervention.[10] Technically challenging, mitral valve repair is preferred over valve replacement to treat acute MR. Treatment strategies for both primary and secondary chronic MR include medical therapy to alleviate symptoms and optimize cardiac function, as well as surgical interventions. GDMT is recommended in patients with MR and hypertension or HF.[10] Cardiac resynchronization therapy, titration of GDMT by a HF specialist, and revascularization of significant CAD is also recommended for patients with secondary MR. Surgical therapy is the treatment of choice for primary MR in a timely manner to ideally avoid LV involvement and decompensation (**Fig. 8**). There is elevated morbidity and mortality due to recurrent HF if intervention is delayed to the point the patient has already decompensated.[10] High risk markers in chronic MR include reduced LVEF less than 60% or LV dilation to LVESD greater than 40 mm and intervention should take place before this point (**Fig. 9**).[10] Mitral transcatheter edge-to-edge repair (TEER) is indicated for both primary and secondary MR in high or prohibitive risk patients who remain symptomatic despite GDMT (**Fig. 10**). In RCTs in a functional MR population, TEER with the MitraClip device was shown to reduce HF hospitalizations

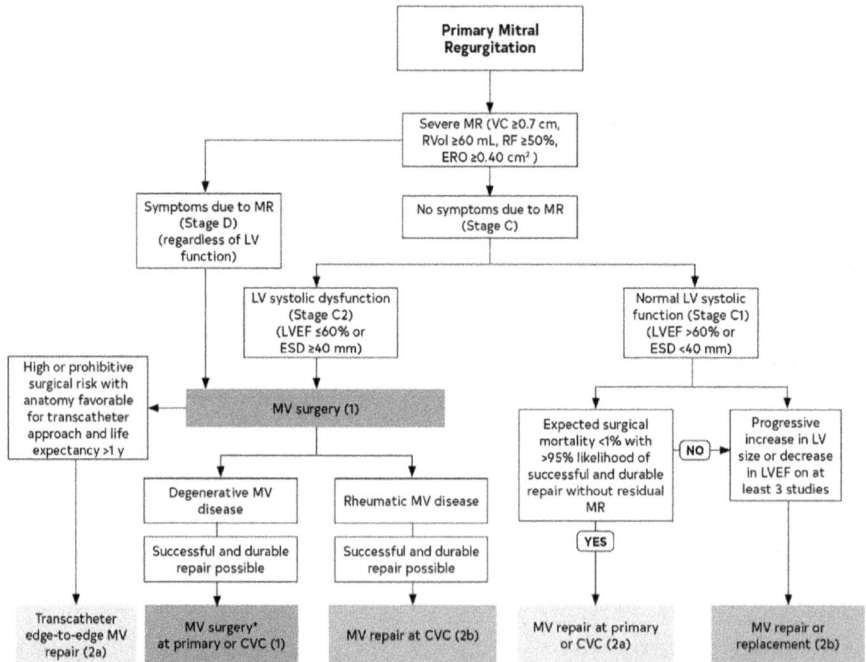

Fig. 8. Primary MR treatment algorithm. (Otto CM, Nishimura RA, Bonow RO, et al. 2020 ACC/AHA Guideline for the Management of Patients With Valvular Heart Disease: A Report of the American College of Cardiology/American Heart Association Joint Committee on Clinical Practice Guidelines. CirculationJ Am Coll Cardiol 2021;7 (4):e25-e197. https://doi.org/10.1016/j.jacc.2020.11.018. With permission from Elsevier Inc.)

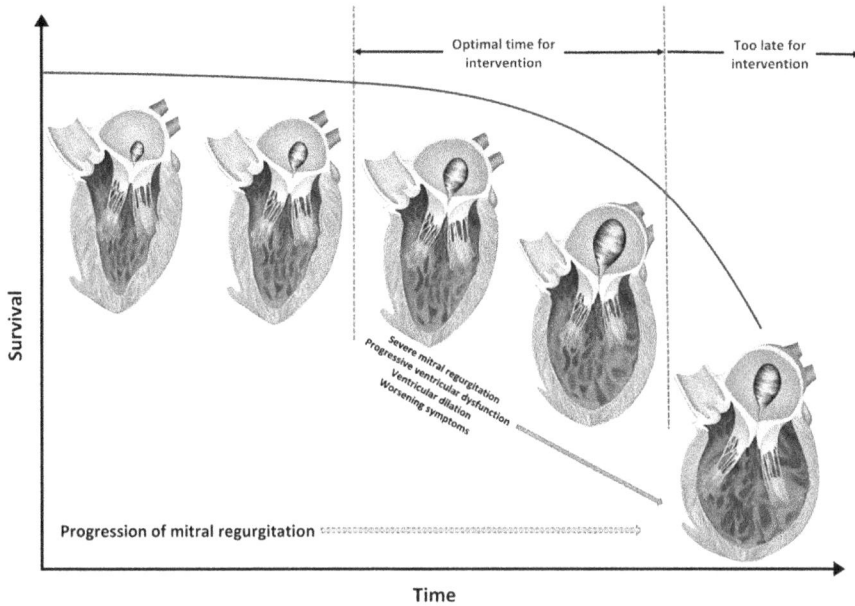

Fig. 9. Optimal timing for mitral valve intervention in functional MR.[10]

and mortality for patients with LVEF between 20% and 50% as well as increased quality of life.[1] Transcatheter mitral valve replacement (TMVR) is a rapidly evolving strategy for patients with MR and is being explored via clinical research trials in the United States.

MITRAL STENOSIS
Background

Mitral stenosis (MS) is characterized by narrowing of the mitral valve orifice restricting blood flow from the left atrium into the left ventricle leading to impaired hemodynamics and increased pressure within the left atrium. Rheumatic fever is the primary cause of MS worldwide and is underdiagnosed in developing countries.[1] In developed countries, MS is the least common left-sided native valve disease.[1] MS typically presents in patients between age 20 and 50 in developing countries.[1] In contrast, rheumatic MS usually manifests after the age of 50 in developed countries.[1] Anatomically, rheumatic MS is associated with commissural fusion and posterior mitral leaflet thickening.[1] Other causes of MS are rare and include congenital MS, inflammatory diseases, infiltrative diseases, carcinoid heart disease, and drug-induced valve disease but commissural fusion is less often seen in these cases.[1]

Diagnosis and Classification

Echocardiography remains the gold standard for confirming the diagnosis and determining severity of MS and guiding treatment. In assessing patients with MS, planimetry using bidimensional echocardiography is the preferred method to measure the mitral valve area (MVA).[1] In addition to MVA, the mean mitral valve gradient and pulmonary artery pressure both at rest and during exercise, are used to determine severity of MS (**Table 8**).

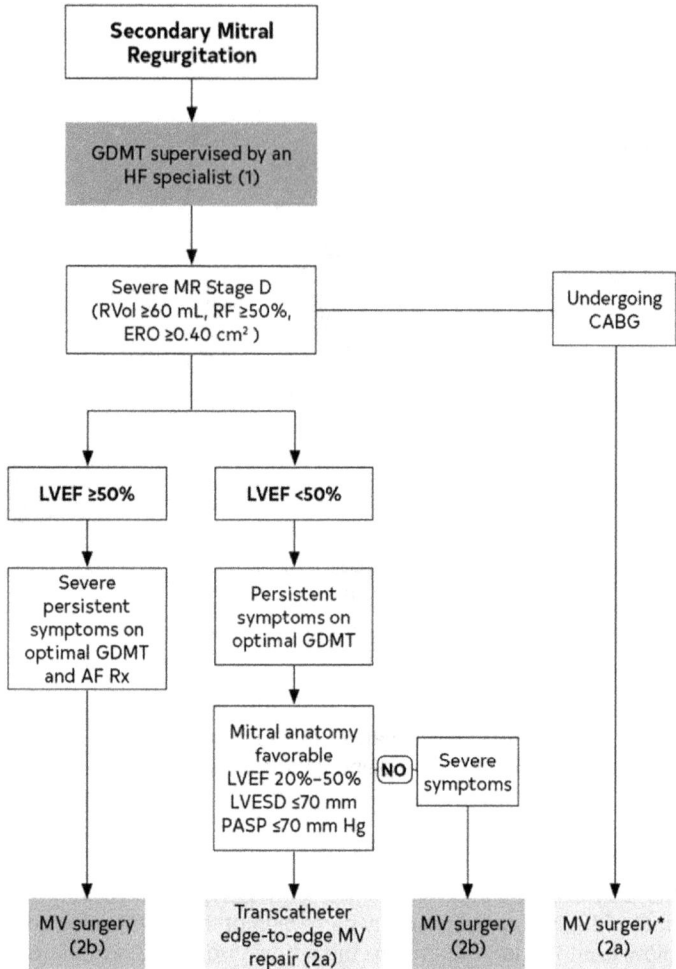

Fig. 10. Secondary MR treatment algorithm. The asterisk refers to chordal-sparing MV replacement may be reasonable to choose over downsized annuloplasty repair. (Otto CM, Nishimura RA, Bonow RO, et al. 2020 ACC/AHA Guideline for the Management of Patients With Valvular Heart Disease: A Report of the American College of Cardiology/American Heart Association Joint Committee on Clinical Practice Guidelines. CirculationJ Am Coll Cardiol 2021;7 (4):e25-e197. https://doi.org/10.1016/j.jacc.2020.11.018. With permission from Elsevier Inc.)

Clinical Presentation

The most common symptoms of MS are dyspnea and fatigue, both of which can be exacerbated by AF if and when present. Shortness of breath can be difficult to assess given the slowly progressive course of the disease. The presence of AF or an embolic event may reveal MS in previously asymptomatic patients. Women can be diagnosed with MS during pregnancy due to the demand for increased cardiac output.

Physical Examination

Upon auscultation, a loud S1 and opening snap in early diastole is heard followed by a holodiastolic rumbling murmur.[1] The murmur of MS can be difficult to detect, however,

Table 8
Echocardiographic assessment of the severity of mitral stenosis and alternative methods[1]

Measurement	Method	Advantages	Disadvantages	Alternative Methods
Valve area (cm²)	Planimetry on 2D/3D parasternal short-axis view	Direct measurement, independent of flow conditions; reference method for rheumatic MS	Experience required; not feasible if there is severe valve deformity or a poor acoustic window	MSCT, CMR, Gorlin formula
	Pressure half-time using CW Doppler	Easy to obtain	Dependence on other factors (regurgitations, chamber compliance, diastolic function)	—
	Continuity equation	Independent of flow conditions; recommended for calcific MS	Errors of measurement (multiple variables); not valid in cases of significant regurgitation	—
	Proximal isovelocity surface	Independent of flow conditions	Technically difficult	—
Mean mitral gradient (mm Hg)	CW Doppler on mitral flow	Easy to obtain	Depends on heart rate and flow conditions	Right + left catheterization
Pulmonary artery pressure (mm Hg)	CW Doppler on tricuspid regurgitant flow	Easy to obtain in cases of tricuspid regurgitation	Arbitrary estimation of right atrial pressure; no estimation of pulmonary vascular resistance	Right catheterization (reference measurement)
Mean gradient and pulmonary artery pressure at exercise (mm Hg)	CW Doppler of mitral and tricuspid regurgitant flow	Objective assessment of exercise tolerance	Lack of validation for decision making	—

Abbreviations: CMR, cardiac magnetic resonance; MS, mitral stenosis; MSCT, multislice computed tomography.

a loud murmur with a thrill suggests severe MS. A holosystolic murmur heard best at the apex and physical examination findings of left-sided HF can be seen. Signs of right HF can be observed in patients who have had long standing, severe MS.

Clinical Course

MS progresses slowly. The prognosis for a symptomatic patient with MS is poor with one study reporting only a 44% survival rate at 5 years for patients without intervention.[1] Asymptomatic patients have a 10-year survival rate greater than 80%, however, one-half of this group becomes symptomatic after 10 years. The leading causes of death for patients with MS are HF or thromboembolic events.[1] AF is frequently associated with rheumatic and calcific MS largely related to left atrial dilation. AF also increases thromboembolic risk for patients with MS secondary to blood stasis in the left atrium.[1]

Timing of Intervention and Treatment Options

Intervention is recommended for patients with an MVA less than 1.5 cm² who are symptomatic.[1] Open surgical mitral commissurotomy requires median sternotomy and cardiopulmonary bypass. Following surgical mitral commissurotomy, 31% to 50% of patients will require reoperation within 15 years and 76% by 20 years.[1] Balloon mitral commissurotomy (BMC), also known as percutaneous mitral balloon commissurotomy, can be utilized for asymptomatic patients with an MVA less than 1.5 cm² who are at elevated risk for thromboembolic events[1] (**Fig. 11**). BMC splits the closed commissures and is therefore only utilized in patients suffering from rheumatic MS.[1] Surgical mitral valve replacement may be the only option for patients who exhibit extensive calcification or greater than moderate MR. TMVR for patients of high or prohibitive risk is currently under investigation through clinical research trials.

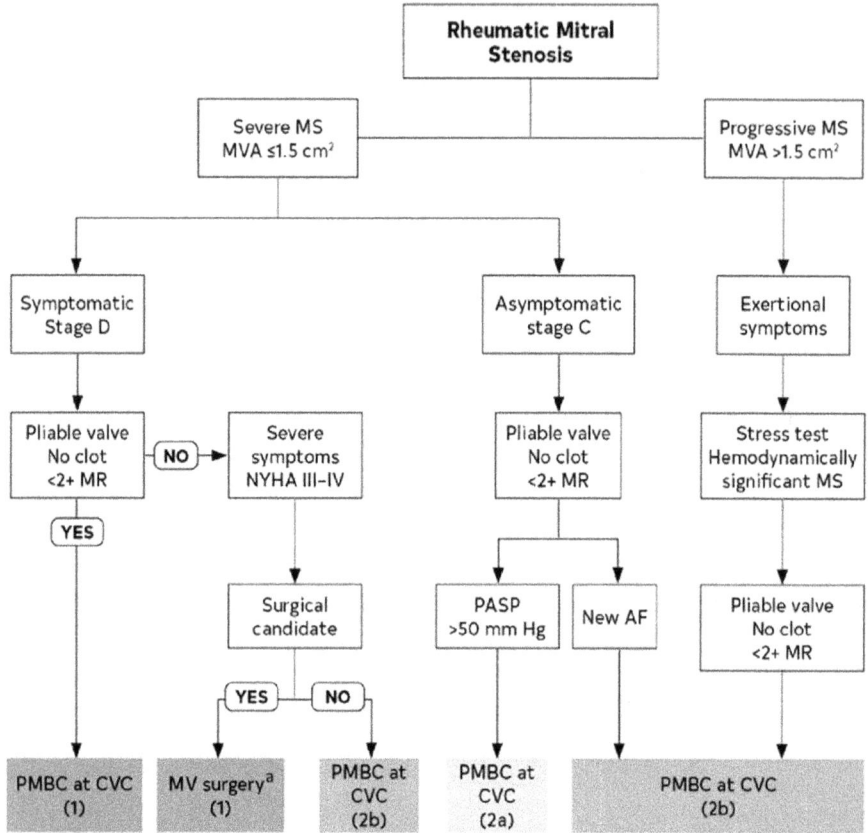

Fig. 11. Intervention for rheumatic MS. [a]Repair, commissurotomy, or valve replacement. (Otto CM, Nishimura RA, Bonow RO, et al. 2020 ACC/AHA Guideline for the Management of Patients With Valvular Heart Disease: A Report of the American College of Cardiology/ American Heart Association Joint Committee on Clinical Practice Guidelines. CirculationJ Am Coll Cardiol 2021;7 (4):e25-e197. https://doi.org/10.1016/j.jacc.2020.11.018. With permission from Elsevier Inc.)

DISEASES OF THE TRICUSPID VALVE
Background

Various conditions affect the structure and function of the tricuspid valve resulting in regurgitation and stenosis. TR occurs when the valve fails to close properly during ventricular systole, allowing the back flow of blood into the right atrium. Primary tricuspid valve regurgitation, a structural valve abnormality, can be caused by rheumatic or carcinoid heart disease, tricuspid valve prolapse, infective endocarditis, trauma, or congenital heart disease.[1] TR is most frequently functional in nature, secondary to a congenital or acquired disease process that produces right ventricular dilation with subsequent tricuspid annular dilation.[1] Right ventricular remodeling due to chronic pressure or volume overload on the right side of the heart can be due to pulmonary hypertension or pulmonary stenosis (**Box 2**).[1]

Tricuspid stenosis (TS) involves a narrowing of the tricuspid valve orifice impeding blood flow from the right atrium to the right ventricle. This can be associated with rheumatic heart disease or carcinoid syndrome and is infrequently seen in isolation.[1] TS is

---

Box 2
Causes of tricuspid valve regurgitation[1]

Congenital causes

    Ebstein anomaly
    Tricuspid valve dysplasia
    Tricuspid valve hypoplasia
    Tricuspid valve cleft
    Double-orifice tricuspid valve
    Unguarded tricuspid valve orifice

Right ventricular disease

    Right ventricular dysplasia
    Endomyocardial fibrosis

Acquired causes

    Annular dilation
    Left-sided valvular heart disease
    Ischemic heart disease with papillary muscle disruption or rupture
    Endocarditis, infectious or marantic
    Trauma
    Tricuspid valve prolapse or flail
    Carcinoid heart disease
    Rheumatic heart disease
    Iatrogenic (eg , irradiation, drugs, biopsy, pacemaker, implantable cardioverter-defibrillator)

Right ventricular dilation

    Pulmonary hypertension
        Primary pulmonary hypertension
        Secondary to left-sided heart disease (eg , valvular heart disease, cardiomyopathy)
    Right ventricular volume overload
    Atrial septal defect
    Anomalous pulmonary venous drainage

---

rare in developed countries, and rheumatic heart disease is responsible for approximately 90% of all cases.[1] There are unusual cases of TS that can be caused by carcinoid heart disease, congenital abnormalities, endocarditis, fibrosis from permanent pacemaker lead, hypereosinophilia, and Whipple disease.[1] We will spend most of this discussion around TR due to its increasing incidence.

Diagnosis and Classification

Transthoracic echocardiogram reveals the presence of TR, however, the severity of TR relies on integrative assessment of multiple parameters including hemodynamics and symptomatology[2] (**Table 9**). The prevalence of TR increases with age and is commonly associated with conditions such as pulmonary hypertension (leading to

Table 9
Stages of tricuspid regurgitation[1]

Stage	Definition	Valve Hemodynamics	Hemodynamic Consequences	Clinical Symptoms and Presentation
B	Progressive TR	Central jet <50% RA Vena contracta width <0.7 cm ERO <0.40 cm² Regurgitant volume <45 mL	None	None
C	Asymptomatic severe TR	Central jet ≥50% RA Vena contracta width ≥0.7 cm ERO ≥0.40 cm² Regurgitant volume ≥45 mL Dense continuous wave signal with triangular shape Hepatic vein systolic flow reversal	Dilated RV and RA Elevated RA with "c-V" wave	Elevated venous pressure No symptoms
D	Symptomatic severe TR	Central jet ≥50% RA Vena contracta width ≥0.7 cm ERO ≥0.40 cm² Regurgitant volume ≥45 mL Dense continuous wave signal with triangular shape Hepatic vein systolic flow reversal	Dilated RV and RA Elevated RA with "c-V" wave	Elevated venous pressure Dyspnea on exertion, fatigue, ascites, edema

Abbreviations: c-V wave, systolic positive wave; ERO, effective regurgitant orifice; RA, right atrial; RV, right ventricular; TR, tricuspid regurgitation.

secondary TR) or IV drug use (which elevates the risk of infectious endocarditis and subsequent primary TR). TR is widely underdiagnosed and undertreated due to its asymptomatic nature in early stages and limited treatment options outside of medical therapy.

Clinical Presentation

TR typically demonstrates an extended asymptomatic latent period and untreated, eventually progresses to right-sided volume overload with right-sided HF signs and symptoms. Patients with significant TR suffer from a dramatically poor quality of life.

Physical Examination

Physical examination findings in TR can vary depending on the severity of the regurgitation and associated conditions. Common manifestations on examination can include jugular venous distention, hepatomegaly, ascites, peripheral edema, and hepatojugular reflux.[1] A holosystolic murmur auscultated along the lower left sternal boarder may increase in intensity during inspiration.

Clinical Course

Untreated severe TR can lead to AF, further right ventricular dilation and dysfunction, and ultimately severe right-sided HF. These complications significantly impact patients' quality of life and increase the risk of morbidity and mortality.[1]

Timing of Intervention and Treatment Options

Medical therapy is indicated to treat symptoms of right HF secondary to severe TR and to reduce pulmonary artery hypertension. Symptoms and volume overload can be treated with diuretics, however, this becomes less effective over time.[1] Tricuspid valve surgery is the only definitive treatment for symptomatic severe TR, and repair is preferred if possible.[1] Isolated surgical tricuspid valve replacement is associated with poor outcomes and increased in-hospital mortality of 8.7%, due in part to late

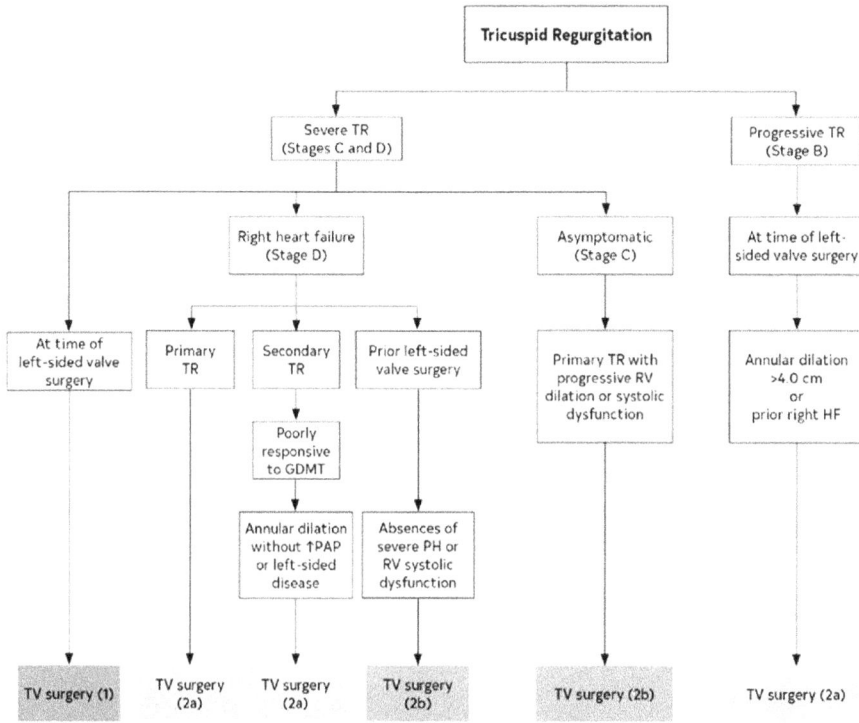

Fig. 12. Intervention for TR. (Otto CM, Nishimura RA, Bonow RO, et al. 2020 ACC/AHA Guideline for the Management of Patients With Valvular Heart Disease: A Report of the American College of Cardiology/American Heart Association Joint Committee on Clinical Practice Guidelines. CirculationJ Am Coll Cardiol 2021;7 (4):e25-e197. https://doi.org/10. 1016/j.jacc.2020.11.018. With permission from Elsevier Inc.)

referral for intervention.[12] The only class I indication for tricuspid valve surgery is for patients undergoing left-sided valve surgery who are found to have concomitant severe TR[2] (**Fig. 12**). Percutaneous therapies including tricuspid TEER and transcatheter tricuspid valve replacement have recently been granted FDA approval for the treatment of certain patient populations with promising future implications.

SUMMARY

Having dedicated my career to valve disease, I have watched the rapid evolution of this field with unwavering excitement and awe. This has been a whirlwind, high-level overview of VHD. Beyond the scope of this article, there is yet much to contemplate: pulmonic valve disease and other congenital valve defects, mixed valve disease, the need for redo valve intervention, VHD in specific populations such as pregnancy, athletes, pediatrics, and more. We have entered an era of personalized treatment plans thanks to the bevy of percutaneous and surgical treatment options. We are only beginning to leverage artificial intelligence to understand disease progression and mitigate procedural complications. Heart valve disease is prevalent, deadly, and treatable. However, to care for patients with valve disease, we must find them. Access to care is an enormous challenge for patients at home and across the globe, and one that clinicians must tackle with staunch dedication and focus. We have come so far, but the work is far from done.

CLINICS CARE POINTS

- Entrust the Multidisciplinary Heart Team to deliver high-quality, team-based, patient-centered care.
- Involve patients in their diagnosis and care plan by utilizing Shared Decision Making to ensure goals and wishes are kept front of mind.
- Develop personalized treatment plans that strive to deliver the best clinical outcome by incorporating guideline-directed recommendations.

DISCLOSURE

Edwards Lifesciences, Employee.

REFERENCES

1. Bonow RO. Valvular heart disease: a companion to Braunwald's heart disease. 5th edition. Philadelphia (PA): Elsevier; 2020.
2. Otto CM, Nishimura RA, Bonow RO, et al. 2020 ACC/AHA guideline for the management of patients with valvular heart disease: executive summary: a report of the American College of cardiology/American heart association Joint Committee on clinical practice guidelines. Circulation 2021;143(5):e35–71.
3. Batchelor WB, Saif A, Dee WD, et al. The multidisciplinary heart team in cardiovascular medicine. JACC Adv 2023;2(1):100160.
4. The Society of Thoracic Surgeons. STS Short-Term/Operative risk calculator: adult cardiac surgery Database – all procedures. Available at: https://acsdriskcalc.research.sts.org/.
5. Royal Papworth Hospital: NHS Foundation. EuroSCORE II calculator. Available at: https://www.euroscore.org/.
6. Akinseye OA, Pathak A, Ibebuogu UN. Aortic valve regurgitation: a Comprehensive Review. Curr Probl Cardiol 2018;43(8):315–34.
7. Ranard LS, Bonow RO, Nishimura R, et al. Imaging methods for evaluation of chronic aortic regurgitation in adults. J Am Coll Cardiol 2023;82(20):1953–66.
8. Siu SC, Silversides CK. Bicuspid aortic valve disease. J Am Coll Cardiol 2010; 55(25):2789–800.
9. Webb JG, Sathananthan J. Transcatheter aortic valve replacement for pure Non-calcific aortic regurgitation is coming, but not yet Primetime. JACC Cardiovasc Interv 2016;9(22):2318–9.
10. Shah M, Jorde UP. Percutaneous mitral valve interventions (repair): current indications and future perspectives. Front Cardiovasc Med 2019;2019(6):88.
11. O'Gara Patrick T, Grayburn Paul A, Vinay B, et al. ACC expert consensus decision pathway on the management of mitral regurgitation. J Am Coll Cardiol 2017;70(19):2421–49.
12. Kawsara A, Alqahtani F, Nkomo VT, et al. Determinants of morbidity and mortality associated with isolated tricuspid valve surgery. J Am Heart Assoc 2021;10(2):e018417.

Cardiovascular Management of Pulmonary Embolism

Caleb Mychael Barrera, PA-C

KEYWORDS

- Pulmonary embolism • PE • Intervention • Thrombolysis • Thrombectomy
- Catheter guided

KEY POINTS

- Pulmonary embolism is the third leading cause of cardiovascular death.
- Medical and interventional treatments are determined by risk stratifying patients into low, intermediate, and high-risk categories.
- Catheter-directed thrombolytic therapy allows for targeted thrombolytic administration at lower doses to treat pulmonary emboli.
- Catheter-directed thrombectomy is a successful interventional approach that is beneficial in many intermediate-risk to high-risk patients, especially those with contraindications to thrombolytics.
- Both interventional approaches to treat pulmonary emboli will benefit from ongoing studies to further clarify the risk benefit ratio compared to standard anticoagulation and systemic thrombolytic therapies.

INTRODUCTION

Venous thromboembolism (VTE) is an overarching diagnosis that includes both deep vein thrombosis (DVT) and pulmonary embolism (PE). Rudolf Virchow helped describe the pathophysiologic factors that lead to clot formation, which include the triad of endovascular endothelial damage, venous stasis, and a hypercoagulable state. A combination of these 3 factors can potentially lead to a VTE, with many potential risk factors playing a role. A diagnosis of VTE is clinically significant as estimates detailed in the American Heart Association (AHA) Heart Disease and Stroke Statistics—2023 Update[1] indicate there were an estimated 393,000 cases of PE and 643,000 cases of DVT for a total of 1,036,000 cases of VTE in the United States in 2019. Additionally, the lifetime risk of VTE in 45 year old adults is estimated to be 8.1%.[2] The American Lung Association estimates that 10% to 30% of individuals with a PE die within 1 month of diagnosis,[3] which is quite profound. This wide range

UPMC Central PA Heart and Vascular Institute, Cardiology, 2808 Old Post Road, Harrisburg, PA 17110, USA
E-mail address: barrerac@upmc.edu

Physician Assist Clin 10 (2025) 333–341
https://doi.org/10.1016/j.cpha.2024.11.014   **physicianassistant.theclinics.com**

Abbreviations	
AHA	American Heart Association
BNP	brain natriuretic peptide
COVID-19	coronavirus disease 2019
CTA	computed tomography angiography
CTEPH	chronic thromboembolic pulmonary hypertension
DVT	deep vein thrombosis
ED	emergency department
ESC	European Society of Cardiology
FDA	Food and Drug Administration
NOACs	novel oral anticoagulants
PE	pulmonary embolism
PERT	Pulmonary Embolism Response Team
RV	right ventricular
sPESI	simplified Pulmonary Embolism Severity Index
VTE	Venous thromboembolism

of estimated incidence is suspected to be due to a portion of PE likely being undiagnosed due to sudden cardiac death prior to diagnostic studies at a health care facility. Of note, in pooled studies that included 3066 patients diagnosed with coronavirus disease 2019 (COVID-19), there was a 15.8% prevalence of PE[4] highlighting the importance of adequate diagnosis and treatment of VTE, especially amid the pandemic.

Anticoagulation has historically been the definitive treatment approach of both DVT and PE. This article will examine utilizing anticoagulation both with and without more novel pharmacomechanical methods of intervention using endovascular access for PE, specifically. These methods include catheter-directed mechanical thrombectomy as well as catheter-directed thrombolysis.

EVALUATION

Acute PE symptoms can be variable and include, but are not limited to, shortness of breath, pleuritic chest pain, cough, and syncope. Some patients may also have a concurrent DVT with symptoms including unilateral calf pain, swelling, or erythema. Risk factors that may be identified during an adequate history taking could include recent immobilization, use of oral contraceptives, recent surgeries, pregnancy, COVID-19, smoking, or active malignancy. Physical examination findings may include tachypnea, tachycardia, fever, or jugular venous distension, and signs associated with DVT.

Laboratory values such as an elevated d-dimer can increase the suspicion for a VTE. Elevated troponin, brain natriuretic peptide (BNP), and lactic acid can also be important in the workup and risk stratification of a PE, as discussed later. A definitive diagnosis of a PE is most commonly made with a computed tomography angiography (CTA) of the chest with intravenous contrast. Alternative imaging modalities, such as ventilation–perfusion (V/Q) scan, are also utilized in clinical practice; however, they are typically limited to use in patients for whom CTA is contraindicated. The gold standard for the diagnosis of PE was previously invasive pulmonary angiography, but a survey of radiologists conducted in 2010 deemed CTA of the chest as the preferred standard.[5]

Once a PE is diagnosed, patients are then risk stratified to guide management. PE severity has been classified into 3 categories by both the AHA and the European Society of Cardiology (ESC) in 2019. The AHA uses low, submassive, and massive risk categories (**Table 1**). The ESC uses low, low-intermediate, high-intermediate, and high-risk categories (**Table 2**). As seen in **Tables 1** and **2**, these organizations have

Table 1
American Heart Association pulmonary embolism severity categorization

Category	Description
Low risk	Without RV strain or hypotension
Submassive risk	RV strain which includes RV:LV ration >0.9, elevated troponin, or elevated BNP Must be without hypotension
Massive risk	Hypotension with SBP <90 mm Hg, drop of >40 mm Hg for at least 15 min, or need for vasopressor support

Data from American Heart Association.9

similar criteria, and the risk assessments can be used interchangeably. Approximately 40% to 60% of all hospitalized patients diagnosed with PE fall into the low-risk category, which has an estimated 1% 30 day mortality rate.[6] These patients are treated with anticoagulation, unless otherwise contraindicated, and they have positive outcomes as highlighted by the relatively low aforementioned mortality rate. Unfortunately, this still leaves the other 40% to 60% of patients with PE as intermediate to massive risk. These patients have higher mortality rates, including up to 22% 30 day mortality for massive pulmonary emboli.[7] In addition to mortality risk, symptomatic pulmonary emboli portend an estimated 3.4% risk for developing chronic thromboembolic pulmonary hypertension (CTEPH) afterward. CTEPH can lead to chronic right ventricular dysfunction and eventually death.[8] This is another important reason for early management of symptomatic PE.

The aforementioned statistics exemplify the importance of risk stratification as all patients with PE are not equal. Risk stratification guides treatment modalities, such as escalating care to catheter-guided approaches. Determining that patients are at intermediate risk requires clinicians to identify patient factors such right ventricular (RV) injury and RV dysfunction. RV injury is typically identified by using an elevated troponin or elevated BNP levels. RV dysfunction can be identified on echocardiography with systolic dysfunction or dilation. RV dilation can be diagnosed with a CTA of the chest, which concurrently identifies PE. RV dilation criteria on both echocardiography and computed tomography is variable by institution but is generally defined as an RV:left ventricle (LV) ratio greater than 0.9[11] or 1.0. In a healthy heart, the left ventricle is generally larger than the right ventricle. With a PE, forward flow of blood through the pulmonary artery is prohibited, and pressure behind the thrombus leads to dilation

Table 2
European Society of Cardiology pulmonary embolism severity categorization

Category	Description
Low risk	Without RV strain or hypotension
Intermediate-low risk	sPESI >1 Either, but not both, signs of RV:LV ratio >0.9 or elevated troponin/BNP
Intermediate-high risk	sPESI >1 Both signs of RV:LV ratio >0.9 and elevated troponin/BNP
High risk	Hypotension with SBP <90 mm Hg, drop of >40 mm Hg for at least 15 min, or need for vasopressor support

Data from European Society of Cardiology.[10]

of the right ventricle. In addition to RV assessment, the ESC utilizes risk stratification with the simplified Pulmonary Embolism Severity Index (sPESI; **Table 3**). sPESI is a 6 point scale derived from the more complex 11 point PESI scale and has been shown to have similar accuracy in determining patient prognosis.[12,13] If a patient meets even 1 of the 6 components of the sPESI scale, they are deemed to be at elevated risk. Of note, a patient with RV dysfunction or elevated cardiac biomarkers despite an sPESI score of 0 is still deemed to be at intermediate risk by the ESC.

MANAGEMENT

Once the patient with an acute PE has been categorized using the AHA/ESC criteria with the assistance of diagnostic studies such as echocardiography, computed tomography, laboratory values, and vital signs, clinicians need to determine the best course of action in terms of treatment. Given the low mortality risk with a low-risk PE, these patients continue to be treated with traditional anticoagulation such as heparin products, vitamin K antagonists, or novel oral anticoagulants (NOACs). In clinical practice, vitamin K antagonists can be challenging for patients due to the need for frequent international normalized ratio (INR) draws. This leads to the utilization of NOACs such as rivaroxaban or apixaban, which are once or twice per day oral medications that do not require laboratory monitoring. Oral anticoagulation treatment duration is 3 months for provoked PE and indefinitely with unprovoked PE. The diagnosis of an unprovoked PE will often lead to a hypercoagulable workup being pursued. Anticoagulation and thrombolysis do have limitations. Contraindications to anticoagulation include active bleeding, coagulopathies, recent major surgeries, acute intracranial hemorrhage, or major trauma.[14] This, along with the high mortality rates associated with an intermediate-massive risk PE, has led to the development of catheter-directed therapies.

DISCUSSION

Catheter-directed therapies can be subdivided into catheter-directed thrombolysis and catheter-directed thrombectomy. Both approaches are typically done in a cardiac catheterization laboratory with an interventional cardiologist. Access of the venous system is obtained via the femoral vein or internal jugular vein using an introducer needle followed by a guide wire that traverses through the inferior vena cava or superior vena cava, into the right atrium, and then the right ventricle before being identified in the pulmonary vasculature using fluoroscopic guidance. The catheters are finally advanced to the proximal portion of the thrombus for treatment.

Patients with a massive PE have historically been treated with systemic thrombolytic therapy, which can lead to an increased risk of major bleeding complications.

Table 3 Simplified Pulmonary Embolism Severity Index	
Age >80 y	+1
History of cancer	+1
History of chronic cardiopulmonary disease	+1
Heart rate >110 bpm	+1
Systolic blood pressure <100 mm Hg	+1
Oxygen saturation <90%	+1

Catheter-directed thrombolysis allows thrombolytic medications, such as alteplase, to be directly administered at the site of the clot through a side port in the catheter. This focal administration leads to decreased doses of the thrombolytic agent[15–17] and, theoretically, decreased major bleeding events. Further prospective studies need to be undertaken to better delineate the bleeding risk complications, but current comparative analysis suggest that major bleeding complications are reduced by half with catheter-directed thrombolysis compared to systemic thrombolysis.[15] The PEITHO trial published in 2014 found that 6.3% of patients treated with systemic thrombolytics had extracranial bleeding and 2.4% had a stroke (majority hemorrhagic) compared to 1.2% and 0.2% in the placebo group, respectively.[18] Reducing these risks with catheter-directed thrombolytics will provide significant improvement in current management.

After the thrombolytic infusion is initiated, it is typically administered for 18 hours along with a heparin infusion before the catheters are removed by medical staff. As the access sites are venous, vascular closure devices are not typically necessary and manual compression is utilized for hemostasis. This treatment is followed by standard anticoagulation. This, again, includes NOACs or vitamin K antagonist oral therapy. The duration of therapy is dependent on the presence of provoking factors previously outlined.

The second approach is a catheter-guided thrombectomy or embolectomy. The venous access approach with ascension to the pulmonary tree remains the same. The catheter designs for the thrombectomy allow the thrombus to be engaged and aspirated. The benefit of this approach is the lack of thrombolytic utilization, which theoretically decreases the risk of major bleeding adverse events. This approach is efficacious and made evident by the FLARE study, which utilized Inari Medical's Flow-Triever System on 106 patients with intermediate-risk PE.[19] Two of the patients were also treated with thrombolytic therapy and evaluated separately. Of the remaining 104 patients, the RV:LV ratio was reduced on average from 1.53 to 1.15 after 48 hours, indicating improved RV function.

These interventional approaches are not without inherent procedural risks. As mentioned previously, catheter-directed thrombolytic therapy still portends a systemic bleeding risk, but further studies need to be carried out to delineate the major bleeding risk reduction with the reduced dose and localized administration of catheter-based versus systemic thrombolytics. For both thrombolytic-based and thrombectomy-based approaches, there are risks associated with catheter utilization that include, but are not limited to, access site complications, vascular injury, arrhythmias, cardiac tamponade, and pulmonary artery rupture. These are clearly not benign procedures, and the risk–benefit ratio needs to be considered.

FUTURE DIRECTIONS

Decision-making, from the risk categorization to a determination of who would benefit from interventional approaches to therapy, for patients with PE is a multimodal effort. Patients generally present to hospitals through the emergency department (ED), where diagnosis is made utilizing a patient's history, physical examination, laboratory studies, and diagnostic imaging as detailed earlier. Therapy can begin in the ED with anticoagulation or systemic thrombolytics, depending on the acuity of the situation. As interventional therapies become more widely used in health care systems, it will be important for ED providers to communicate with interventional cardiologists as well as pulmonary critical care teams. Joint decision-making can be utilized to identify patients who would benefit most, with the least risk, from being taken to the catheterization laboratory for catheter-directed thrombolysis or thrombectomy. These multidisciplinary cohorts are commonly labeled as a Pulmonary Embolism Response Team (PERT). Hospital systems will benefit from the development of algorithms to streamline this process, an example of which is seen in **Fig. 1**.

A majority of the studies that have brought about the Food and Drug Administration (FDA)-approval for catheter-directed treatments of PE have been single-armed

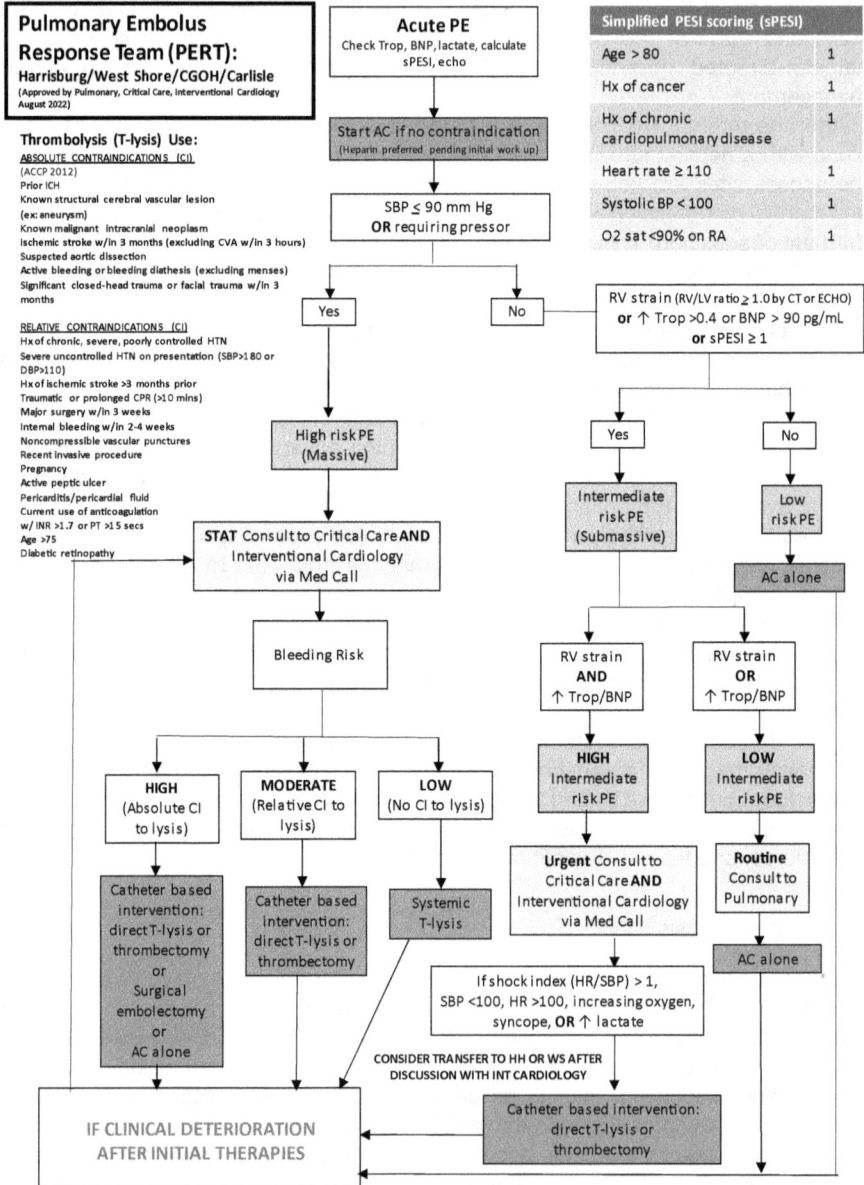

Pulmonary Embolus Response Team (PERT):
Harrisburg/West Shore/CGOH/Carlisle
(Approved by Pulmonary, Critical Care, Interventional Cardiology August 2022)

Thrombolysis (T-lysis) Use:

ABSOLUTE CONTRAINDICATIONS (CI)
(ACCP 2012)
Prior ICH
Known structural cerebral vascular lesion (ex: aneurysm)
Known malignant intracranial neoplasm
Ischemic stroke w/in 3 months (excluding CVA w/in 3 hours)
Suspected aortic dissection
Active bleeding or bleeding diathesis (excluding menses)
Significant closed-head trauma or facial trauma w/in 3 months

RELATIVE CONTRAINDICATIONS (CI)
Hx of chronic, severe, poorly controlled HTN
Severe uncontrolled HTN on presentation (SBP>180 or DBP>110)
Hx of ischemic stroke >3 months prior
Traumatic or prolonged CPR (>10 mins)
Major surgery w/in 3 weeks
Internal bleeding w/in 2-4 weeks
Noncompressible vascular punctures
Recent invasive procedure
Pregnancy
Active peptic ulcer
Pericarditis/pericardial fluid
Current use of anticoagulation w/ INR >1.7 or PT >15 secs
Age >75
Diabetic retinopathy

Acute PE
Check Trop, BNP, lactate, calculate sPESI, echo

Start AC if no contraindication
(Heparin preferred pending initial work up)

SBP ≤ 90 mm Hg
OR requiring pressor

Yes → High risk PE (Massive)

No

STAT Consult to Critical Care **AND** Interventional Cardiology via Med Call

Bleeding Risk

HIGH (Absolute CI to lysis)
Catheter based intervention: direct T-lysis or thrombectomy or Surgical embolectomy or AC alone

MODERATE (Relative CI to lysis)
Catheter based intervention: direct T-lysis or thrombectomy

LOW (No CI to lysis)
Systemic T-lysis

Simplified PESI scoring (sPESI)	
Age > 80	1
Hx of cancer	1
Hx of chronic cardiopulmonary disease	1
Heart rate ≥ 110	1
Systolic BP < 100	1
O2 sat <90% on RA	1

RV strain (RV/LV ratio ≥ 1.0 by CT or ECHO) or ↑ Trop >0.4 or BNP > 90 pg/mL or sPESI ≥ 1

Yes → Intermediate risk PE (Submassive)

No → Low risk PE → AC alone

RV strain **AND** ↑ Trop/BNP → **HIGH** Intermediate risk PE → **Urgent** Consult to Critical Care **AND** Interventional Cardiology via Med Call

RV strain **OR** ↑ Trop/BNP → **LOW** Intermediate risk PE → **Routine** Consult to Pulmonary → AC alone

If shock index (HR/SBP) > 1, SBP <100, HR >100, increasing oxygen, syncope, **OR** ↑ lactate

CONSIDER TRANSFER TO HH OR WS AFTER DISCUSSION WITH INT CARDIOLOGY

Catheter based intervention: direct T-lysis or thrombectomy

IF CLINICAL DETERIORATION AFTER INITIAL THERAPIES

Fig. 1. PERT algorithm. (Used with permission from T.R. Schmidt DO, FACC, FSCAI, Director, Pulmonary Embolism Interventional Program, UPMC Heart and Vascular Institute.)

studies. These include the SEATTLE II, which assisted with gaining FDA-approval of catheter-directed thrombolytic EKOSonic and FLARE, which led to FDA-approval of the catheter-directed thrombectomy device, FlowTriever. There has been clear benefit of utilizing these approaches with major bleeding risk reduction; however, the fact they are single-arm studies makes comparison to standard of care anticoagulation challenging to derive.

With that being said, the ULTIMA trial was a small (n = 59) randomized control trial comparing unfractionated heparin to catheter-directed thrombolysis in patients with an acute PE and RV:LV ratio of 1.0 or greater. This study found that the thrombolytic arm was superior to anticoagulation monotherapy in RV dilation improvement with no major increase in bleeding risk.[15] Further randomized control trials need to be pursued for a greater understanding of the benefit.

There are 2 trials that are ongoing to further study catheter-directed thrombectomy. The PEERLESS study is a randomized control trial comparing catheter-directed thrombectomy to catheter-directed thrombolytics.[20] At present time, decisions on pursuing thrombectomy versus thrombolytic therapy by an interventional cardiologist can be based on whether patients have absolute contraindications to thrombolytic therapy, but operator preference may also play a role in the decision. The primary endpoints in the PEERLESS study include all-cause mortality, major bleeding, intracranial hemorrhage, and clinical deterioration, which will lead to safety profile comparisons to guide decision-making. Results are yet to be published at the time of this writing. In addition to the PEERLESS study, PEERLESS II is also on the horizon as a randomized control trial that compares catheter-directed thrombectomy to anticoagulation such as heparin, NOACs, and vitamin K antagonists.[21] This study will also allow the cardiology community to better understand the safety profile in addition to the clinical benefit of the catheter-directed thrombectomy, as the primary endpoints include clinical deterioration, dyspnea at 48 hours, bailout therapy, and 30 day hospital readmission. Results of this study are also yet to be published; however, these randomized control trials will guide future decisions on both interventional versus medical therapy as well as catheter-directed thrombectomy versus catheter-directed thrombolytic therapy.

SUMMARY

PE management has traditionally been undertaken by primary care, pulmonology, and hematology. Cardiology, specifically interventional cardiology, is now poised to play a major role as anticoagulation and systemic thrombolytic therapies are no longer the sole ways to approach treatment. Catheter-directed thrombectomy and catheter-directed thrombolysis have both shown clear benefit, specifically for intermediate and high-risk patients as categorized by AHA and ESC guidelines. These catheter-based approaches, while coming with their own inherent procedural risks, have not been found to increase major bleeding, which is a primary concern of current treatment methods. Future studies will continue to create a foundation onto which health care professionals can swiftly decide the best treatment method for a patient who presents with a PE using a multispecialty approach.

CLINICS CARE POINTS

- PE is the third leading cause of cardiovascular mortality.
- A low-risk sPESI score of 0 portends a 1% 30 day mortality risk while a high-risk sPESI score of 1 or greater estimates 10.9% 30 day mortality risk.

- Anticoagulation is the mainstay of therapy for patients with PE but an intermediate to high-risk patient has a higher risk of mortality than low-risk patients when treated with anticoagulation alone.
- Catheter-directed thrombolytic therapy reduces the necessary dose of thrombolytic medications while effectively reducing RV dysfunction and improving pulmonary artery systolic pressures without increasing bleeding risk based on SEATTLE II study.
- Catheter-directed thrombectomy reduces RV dysfunction with only a 1.9% risk of significant adverse events based on the FLARE study and is a consideration for intermediate to high-risk patients with a PE and contraindications to thrombolytic therapy.

DISCLOSURE

The author has no financial disclosures.

REFERENCES

1. Tsao C, Aday A, Almarzooq Z, et al. Heart Disease and stroke statistics – 2023 update: a report from the American heart association. Circulation 2023;147: e93–621.
2. Bell EJ, Lutsey PL, Basu S, et al. Lifetime risk of venous thromboembolism in two cohort studies. Am J Med 2016;129:339.e19–26.
3. Association AL. Learn about pulmonary embolism. American Lung Association. Available at: https://www.lung.org/lung-health-diseases/lung-disease-lookup/pulmonary-embolism/learn-about-pulmonary-embolism. Accessed January 30, 2024.
4. Desai R, Gandhi Z, Singh S, et al. Prevalence of pulmonary embolism in COVID-19: a pooled analysis. SN Comprehensive Clinical Medicine 2020;2(12):2722–5.
5. Estrada-Y-Martin RM, Oldham SA. CTPA as the gold standard for the diagnosis of pulmonary embolism. Int J Comput Assist Radiol Surg 2011;6(4):557–63.
6. Jiménez D, Kopecna D, Tapson V, et al. Derivation and validation of multimarker prognostication for normotensive patients with acute symptomatic pulmonary embolism. Am J Respir Crit Care Med 2014;189:718–26.
7. Becattini C, Agnelli G, Lankeit M, et al. Acute pulmonary embolism: mortality prediction by the 2014 European Society of Cardiology risk stratification model. Eur Respir J 2016;48:780–6.
8. Simonneau G, Torbicki A, Dorfmüller P, et al. The pathophysiology of chronic thromboembolic pulmonary hypertension. Eur Respir Rev 2017;26:160112.
9. Giri J, Sista AK, Weinberg I, et al. Interventional therapies for acute pulmonary embolism: current status and principles for the development of novel evidence: a scientific statement from the American Heart Association. Circulation 2019; 140(20):e774–801.
10. Konstantinides SV, Meyer G, Becattini C, et al. ESC guidelines for the diagnosis and management of acute pulmonary embolism developed in collaboration with the European Respiratory Society (ERS). Eur Respir J 2019;54(3):1901647.
11. Frémont B, Pacouret G, Jacobi D, et al. Prognostic value of echocardiographic right/left ventricular end-diastolic diameter ratio in patients with acute pulmonary embolism: results from a monocenter registry of 1,416 patients. Chest 2008;133: 358–62.
12. Jiménez D, Aujesky D, Moores L, et al. Simplification of the pulmonary embolism severity index for prognostication in patients with acute symptomatic pulmonary embolism. Arch Intern Med 2010;170(15):1383–9.

13. Zhou XY, Ben SQ, Chen HL, et al. The prognostic value of pulmonary embolism severity index in acute pulmonary embolism: a meta-analysis. Respir Res 2012; 13(1):111.
14. Umerah C o. Anticoagulation. StatPearls. 2023. Available at: https://www.ncbi. nlm.nih.gov/books/NBK560651/. Accessed March 21, 2024.
15. Kucher N, Boekstegers P, Müller OJ, et al. Randomized, controlled trial of ultrasound-assisted catheter-directed thrombolysis for acute intermediate-risk pulmonary embolism. Circulation 2014;129:479–86.
16. Piazza G, Hohlfelder B, Jaff MR, et al. A prospective, single-arm, multicenter trial of ultrasound-facilitated, catheter-directed, low-dose fibrinolysis for acute massive and submassive pulmonary embolism: the SEATTLE II study. JACC Cardiovasc Interv 2015;8:1382–92.
17. Chatterjee S, Chakraborty A, Weinberg I, et al. Thrombolysis for pulmonary embolism and risk of all-cause mortality, major bleeding, and intracranial hemorrhage: a meta-analysis. JAMA 2014;311:2414–21.
18. Meyer G, Vicaut E, Danays T, et al. Fibrinolysis for patients with intermediate-risk pulmonary embolism. N Engl J Med 2014;370(15):1402–11.
19. Tu T, Toma C, Tapson VF, et al. A prospective, single-arm, multicenter trial of catheter-directed mechanical thrombectomy for intermediate-risk acute pulmonary embolism: the FLARE study. JACC Cardiovasc Interv 2019;12(9):859–69.
20. The peerless study - full text view. ClinicalTrials.gov. Available at: https://classic. clinicaltrials.gov/ct2/show/NCT05111613. Accessed February 10, 2024.
21. The peerless II study - full text view. ClinicalTrials.gov. Available at: https://classic. clinicaltrials.gov/ct2/show/NCT06055920. Accessed February 10, 2024.

Infectious and Inflammatory Disorders of the Heart

Myocarditis, Endocarditis, and Pericardial Disease

Clay W. Walker, MSPA, PA-C, CPAAPA[a,b,*]

KEYWORDS

- Myocarditis • Endocarditis • Pericarditis • Primary care

KEY POINTS

- Prompt recognition and treatment of myocarditis, endocarditis, and pericarditis are vital to prevent severe cardiac complications and improve patient outcomes.
- Despite similar inflammatory features, each condition requires distinct management: supportive care for myocarditis, antibiotics for endocarditis, and anti-inflammatories for pericarditis.
- Prognosis varies, with pericarditis often resolving completely, while myocarditis and endocarditis can lead to serious complications, particularly in severe cases.

INTRODUCTION

This article presents a comprehensive overview of diagnosing, evaluating, and treating 3 inflammatory and infectious cardiac disorders: myocarditis, endocarditis, and pericarditis. Inflammatory and Infectious heart diseases represent significant clinical diseases that impact the myocardium, endocardium, and pericardium, respectively. These conditions share common features of inflammation and can lead to significant cardiac complications if not appropriately diagnosed and managed timely.

These diseases' overlapping symptoms and potentially life-threatening nature highlight the significance of early diagnosis and appropriate management. This article will discuss the underlying etiology, epidemiology, pathophysiology, history and physical findings, differential diagnoses, evaluation and management, and prognosis of these

[a] Department of Family Medicine, Mayo Clinic, 5777 E Mayo Boulevard, Phoenix, AZ 85054, USA; [b] Department of Physician Assistant Studies, A.T. Still University, 5850 E. Still Circle, Mesa, AZ 85206, USA
* Department of Family Medicine, Mayo Clinic, 5777 E Mayo Boulevard, Phoenix, AZ 85054; Department of Physician Assistant Studies, A.T. Still University, 5850 E. Still Circle, Mesa, AZ 85206
E-mail addresses: cwalkerpac@gmail.com; claywalker@atsu.edu; clay.walker@mayo.edu

Physician Assist Clin 10 (2025) 343–357
https://doi.org/10.1016/j.cpha.2024.11.007
physicianassistant.theclinics.com
2405-7991/25/© 2024 Elsevier Inc. All rights are reserved, including those for text and data mining, AI training, and similar technologies.

Abbreviations	
CRP	C-reactive protein
EKG	Electrocardiogram
ECG	Electrocardiogram
NSAID	nonsteroidal anti-inflammatory drugs
HIV	human immunodeficiency virus
ACE	Angiotensin converting enzyme
IV	Intravenous
JVD	Jugular venous distension

conditions. By understanding these distinct yet interconnected diseases, health care professionals can better manage and mitigate the impact on their patients and overall health.

MYOCARDITIS

Myocarditis is the inflammation of the myocardium, with consequential tissue degeneration or necrosis. Myocarditis can be classified in a temporal pattern of acute, fulminant, chronic active, or chronic persistent cases.[1,2] Acute myocarditis comprises the majority of myocarditis cases, accounting for around 65%, and is most commonly due to a viral etiology.[1] The clinical manifestation of myocarditis can be variable in each patient case, potentially including arrhythmias, chest pain, heart failure, febrile illness, cardiogenic shock, or death.[1,2] Confirming myocarditis diagnosis is often difficult, but overall treatment is mainly supportive.[3]

ETIOLOGY

The etiology of acute myocarditis is mainly divided into infectious and noninfectious causes. In roughly half of the cases, no etiology can be identified, falling into the class of idiopathic myocarditis.[1,2] The most commonly involved underlying etiology in patients with a found cause is due to a viral infection.[1] Potential underlying infectious causes of myocarditis can be seen in **Table 1**.

There are several noninfectious causes of myocarditis. These range from iatrogenic to postcardiovascular transplantation complications and underlying systemic disease. Potential underlying infectious causes of myocarditis can be seen in **Box 1**.

EPIDEMIOLOGY

Due to the variable manifestations and difficulty with clinical diagnosis, the exact prevalence of myocarditis is not known. Acute myocarditis is more common in younger patients and appears to affect both sexes equally.[2] As per the Global Burden of Disease

Table 1 Potential infectious causes of myocarditis[2]	
Virus	Coxsackie virus, echovirus, HIV, adenovirus, hepatitis B and C, parvovirus B19, poliovirus, Epstein-Barr virus
Bacteria	*Legionella, Staphylococcus, Salmonella, Shigella, Streptococci, Clostridium, Mycobacterium tuberculosis*
Parasites	*Trichinella* genus, *Schistosoma*
Protozoa	*Trypanosoma cruzi, Toxoplasmosis gondii*
Spirochetes	*Borrelia burgdorferi*

Box 1
Potential noninfectious causes of myocarditis[2]
Eosinophilic myocarditis
Collagen vascular diseases • Systemic lupus erythematosus, polymyositis, dermatomyositis
Cardiotoxic drugs • Anthracyclines, alkylating agents, antimetabolites, monoclonal antibodies, taxanes, antiretroviral agents, antidiabetic agents, illicit drugs
Systemic diseases • Sarcoidosis, inflammatory bowel disease, giant cell arteritis, acute rheumatic fever
Chemical exposure • Hydrocarbons
Cellular rejection after cardiac transplantation

Report, the approximate rate of myocarditis is 6.1 per 100,000; however, some estimations have reported the incident to be 10 to 22 per 100,000 cases with an estimated 1.5 million cases worldwide.[2]

PATHOPHYSIOLOGY

Acute myocarditis is an inflammatory cardiomyopathy that is initiated most commonly after the entry of a virus into the myocardial cells. This leads to the activation of an innate immune response, which is then followed by an adaptive immune response over 1 to 4 weeks.[2] During the chronic stage of myocarditis, inflammation and remodeling of the myocardium eventually lead to dilation of the heart and subsequent cardiomyopathy.[2]

The cellular damage caused by a viral infection leads to the release of interleukin and damage-associated molecular patterns, which leads to the recruitment of inflammatory cells of the immune system.[2] This leads to the release of myeloid progenitor cells, leading to these cells aggregating to the damaged myocardium. This profound inflammatory response due to the viral damage of the myocardium leads to chronic inflammation, myocardial remodeling, and subsequent ventricular dysfunction.[2]

In cases of myocarditis due to an underlying autoimmune condition, autoantibodies against the myosin chain in the cardiac tissue are found in half of the cases, which are believed to have an underlying pathophysiologic role in myocarditis.[2]

HISTORY AND PHYSICAL

The presentation of acute myocarditis can be variable, with some patients being asymptomatic or having a mild febrile illness, to more severe cases where patients present with cardiogenic shock and sudden cardiac death.[2]

Patients may present with fatigue, palpitations, orthopnea, fever, malaise, chest pain, dyspnea, presyncope, or syncope. The chest pain associated with acute myocarditis can pattern that of pericarditis or occasionally be more centralized, mimicking the pain of a myocardial infarction.[2] In around 60% of patients with acute myocarditis, there will be historical findings of a recent upper respiratory tract infection proceeding the acute myocarditis.[2]

Physical examination in a patient with acute myocarditis may reveal evidence of heart failure with pulmonary rales, peripheral edema, and an S3 gallop. Additionally, a pericardial friction rub may be heard on auscultation in patients with pericardial involvement, and patients with ventricular dilation may also have a mitral regurgitation murmur on auscultation.[2]

Patients can also have evidence of underlying systemic disease, which may be the etiology of myocarditis. Patients may have lymphadenopathy in sarcoidosis, dysphagia in Chagas disease, a maculopapular rash in eosinophilic myocarditis, or erythema marginatum, polyarthralgia, and subcutaneous nodules in acute rheumatic fever.[2] Additionally, patients who have an underlying diphtheria infection may manifest with neurologic symptoms.[2]

EVALUATION

Due to the myriad of ways that myocarditis may present, as well as the overlap in the manifesting symptoms of myocarditis, confirming the diagnosis can be challenging. Acute myocarditis should be considered in a patient with signs and symptoms of the disease who has no risk factors for coronary artery disease, especially in the younger population.[2,3] Additionally, a preceding upper respiratory infection, viral syndrome, or a history of underlying autoimmune disease should make myocarditis a more suspicious underlying etiology.[2,3]

The evaluation of myocarditis and potential underlying etiologies can include blood laboratory testing and diagnostics such as an EKG showing nonspecific ST changes, chest X ray, echocardiogram, and cardiac magnetic resonance imaging.[3] Additionally, more invasive testing with coronary angiography and endomyocardial biopsy can be considered in the diagnostic evaluation of myocarditis.[3]

Endomyocardial biopsy is the gold standard for diagnosing myocarditis; however, it has its inherent risk as a more invasive diagnostic method.[3] Indications for an endomyocardial biopsy include the presence of new-onset heart failure with preserved ventricular dimensions but compromised hemodynamics, new onset heart failure of 2 weeks to 3 months duration with dilated ventricles, evidence of tachyarrhythmia or bradyarrhythmia, and failure to respond to standard therapy in 1 to 2 weeks.[3] Finally, patients with potential underlying anthracycline toxicity, restrictive cardiomyopathy, or with no underlying identified cause but continued clinical worsening would be candidates for endomyocardial biopsy.[3] **Box 2** reviews underlying diagnostic modalities in the evaluation of myocarditis.

TREATMENT/MANAGEMENT

The overall management of myocarditis is mainly supportive. For those patients with heart failure symptoms, medications including beta-blockers, angiotensin-converting enzyme inhibitors, angiotensin receptor blockers, mineralocorticoid receptor antagonists, sodium-glucose cotransporter-2 inhibitors, and diuretics can be beneficial.[3] In more severe cases, mechanical support devices such as a left ventricular assist device or an intra-aortic pump may also be required.[3]

For underlying arrhythmias associated with acute myocarditis, patients may be started on beta-blockers, amiodarone, or dofetilide, with the latter medications used for sustained ventricular arrhythmias.[3] Temporary pacemakers or implantable cardioverter-defibrillators may be indicated in patients with persistent arrhythmias.

Immunosuppressive therapy is not shown to provide clinical benefit for patients with myocarditis; thus, it would not be used routinely. Cases where immunosuppressive therapy may be warranted would be in patients with underlying autoimmune or

---

Box 2
Diagnostic testing in the evaluation of myocarditis[3]

Complete blood count
• Leukocytosis, eosinophilia (in eosinophilic myocarditis)

Inflammatory makers
• Elevated C-reactive protein, erythrocyte sedimentation rate, interleukin, and interferon levels

Cardiac markers
• Elevated troponin-I and troponin-T levels, elevated pro-brain natriuretic peptide

EKG
• Nonspecific ST segment changes, sinus tachycardia, ventricular arrhythmias, bradyarrhythmia

Chest X ray
• Cardiomegaly, pulmonary vascular congestion, pulmonary edema, pleural effusions

Echocardiogram
• Assess for valvular heart disease, intracardiac thrombus, septal wall thickness

Cardiac magnetic resonance imaging
• T1 imaging revealing showing increased T1 relaxation time, T2 imaging showing raised T2 relaxation time or signal intensity

Coronary angiography
• Gold standard test to rule out coronary artery disease as an underlying potential etiology

Viral antibody testing
• Infrequently used with low specificity and result in delay of diagnosis. If used the titers for the specific underlying virus are typically elevated at least 4-fold

Endomyocardial biopsy
• Gold standard for diagnosis myocarditis

---

granulomatous inflammatory diseases as the cause of myocarditis.[3] Antiviral treatment, as well as NSAIDs, should be avoided in cases of acute myocarditis due to the lack of evidence of benefit and the potential to impair the recovery of the myocardium, respectively.[3] Anticoagulation therapy may be indicated in patients who have been found to have evidence of atrial or ventricular thrombus or the presence of atrial fibrillation.

Activity restriction is recommended in patients with acute myocarditis. The patient should not participate in competitive sports for at least 3 to 6 months with continued clinical, Holter monitor, and echocardiogram monitoring to assess safety for return to activity.[3]

PROGNOSIS

Given the variation in disease severity and underlying etiology in the presentation of acute myocarditis, the prognosis is also variable. Generally, patients who have acute decompensated heart failure, reduction of the left ventricular ejection fraction, sustained arrhythmias, or who require treatment with vasopressors, inotropes, or mechanical cardiac support are typically more prone to adverse cardiovascular outcomes.[2,3] Around 50% of patients with acute myocarditis will develop cardiomyopathy on long-term follow-up, with the 1-year mortality rate being 20% and increasing to 56% at 4 years follow-up.[2,3]

ENDOCARDITIS

Infectious endocarditis is the inflammation of the heart's inner lining and valves. Endocarditis is primarily due to bacterial etiologies, which subsequently lead to a variety of manifestations clinically as well as complications. Significant cardiac and extra-cardiac complications can occur without the early identification of endocarditis and subsequent appropriate treatments. Careful evaluation, including a complete history and physical examination, can help identify infectious endocarditis cases and lead to timely evidence-based management, reducing the risk of morbidity and mortality.

ETIOLOGY

Most cases of infective endocarditis are due to bacterial etiologies, specifically gram-positive streptococci, staphylococci, and enterococci.[4] Altogether, these afore-mentioned bacteria comprise 80% to 90% of all cases, with *Staphylococcus aureus* specifically accounting for around 30% of cases worldwide.[4]

Other common bacteria within the oropharynx, such as the HACEK organisms (Hae-mophilus, Actinobacillus, Cardiobacterium, Eikenella, and Kingella), can less frequently be the etiology of infectious endocarditis.[4,5] A myriad of other bacteria have previously been identified as potential causes of bacterial endocarditis, but these only assume around 6% of total cases.[4,5] Lastly, fungal endocarditis occurs in around 1% of cases but, unfortunately, can be a complication of systemic Candida and Aspergillus infection in the immunocompromised patient, which can lead to increased mortality.[5]

Patients' risk factors with potential environmental exposures, and whether the bac-terial infection was acquired in a health care setting versus in the community, can pro-vide direction toward potential underlying etiologies. In cases where a patient has bacterial endocarditis of a prosthetic heart valve or following recent vascular catheter-ization, hemodialysis, or hospitalization, the most likely etiology is *Staphylococcus aureus*, which has been found to be responsible for around 50% of the cases.[5]

The less infectious coagulase-negative staphylococci, *Staphylococcus epidermis*, can lead to infectious endocarditis arising from an indwelling vascular device or recently implanted prosthetic valve.[5] Enterococcus infections leading to endocarditis appear to be similarly common with health care-associated infections as well as community-acquired infections, accounting for 15% and 18% of cases, respectively.[5]

Community-acquired infections leading to infective endocarditis often occur in pa-tients that have underlying immunocompromised conditions, poor dentition, known rheumatic heart disease or degenerative valve disease, or with intravenous drug us-age. Intravenous drug use, which is known to be the underlying risk factor in almost 10% of infectious endocarditis cases, points toward repeated exposure to skin flora such as *Staphylococcus aureus* and *Streptococcus epidermidis*, with *Staphylococcus aureus* more often affecting the tricuspid valve.[4,5]

Streptococcus viridans less commonly comprises around 20% of community-acquired bacterial endocarditis cases.[4,5] Classically, bacterial endocarditis with *Streptococcus gallolyticus* as the underlying etiology should clinically raise concern for underlying colon cancer as a potential confounding condition.[5]

EPIDEMIOLOGY

Overall, infectious endocarditis is an uncommon condition with an estimated yearly incidence of 3 to 10 cases per 100,000 people.[5] Infective endocarditis has shown a greater predominance for males with a ratio of nearly 2-1, and the average age being greater than 65 years.[5] The increase in risk for endocarditis in the elderly population is likely due to the increased prevalence of risk factors such as indwelling cardiac de-vices, hemodialysis, diabetes mellitus, acquired valvular disease, or prosthetic valves.[4,5] Another significant risk factor, which now accounts for around 10% of all infectious endocarditis cases, is due to recreation or intravenous drug use, which represents a continued growing risk factor.[5]

PATHOPHYSIOLOGY

The development of infectious endocarditis often requires an initial injury to the endocardial surface, which allows a point of access for bacterial seeding. This initial injury to the endocardial surface can have multiple in etiologies, such as due to a direct mechanical trauma caused by a catheter or electrode insertion, or due to repetitive valvular trauma by injected particulate matter from recreational intravenous drug use.[5] Once injury to the endocardial surface has occurred, subsequent bacteremia allows colonization to occur, primarily on the undersurface of the affected valve.[5]

HISTORY AND PHYSICAL EXAMINATION

A patient presenting with infective endocarditis may reveal a myriad of signs and symptoms that are nonspecific. Thus, a clinician should consider this diagnosis in any patient with risk factors and a fever or underlying sepsis.[4,5] Patients may often describe slow onset chills, fatigue, and fevers that lead them to seek medical care. However, patients who are older, who are immunosuppressed, or those who have used antipyretics or previous antibiotics, may not manifest as fulminant of symptomatology.[5]

Additional nonspecific symptoms of systemic infection may include generalized weakness, anorexia, or headache, as well as other cardiopulmonary symptoms such as decreased exercise tolerance, orthopnea, chest pain, dyspnea, and paroxysmal nocturnal dyspnea. If underlying cardiac symptoms are present, this should raise concern for potential underlying valvular pathology, such as aortic or mitral insufficiency.[5]

During history taking, an underlying predisposing condition or risk factors such as intravenous drug use, history of prosthetic valve placement, recent pacemaker placement, or current or previous indwelling catheterization are often revealed. Additionally, clinicians should inquire about known degenerative valve disease such as aortic stenosis or mitral valve prolapse, which occurs in around 30% of cases of infectious endocarditis.[5] Rheumatic heart disease was previously a significant risk factor for endocarditis; however, in the United States, this condition is less common and only comprises around 5% of all infective endocarditis cases in the developed world.[5] Physical examination in a patient with infective endocarditis may reveal evidence that reinforces the diagnosis as well as potential underlying complications such as peripheral embolization. In patients that have underlying valvular insufficiency or systemic infection, tachycardia and tachypnea are commonly present, as well as potential fever and hypotension either secondary to cardiogenic shock or sepsis.[5] Although commonly described in education as being associated with infective endocarditis, a new worsening murmur is present in less than half of cases of new infective endocarditis.[5]

The skin examination may reveal immunologic as well as hemorrhagic findings consistent with infective endocarditis, such as subungual splinter hemorrhages, painless hemorrhagic plaques on the palms and soles known as Janeway lesions, or painful subcutaneous nodules typically found in the palms known as Osler nodes. Each dermatologic finding is seen in less than 10% of all cases of infective endocarditis.[5]

EVALUATION

Due to the variety of symptoms that a patient may present with during infective endocarditis, the initial evaluation workup must be broad. Patients who present with chest pain or shortness of breath should be evaluated for potential life-threatening cardiac and pulmonary diseases such as pneumonia, pulmonary embolism, or myocardial infarction. In contrast, patients who present with sepsis should undergo rapid evidence-based directed evaluation following validated protocols.[5]

For patients who present with dyspnea or chest pain, an initial 12-lead EKG should be completed to evaluate for any underlying arrhythmias, structural heart disease, or ischemia. In cases of infective endocarditis, the EKG most often appears normal.[5] A chest X ray can identify evidence of pulmonary infiltrates, effusion, or abscesses, and in severe valvular insufficiency due to infective endocarditis can identify pulmonary edema, cardiomegaly, or cephalization of the pulmonary vasculature.[5] Investigation for further pulmonary complications such as a pulmonary artery embolization, pulmonary parenchymal disease, or empyema may require more advanced imaging of the chest with a computed tomography scan or computed tomography angiography. In patients with endocarditis who present with signs or symptoms concerning for myocardial ischemia or myocarditis, cardiac biomarkers with troponin I and troponin T should be completed to assess for any underlying infarction. Additional initial laboratory work that should be considered includes a complete blood count, often demonstrating leukocytosis, inflammatory markers such as erythrocyte sedimentation rate and C-reactive protein (CRP), often elevated in 60% of cases, and a metabolic panel to identify any electrolyte derangements.[5]

After completion of the initial evaluation, diagnostics, and exclusion of life-threatening etiologies, a diagnosis of infective endocarditis is based on both microbiologic as well as echocardiogram results. The diagnosis of infective endocarditis is made by the Modified Duke Criteria, as seen in **Table 2**. The Modified Duke Criteria is divided into major and minor criteria, in which the definite diagnosis requires either 2 major criteria, 1 major and 3 minor criteria, or 5 minor criteria all be met.[5] A diagnosis of possible infective endocarditis can be made if 1 major and 1 minor criterion are positive, or 3 minor criteria are positive.

Table 2
Modified Duke Criteria for diagnosis of infective endocarditis

Major Criteria	Minor Criteria
Positive blood cultures for typical organisms (ie, *Staphylococcus aureus, Enterococcus, Streptococcus viridans*) on 2 separate blood cultures	Fever >38 degrees Celcium
Echocardiogram showing valvular vegetation	Predisposing heart condition or injection drug usage
	Vascular phenomena • Arterial emboli, septic pulmonary infarction, mycotic aneurysm, intracranial hemorrhage, conjunctival hemorrhages, and Janeway lesions
	Immunologic phenomena • Glomerulonephritis, Osler nodes, Roth spots, and positive rheumatoid factor
	Microbiologic evidence • Positive blood culture but does not meet a major criterion as noted earlier, or serologic evidence of active infection with organism consistent with infective endocarditis

MANAGEMENT

Effective and timely treatment of infective endocarditis can reduce the risk of secondary complications. However, patients who present with the complications of infective endocarditis such as acute decompensated heart failure, stroke, or septic shock require stabilization and resuscitation and once stabilized, followed with subsequent measures for bacterial cycle antibiotic regimens and potential cardiothoracic surgical intervention.[5]

Antimicrobial treatment duration and selection depend on the nature of the valve involved as well as the resistance pattern of the infecting organism. In cases of native valve endocarditis with penicillin-susceptible *Streptococcus viridans* or *Staphylococcus gallolyticus*, treatment may include ceftriaxone plus gentamicin or penicillin G.[5]

Treatment courses with nafcillin or cefazolin are appropriate for patients at risk for staphylococcal infection, such as methicillin-sensitive *Staphylococcus aureus*. In instances of methicillin-resistant *Staphylococcus aureus*, vancomycin or daptomycin can be used for antimicrobial therapy.[5]

Treatment with gentamicin plus rifampin and rifampin can be considered in patients with prosthetic valve infection with methicillin-sensitive *Staphylococcus aureus*. In patients with prosthetic valve infection who have methicillin-resistant *Staphylococcus aureus* in addition to vancomycin, they should also receive gentamicin and rifampin therapies.[5]

Patients with enterococcal infections with either native valve or prosthetic infection can be treated with ampicillin or penicillin G plus an aminoglycoside therapy such as gentamicin.[5] Overall, antimicrobial treatment guidelines remain ever-changing and are frequently updated with new evidence, and thus, the antibiotic regimen should be routinely reviewed in clinical practice.

Early surgical intervention may be recommended, including valvular repair versus replacement in indicated cases, such as those with acute heart failure, extensive infection with localized complications, and recurrent arterial embolization.[5]

PROGNOSIS

The prognosis of the patient with infective endocarditis can widely vary depending on the infective pathogen, pre-existing comorbidities, presence of native versus prosthetic valve infection, as well as the emergence of secondary complications. The in-hospital mortality rate is around 18%, with a 1-year mortality rate reaching up to 40%.[5] Cases of infective endocarditis affecting a newly placed prosthetic valve within 60 days have the highest subset of mortality rates of around 30%.[5] Although around half of patients with infective endocarditis either undergo in-hospital or outpatient surgical intervention, in itself, the surgical intervention does not appear to increase overall mortality rates.[5]

PERICARDITIS

Pericarditis, or inflammation of the pericardium, has a myriad of different etiologies and often clinically leads to a characteristic pleuritic chest pain. Pericarditis can be further narrowed into acute pericarditis, subacute pericarditis, chronic pericarditis, and recurrent pericarditis.[6] Pericarditis may also be associated with other conditions of the pericardium, such as cardiac tamponade, constrictive pericarditis, or pericardial effusion.[7]

ETIOLOGY

The 2015 European Society of Cardiology pericarditis guidelines divide the underlying potential etiologies of acute pericarditis into 2 main groups: infectious and noninfectious causes (**Table 3**).[6] Viruses are known to be the most common infectious causes of pericarditis, including adenovirus, Coxsackie virus A and B, influenza, HIV, parvovirus B19, Epstein-Barr virus, and cytomegalovirus.[7] Bacterial etiologies of pericarditis are more infrequent; however, tuberculosis is still quite prevalent in developing countries and is the most common cause of pericarditis in endemic regions.[8] Less common other forms of bacteria can lead to pericarditis, such as Meningococcus, Staphylococcus, Pneumococcus, Streptococcus, and Coxiella. In rare cases, pericarditis can be due to fungal or parasitic organisms such as Candida, Coccidioides, Blastomyces, or histoplasmosis, as well as toxoplasmosis or Echinococcus.[8] In instances where these more rare etiologies are encountered as the cause of pericarditis, an immunocompromised state should be considered, as many of these organisms are opportunistic in nature, and have been described predominantly in patients with inadequately treated HIV.[7,8]

Noninfectious etiologies of pericarditis are numerous, including malignancy, metabolic conditions such as uremia and myxedema, as well as connective tissue diseases such as systemic lupus erythematosus, Bechet's disease, and rheumatoid arthritis. Trauma may also lead to pericarditis, occurring either as early onset following an injury or as a delayed inflammatory reaction. Dressler syndrome, also known as late postmyocardial infarction syndrome, is a well-known postcardiac injury where pericarditis occurs after a recent myocardial infarction, typically occurring several weeks after the inciting event.[7,8]

Dressler syndrome is thought to occur due to formed antibodies against the myocardium as a delayed autoimmune process leading to pericarditis symptoms.[8] Initially, when Dressler syndrome was identified, its prevalence was estimated to occur in 5% to 7% of patients with myocardial infarction; however, with improvements in the management of myocardial infarctions, as well as with a goal of early revascularization, the frequency has now become uncommon.[8]

Several medications have been found to lead to drug-induced pericarditis. Although the list of medications is significant, the incidence of medication-induced pericarditis remains rare.[8] Procainamide, isoniazid, and hydralazine have been classically known to lead to medication-induced systemic lupus erythematosus, leading to serositis with

Table 3
Common etiologies of pericarditis

Infectious	Noninfectious
Viral	*Metabolic conditions*
• Adenovirus, Coxsackie virus A and B, influenza, HIV, parvovirus B19, Epstein-Barr virus, and cytomegalovirus	• Uremia and myxedema
Bacterial	*Connective tissue disease*
• Tuberculosis, Meningococcus, Staphylococcus, Pneumococcus, Streptococcus, and Coxiella	• Systemic lupus erythematosus, Bechet's disease, and rheumatoid arthritis
Fungal	*Medications*
• Candida, Coccidioides, Blastomyces, or histoplasmosis	• Procainamide, isoniazid, nivolumab, ipilimumab, and hydralazine
Parasitic	*Malignancy*
• Toxoplasmosis or Echinococcus	*Trauma*
	• Dressler syndrome
	Amyloidosis and Sarcoidosis

pericardial involvement.[8] More commonly, checkpoint inhibitors, such as nivolumab and ipilimumab, have been increasingly identified as causes of cardiac toxicity, including myocarditis and pericarditis.[6]

Other conditions, such as sarcoidosis and amyloidosis, are rare causes of pericarditis but can be considered when a patient has pericarditis with other systemic findings of these conditions. Unfortunately, in up to 90% of cases of pericarditis, no clear cause is identified, and a diagnosis of idiopathic acute pericarditis is made.[6–8]

EPIDEMIOLOGY

Acute pericarditis is one of the most common forms of pericardial disease and a common cause of chest pain. In one study, acute pericarditis was found in 4.4% of patients who were seen in the emergency department that were found to have nonischemic chest pain and was found to account for 0.2% of all cardiovascular hospital admissions.[6] However, due to most cases of pericarditis being mild, and resolving without patients presenting for care, it is difficult to estimate the exact incidence.

Pericarditis mostly occurs in the adult population, with a mean age being in the 50s.[6] Data suggest that men are more likely than women to be affected by pericarditis, with an incidence ratio of roughly 2:1.[6] Despite more advanced diagnostic testing, more than half of episodes of pericarditis are idiopathic, presumed to be due to a viral infection.[6] In endemic areas, tuberculosis has been found to account for up to 70% of cases of pericarditis, but in nonendemic areas, it was a rare etiology.[6]

PATHOPHYSIOLOGY

The pericardium is a fibrous sac surrounding the heart, which can become inflamed due to several different causes, such as infectious and noninfectious etiologies. The pericardium's parietal layer is known to have significant nervous innervation, in which any inflammatory process, whether caused by an autoimmune, traumatic, or infectious etiology, can lead to significant retrosternal chest pain.[6,8] In instances with a pericardial effusion, the compliance of the pericardium can increase due to the accumulating fluid, which may allow the pericardial sac to increase in size without leading to compression on the atria and ventricles. This means that the rate at which fluid accumulates is more critical than the fluid volume in determining the hemodynamic complications that may affect the heart.[6]

Due to this, a small pericardial effusion can lead to complications such as cardiac tamponade if it accumulates quickly, whereas a slower formation fluid, such as due to underlying malignancy, can create a large pericardial effusion to form over weeks without leading to significant compressive physiology over the cardiac structures.[6,8]

HISTORY AND PHYSICAL EXAMINATION

Pericarditis is divided into 3 categories: acute pericarditis lasting less than 4 to 6 weeks, incessant pericarditis lasting more than 6 weeks but less than 3 months, and chronic pericarditis lasting more than 3 months.[6–8] Additionally, if a patient has 2 separate cases of pericarditis separated by a symptom-free interval of 4 to 6 weeks, they would be categorized as having recurrent pericarditis.[6–8]

Acute pericarditis accounts for 5% of emergency department visits due to chest pain, manifesting with low-grade fever, with sharp, centralized chest pain that is worse with inspiration (pleuritic) and improves by sitting up and leaning forward (positional) that is characterized as severe.[6] The pain associated with pericarditis may also radiate outside of the precordium area, involving the area of the trapezius muscles if the phrenic nerve is inflamed.[8]

On examination with auscultation over the heart, a pericardial friction rub may be heard.[8] A pericardial friction rub is highly specific for pericarditis but can be transient; it is best heard with the diaphragm of a stethoscope at the left sternal border region.[8] Determining if a friction rub is from a pericardial versus a pleural source can be challenging clinically. Asking the patient to hold their breath while auscultating can be a key clinical maneuver to help distinguish the presence of a pericardial friction rub, which would be present with both breathing and not breathing by the patient.[8] Additionally, if there are complications of pericarditis, such as cardiac tamponade, a patient may present with jugular venous distention, muffled heart sounds, and hypotension, best known as Beck's triad.[6]

The pain from pericarditis is often differentiated from ischemia cardiac pain, the latter worsened by exertion and improved with rest or with nitroglycerin administration.[8] Additionally, chest pain that is ischemic in etiology is typically not affected by position and is nonpleuritic. If a patient has pleuritic chest pain but it does not improve with positional change and is associated with cough or sputum production, the symptoms may be associated with pulmonary disease instead of pericarditis.

Additionally, lower chest pain that improves with leaning forward is nonpleuritic and is associated with food intake. It should point toward an abdominal cause of the symptoms, such as acute pancreatitis, gastroesophageal reflux, or esophagitis.[8] **Table 4** illustrates common differential diagnoses in a patient presenting with symptoms concerning for pericarditis (pleuritic chest pain).

EVALUATION

The differential diagnosis for chest pain is quite broad, and in the acute setting, it is critical to rule out life-threatening causes before evaluating for acute pericarditis when the underlying diagnosis is uncertain.[8] More than half of patients with pericarditis will develop changes in their EKG that evolve through 4 stages over a period of weeks.

In the first stage, the EKG will reveal diffuse concave-up ST-segment elevation, potentially with associated reciprocal ST segment depression and PR segment elevation in the lead AVR.[8] These findings can help to accurately distinguish acute pericarditis from myocardial infarction. In stage 2, the ST and PR segments are normalized, which typically occurs within the first week after symptoms begin. Stage 3 is categorized by a widespread T-wave inversion throughout the EKG, which is followed by stage 4 characterized by normalization of the EKG.[8] The European Society of Cardiology 2015 guidelines require 2 out of 4 criteria to be present to diagnose acute pericarditis. These criteria include the presence of[8]:

Table 4 Differential diagnoses for patient's presenting with pericarditis symptoms	
Pleurisy	Rib pain/bone lesion
Pneumonia	Costochondritis
Acute myocardial infarction	Angina
Pulmonary embolism	Pneumothorax
Aortic dissection	Postpericardiotomy syndrome
Epicardial fat necrosis	

1. Pericardial chest pain
2. Pericardial rubs
3. New widespread ST segment elevation or PR segment depression on EKG
4. Pericardial effusion

Additional supporting findings on diagnostic testing include an elevated erythrocyte sedimentation rate, CRP, and evidence of acute leukocytosis.[8] Pericardial inflammation on imaging such as echocardiogram, cardiac magnetic resonant imaging, or cardiac computed tomography can indicate pericarditis and assess for small pericardial effusions.[8] In the evaluation of chest pain, a chest X ray can also be included to assess for potential underlying etiologies of chest pain, such as pneumonia or evidence of widened mediastinum.[8] In the underdeveloped world, where tuberculosis may be more commonly seen, further diagnostic testing with QuantiFERON gold may be warranted.[8]

Certain historical or examination clues may suggest the underlying cause when assessing the etiology of acute pericarditis. Viral pericarditis may be associated with a flu-like prodrome with fever and upper respiratory symptoms, whereas autoimmune and inflammatory etiologies may have associated systemic symptoms.[6,8] In cases of autoimmune and inflammatory etiologies, the patient may have polyarthritis associated with rheumatoid arthritis, skin and kidney infections associated with systemic lupus erythematosus, or encephalopathy and asterixis caused by uremia.[6,8]

In select patients, viral serology testing, as well as blood cultures, should be completed along with HIV testing if the patient is found to be immunocompromised or has an opportunistic infection.[6–8] If there is clinical concern for an underlying autoimmune etiology, testing with antinuclear antibody serology or angiotensin-converting enzyme level for underlying sarcoidosis may be considered.[8]

If there is concern about constrictive pericarditis, cardiac catheterization may be considered to evaluate the diastolic pressure for equalization and respiratory interventricular dependence.[8] This testing, however, is not recommended for diagnostic purposes of patients with suspected acute pericarditis only.[8]

MANAGEMENT

In emergent cases of pericarditis with cardiac tamponade, patients should undergo an emergent pericardiocentesis. In cases of smaller pericardial effusions without cardiac tamponade, a pericardiocentesis can be performed less urgently with a chest tube left in place for several days until the effusion dissipates.[8] On the fluid collected from the pericardiocentesis, fungal, tuberculosis, and bacterial fluid studies can be completed along with viral PCR and blood cultures to assess for an underlying etiology. Cytology of the pericardial fluid aspirate can be considered to evaluate for malignant pericardial disease. If cytology is abnormal, further testing, including a pericardial biopsy and tumor marker testing such as carcinoembryonic antigen and CA-19, can be completed for evaluation.[8]

In nonemergent cases of acute pericarditis, management starts by identifying and addressing the underlying cause. Patients with uremic pericarditis should undergo more frequent dialysis sessions, while patients with tuberculosis or malignancy should complete disease-directed therapy.[6–8] The majority of patients will be found to have idiopathic acute pericarditis, which primarily can be managed on an outpatient basis with medical therapy. Activity restriction beyond sedentary activity is advised for patients until their symptoms have resolved.[8] Empiric treatment with anti-inflammatory agents in addition to colchicine therapy is recommended, with the duration of therapy

Table 5
Potential regimens for anti-inflammatory medications in the treatment of acute pericarditis[8]

Ibuprofen	600 mg every 8 h
Indomethacin	25–50 mg every 8 h
Naproxen	500–1000 mg every 12 h
Aspirin	100 mg every 6–8 h
Prednisone	0.2–0.5 mg/kg/d or equivalent with tapering

continuing until symptoms have resolved, typically between 3 and 14 days.[8] Potential anti-inflammatory dosing regimens of medications can be viewed in **Table 5**.

Low- to moderate-dose oral steroids with a slow taper may also be used if a regimen of aspirin, NSAIDs, and colchicine is contraindicated. While steroids can offer quick clinical improvement of the patient's symptoms with pericarditis, there is known evidence that steroids can increase the risk for recurrent pericarditis after discontinuation.[8] Thus, corticosteroids are not recommended as first-line therapy for most patients without contraindications to other medications.[8]

Response to therapy, whether with corticosteroids, NSAIDs, aspirin, or colchicine, is based mainly on the patient's symptomatic improvement. However, serial CRP measurements can also be helpful, with the CRP level trending back to normal as a clinical indicator of improvement.[8]

PROGNOSIS

The overall prognosis of acute pericarditis is promising, with the majority of patients recovering fully. Recurrent pericarditis can occur in up to 1/3 of patients who go without seeking medical care and undergoing treatment.[8] Constrictive pericarditis is quite rare following acute pericarditis, occurring in less than 1% of cases; however, the risk increases with specific etiologies such as purulent bacterial or tuberculosis pericarditis.[8] Cardiac tamponade is the most severe complication, which is seen rarely in idiopathic cases; however, it is more commonly identified in patients who have acute pericarditis due to underlying malignancy and infectious etiologies.[8]

CLINICS CARE POINTS

Myocarditis:
- Consider myocarditis in young patients with unexplained heart failure or arrhythmias, especially after a recent viral illness.
- Prompt diagnosis and supportive care are crucial; the use of beta-blockers and ACE inhibitors can help manage heart failure symptoms of myocarditis.
- Avoid NSAIDs and steroids in acute myocarditis, as they may worsen myocardial injury.
- Relying solely on biomarkers; troponin may not be elevated in all cases, requiring further imaging or biopsy for confirmation.

Endocarditis:
- Early use of echocardiography and blood cultures is essential for a timely diagnosis, guided by the Modified Duke Criteria.
- Delaying treatment in patients with risk factors (eg, prosthetic heart valves, IV drug use) can lead to serious complications like emboli or valvular damage.
- Empirical antibiotics should cover staphylococci, streptococci, and enterococcus until cultures are finalized.
- Underestimating the need for surgical intervention; in some cases, antibiotics alone may not resolve valvular infections or prevent embolic events.

Pericardial Disease (Pericarditis):
- Recognize the characteristic chest pain relief by sitting up and leaning forward; a friction rub on auscultation is highly specific.
- Failing to rule out cardiac tamponade, especially in cases with hypotension, JVD, and muffled heart sounds (Beck's triad).
- NSAIDs combined with colchicine are effective first-line therapies; corticosteroids are reserved for refractory or contraindicated cases.
- Misinterpreting ECG findings as a myocardial infarction; diffuse ST elevation in pericarditis is often concave, not convex.

DISCLOSURE

Physician Assistant for Mayo Clinic. Advisory Board Member on GSK Panel for Management of Uncomplicated UTIs.

REFERENCES

1. Kang M, Chippa V, An J. Viral myocarditis. In: StatPearls. Treasure Island (FL): StatPearls Publishing; 2023.
2. Al-Akchar M, Shams P, Kiel J. Acute myocarditis. In: StatPearls. Treasure Island (FL): StatPearls Publishing; 2023.
3. Ammirati E, Moslehi JJ. Diagnosis and treatment of acute myocarditis: a review. JAMA 2023;329(13):1098–113.
4. Khaledi M, Sameni F, Afkhami H, et al. Infective endocarditis by HACEK: a review. J Cardiothorac Surg 2022;17(1):185.
5. Yallowitz AW, Decker LC. Infectious endocarditis. In: StatPearls. Treasure Island (FL): StatPearls Publishing; 2023.
6. Peterson TA, Turner SP, Dolezal KA. Acute pericarditis: rapid evidence review. Am Fam Physician 2024;109(5):441–6.
7. Lazarou E, Tsioufis P, Vlachopoulos C, et al. Acute pericarditis: update. Curr Cardiol Rep 2022;24(8):905–13.
8. Dababneh E, Siddique MS. Pericarditis. In: StatPearls. Treasure Island (FL): StatPearls Publishing; 2023.

Coronavirus Disease 2019 and Associated Cardiovascular Complications
Acute and Chronic

Julie A. Jones, MS-PAS, PA-C[a,1], Marie Shaner, MMS, PA-C[a,2],
Catherine Roden, MHS, PA-C[a,]*, Marnie O'Donnell, MHS, PA-C[a,3]

KEYWORDS

- Post-covid POTS • Covid-19 arrhythmia • Covid-19 myocarditis
- mRNA Covid-19 vaccine myocarditis • Coronary artery aneurysm in MIS-C
- Coronary artery dilatation in MIS-C

KEY POINTS

- Acute Covid-19 (coronavirus disease 2019) has several cardiac complications including arrhythmias and myocarditis.
- Sub-acute Covid-19 cardiac manifestations include postural orthostatic tachycardia syndrome (POTS), arrhythmias, multisystem inflammatory syndrome in children (MIS-C).
- POTS is a long Covid complication
- A MIS-C finding is coronary dilation or aneurysm; correct measurement of the dominant coronary artery is crucial.

SEVERE ACUTE RESPIRATORY SYNDROME-CORONAVIRUS DISEASE 2019 ACUTE/SUBACUTE MYOCARDITIS AND SEVERE ACUTE RESPIRATORY SYNDROME-CORONAVIRUS DISEASE 2019 mRNA VACCINE-INDUCED MYOCARDITIS

Myocarditis predominately presents acutely following a viral infection. Etiologies other than a virus are associated with myocarditis including bacteria, toxins, venom, autoimmune disease, and immune stimulation. Males are twice as likely to contract myocarditis and it most commonly affects young males (puberty—4th decade of

[a] Department of Congenital Heart Center, Penn State Health, Hershey, PA, USA
[1] Present address: 990 Miller Road, Strasburg, PA 17579.
[2] Present address: 1706 Falls Road, Breinigsville, PA 18031.
[3] Present address: 118 Wheatland Road, Lewisberry, PA 17339.
* Corresponding author. Penn State Health Milton S Hershey Medical Center, Congenital Heart Center, 500 University Drive, Hershey, PA 17033.
E-mail address: croden@pennstatehealth.psu.edu

Physician Assist Clin 10 (2025) 359–370
https://doi.org/10.1016/j.cpha.2024.11.008   physicianassistant.theclinics.com
2405-7991/25/© 2024 Elsevier Inc. All rights reserved, including those for text and data mining, AI training, and similar technologies.

Abbreviations	
AV block	atrioventricular block
BNP	brain natriuretic peptide
CA	coronary artery
CAG	coronary angiography
CCTA	coronary computed tomography angiography
Covid-19	coronavirus disease 2019
IAS	inherited arrhythmia syndromes
IVCD	intraventricular conduction delay
KD	Kawasaki disease
LCA	left coronary artery
LQTS	long QT syndrome
MCS	mechanical circulatory support
MIS-C	multisystem inflammatory syndrome in children
POTS	postural orthostatic tachycardia syndrome
RCA	right coronary artery
SARS	severe acute respiratory syndrome
SCA	sudden cardiac arrest
SCD	sudden cardiac death

life). The contents of this presentation will focus on viral myocarditis and myocarditis associated with the mRNA vaccine for SARS-Covid (severe acute respiratory syndrome coronavirus disease).

Etiology

Myocarditis is the inflammation of the myocardium. The inflammation is triggered by a secondary immune response from the virus. A cascade of inflammatory agents such as cytokines, macrophages, monocytes, neutrophils, and B and T cells are released and can target the heart, lungs, kidney, and brain, causing cell death and damage. An acute and fulminant presentation can occur hours to days from when a patient had the onset of viral symptoms. Subacute presentation can occur within a few weeks or months following the virus.

Symptoms

The most common presentation of patients with myocarditis is chest pain (95%) followed by dyspnea/tachypnea (45%), syncope, arrhythmias, and respiratory distress. A recent history of a respiratory or gastrointestinal illness is common. In some cases, there may not be a recent history of symptoms, but recent high exposure to a virus is present, presuming the patient had a subclinical case of the virus.[1]

EVALUATION

As with any patient that presents with chest pain, a 12-lead ECG (electrocardiogram) is the standard of care. ST segment changes can be seen (47%) with acute myocarditis as well as ectopy and dysrhythmia. A chest x-ray may demonstrate pulmonary edema, cardiomegaly, or pleural effusion. Serum laboratory troponins are likely to be elevated (83%–89%).[2] Inflammatory markers, such as erythrocyte sedimentation rate and c-reactive protein, are likely to be elevated as well. A brain natriuretic peptide (BNP) can be useful to trend the severity of heart failure. Viral studies can be evaluated but may have limited value as standard hospital panels only test for the most prevalent viruses in a community. Transthoracic echocardiography is used to evaluate ventricular function and regional wall motion abnormalities. The gold standard of diagnosis is cardiac MRI with late enhancement with gadolinium.

Treatment

Uncomplicated viral myocarditis has an excellent prognosis and only requires supportive care during the initial presentation. Most cases of viral myocarditis present in young healthy males without any comorbidities, which contributes to this good outcome. Older age and comorbidities increase mortality. Patients who are hemodynamically stable but have signs and symptoms of heart failure should be managed with traditional heart failure therapies: ACEI, ARB, BB, aldosterone antagonists, and diuretics. The majority of patients may only require short-term treatment. A minority of patients may require intensive care level support with inotropic agents, cardiorespiratory support, mechanical circulatory support (MCS) (eg, ventricular assist devices or extracorporeal membrane oxygenation).

MYOCARDITIS AND SEVERE ACUTE RESPIRATORY SYNDROME CORONAVIRUS DISEASE

In the first year of the pandemic, there was a significant increase in the diagnosis of myocarditis. Myocarditis inpatient encounters were 42.3% higher in 2020 compared with year 2019. Covid-19 myocarditis was 16 times higher than all other causes of myocarditis. The data was compiled prior to the public mass vaccination with mRNA vaccines.[1]

Covid-19 myocarditis presents within 2 weeks after experiencing Covid-19 symptoms. Covid-19 myocarditis presents similarly to other forms of viral myocarditis and pericarditis, with symptoms including chest pain/pressure, dyspnea, palpitations, syncope, fatigue, or abdominal symptoms. In one multicenter study, the average age was around 40 years, and as with other viruses, prevalence was greater in males than females. Approximately 70% required ICU-level care and 39% required inotropic support or MCS. The estimated mortality was 6.6% at 120 days.[2]

MYOCARDITIS AND mRNA VACCINE CORONAVIRUS DISEASE 2019

Shortly after the availability of the mRNA Covid-19 vaccine, myocarditis was noted as an adverse event, first in the adult population and then in pediatric patients once the use was of the vaccine was authorized in that population. The Vaccine Adverse Event Reporting System has documented adverse events since 1990. Myocarditis has been a known adverse event in several live vaccines, such as smallpox and anthrax. The most affected population continues to be young males.[3]

All studies agree the greatest risk of developing myocarditis occurs after the second vaccine dose in young men aged 12 to 39 years. People greater than 50 years had few reports of vaccine-associated myocarditis, similar to pre- and COVID-19–associated myocarditis.

Signs and symptoms of COVID-19 vaccine–associated myocarditis include shortness of breath, chest pain or pressure, palpitations, malaise, or fatigue, similar to other forms of myocarditis.

Most cases of myocarditis associated with vaccines have been reported to be mild and of short duration. Most patients are hospitalized only to monitor for arrhythmias and heart failure, rather than for severe signs and symptoms.[4] Most individuals were considered recovered by 3 months of the onset of myocarditis and quality-of-life measures were comparable to those of pre-pandemic populations.

In analysis of mRNA Covid-19 vaccine mortality, there was a small but statistically significant association between the vaccine and cardiac related mortality. Male gender was recognized as the most important risk factor.[5]

Despite the small risk of mRNA vaccine-induced myocarditis, vaccination continues to be safe and recognized as the best prevention of Covid-19. **Table 1** demonstrates risks of myocarditis before the Covid-19 pandemic, during the pandemic but before vaccine availability, with the initial 2 doses of mRNA vaccine, and with the booster dose.

CONSIDERATION OF CORONARY ARTERY DOMINANCE WHEN EVALUATING CORONARY ANEURYSM IN MULTISYSTEM INFLAMMATORY SYNDROME IN CHILDREN

Although Covid-19 infection in children presents as asymptomatic to mild illness, there is a described illness of hyperinflammation and multi-organ involvement following the SARS-COV-2 viral infection. It is a multisystem inflammatory syndrome with findings that occur several weeks after the viral infection. The condition is known as multisystem inflammatory syndrome in children (MIS-C). The clinical findings overlap with the inflammatory syndrome of Kawasaki disease (KD), involving severe immune-mediated response characterized by fever, tissue damage, and multiple organ failure.[9]

Clinically, MIS-C is expressed through inflammation involving organ systems, including cardiac, neurologic, gastrointestinal, pulmonary, and hematologic. Cardiac involvement is prevalent. Children can present with cardiogenic shock, myocardial dysfunction, hypotension, myocarditis, and pericarditis. Coronary artery (CA) involvement is highly evident, with dilatation and aneurysms reported in several cases.[9] Dilatation of the CA is one of the findings that is similar between MIS-C and KD. Therefore, a review of some points of consideration for CA measurement is important.

A CA aneurysm is defined as a 50% or greater increase in CA diameter compared with adjacent arterial segments. It is essential to recognize that an arterial segment dilated more than 1.5 times its baseline caliber represents a fusiform aneurysm or aneurysmal dilatation.[10]

The most reasonable way to primarily assess CA in children is by echocardiography rather than by coronary computed tomography angiography (CCTA), which involves radiation exposure, or by a more invasive procedure like coronary angiography (CAG). Therefore, the use of CCTA and CAG in children is limited. Echocardiography has high sensitivity and specificity for detecting abnormalities of the CA segments.[10,11] CA measurement and the assessment of dilatation in children needs to take into consideration a z score (standard deviation units from the mean) determined by (1) body surface area and (2) age-specific absolute values or the ratio to the caliber of the surrounding artery; these are based on regression equations to contribute to a standardization across time and populations.[12]

In previous assessments of the measurement of CA in KD, even if CA caliber values using z-score are used, there are other considerations for interpreting the measurements of the CA diameters. One area of importance is variations in patients' right coronary

Table 1 Risk of myocarditis per 100,000			
Non-COVID Prior to 2020 (USA)	SARS-COVID Unvaccinated (2020–2021 USA)	mRNA Vaccine (Initial 2 Doses USA)	mRNA Vaccine (Booster Dose Nordic Nations)
1–10[6]	150[7]	4–8[8]	.8–2[8]

artery (RCA) and left coronary artery (LCA) measurements based on CA dominance.[11–14] The artery that supplies the posterior descending artery and the posterolateral branch determines the pattern of coronary dominance.[11,14] RCA dominance is more common in adults as well as children, occurring in about 70% to 90%.[10,12–14]

Using echocardiography to determine CA dominance by imaging can be difficult even in children. Using CA indices is more useful than direct assessment of the posterior descending artery (PDA) distribution. Lee and colleagues showed that using CA indices can assist with determining the CA dominance. The diameter ratio of the LCA to RCA with left coronary dominance is 1.62.[10,11,15] This value was a similar finding by Dodge and colleagues.[15] If the diameter ratio is less than 1.62, then the dominance can be inferred to be on the left side despite not knowing the exact CA distribution of the left ventricular posterior wall.[10,11,16–18] The studies done using the coronary-aorta index (CA-to-aortic-annulus ratio) or normal CA dimensions established reference ranges for CA in children that varied, but they did not take CA dominance into account.[11,16,17]

In KD, early dilatations were ipsilateral (dominance-related) at acute diagnosis compared to contralateral dilatations in which the peak z-scores were at 2 weeks after acute onset, with ipsilateral regression.[12,13,16]

This leads to another topic regarding the assessment of CA dilatation and measurement in KD and consideration for MIS-C, which includes the timing of the CA dilatation as determined by echocardiography. In KD, early dilation in the ipsilateral CA may be due to a physiologic increase in CA blood flow during the acute febrile period whereas the contralateral dilatation-increase in z-score at 2 weeks from fever onset may be due to diffuse vasculitis. Therefore, a portion of patients with ipsilateral dilatation may be falsely diagnosed with CA complications. Based on children with RCA dominance, which is most common, this may explain the higher prevalence of LCA dilatation in patients with LCA dominance in the acute febrile state.[11,12,18]

Accordingly, a peak CA dilatation 2 weeks from the onset of the acute onset may be the actual reflection of true dilatation secondary to vasculitis, as opposed to the onset CA dilatation followed by regression of CA z-score, which may be attributed to vaso-dilatation as a physiologic response to carditis. This means that associated inflammatory markers may be valuable to determine the true cause of dilatation of the CA and assist in determining CA function later in life.[12]

Essentially, patients with maximal dilatation at the time of diagnosis followed by early CA diameter normalization could be considered at lower risk compared with patients who develop CA dilatation at the 2-week follow-up or later.[12]

Follow-up may help to stratify patients between dominance-related coronary dilatation and vasculitis-induced dilatation.[12] In addition, it currently remains unclear whether there are irreversible complications or long-term sequelae associated with MIS-C. Appropriate ongoing surveillance is needed longer term.[19]

Given the overlap of the inflammatory properties between KD and MIS-C, it may be clinically relevant to consider these presented points that have been previously considered in KD as clinical relevance for assessment of MIS-C.

CORONAVIRUS DISEASE AND POST-CORONAVIRUS DISEASE CARDIAC ARRHYTHMIA
Introduction

Cardiac arrhythmia as a manifestation of Covid-19 in pediatric patients includes non-sustained ventricular tachycardia, supraventricular tachycardia, first-degree and second-degree atrioventricular block (AV block), bundle branch block, and intraventricular conduction delay (IVCD). Covid-arrhythmias and post-Covid arrhythmias are associated with multisystem inflammatory syndrome (MIS-C), myocarditis, electrolyte imbalance, inflammation, demand ischemia, QT prolonging and pro-arrhythmic medications used to treat Covid, and underlying heart conditions such as congenital heart defects and inherited arrhythmia syndromes (IAS).

Pathophysiology

The complete pathogenesis and molecular mechanism for cardiac conduction disease and arrhythmia from SARS-CoV-2 is not entirely understood and continues to be studied. SARS-CoV-2 has been associated with an overproduction and upregulation of pro-inflammatory cytokines including IL-6 and TNF-α. Some synergistic effects of IFN-γ and TNF-α have been shown to precipitate systemic inflammation and cell death, ultimately leading to cardiac tissue insult.[20] The pathophysiologic mechanism of SARS-CoV-2 in the heart may be attributed to the angiotensin converting enzyme, which acts as a functional cell receptor through which SARS-CoV-2 can easily enter, causing immune dysregulation, increase in cytokines, inflammation, and myocardial injury.[21] Upregulation of certain genes associated with cytokine activation and inflammation may also contribute to the effects of SARS-CoV-2 and cardiomyocyte apoptosis.[22]

Screening/Clinical Presentation

Detecting arrhythmia in the post-Covid pediatric patient with proper risk stratification and treatment is imperative for reducing the risk of tachycardia-induced cardiomyopathy, sudden cardiac arrest (SCA), and death. The student athlete with Covid-19 and post-Covid-19 arrhythmia may be at an increased risk for adrenaline-sensitive arrhythmia. This unique population should have proper screening, diagnosis, risk stratification, and optimal treatment, with possible sports restrictions.

The pediatric population, in general, is spared severe and critical manifestations of Covid-19. However, pediatric patients may be predisposed to developing Covid-arrhythmia or post-Covid arrhythmia if they have congenital heart disease, history of cardiac repair or intervention, or a personal history or family history of SCA, cardiomyopathy, or IAS. A comprehensive past medical history, family history, and physical examination are imperative for proper diagnosis and treatment.

Patients with a history of congenital heart disease and/or a history of cardiac intervention or repair with suspected or confirmed Covid-19 should be referred to a pediatric cardiology team for evaluation to determine if inpatient monitoring, fluid resuscitation, supportive care, or Covid-19 treatment is warranted.

Family history inquiry should include knowledge of maternal and paternal first-degree and second-degree families with concerns for congenital deafness, sudden cardiac death (SCD) or SCA, infant death, cardiomyopathy, aortic aneurysm, early CA disease or stroke, and IAS such as Long QT syndrome (LQTS), Wolff-Parkinson-White syndrome, arrhythmogenic right ventricular cardiomyopathy, catecholaminergic polymorphic ventricular tachycardia and Brugada syndrome. Pediatric patients with a suspected or confirmed SARS-CoV-2 infection with a concerning cardiac family history should be referred to pediatric cardiology for evaluation.

Pediatric patients with suspected or confirmed SARS-CoV-2 infection may present without clinical signs of a respiratory illness. Therefore, if a pediatric patient presents with complaints of exercise-induced chest pain, palpitations, exercise intolerance, dyspnea, or syncope (with and without stress), a past or current Covid-19 infection may be considered and cardiac screening should be performed, regardless of a known personal history of or exposure to Covid-19.

Screening pediatric patients with a concerning family history and/or those with cardiac symptoms includes obtaining a 12-lead ECG. Patients with signs of ectopy, axis deviation, pre-excitation, QT prolongation, ST segment abnormality, nonspecific T wave abnormality (strain pattern), AV block, bundle branch block, IVCD, or ventricular hypertrophy should have a pediatric cardiology consultation for further cardiac workup. Serum biomarkers markers, including troponin, creatinine kinase-MB, BNP, erythrocyte sedimentation rate, C-reactive protein, complete blood count, basic metabolic panel, transaminases, and echocardiogram, should be considered. Further testing may include rhythm surveillance with a holter monitor, event monitor, or loop monitor. Stress testing to evaluate for adrenaline-sensitive arrhythmia and endomyocardial biopsy and cardiac MRI to evaluate for myocarditis may also be considered.

Diagnosis

Myocarditis and cardiac arrhythmia

Pediatric patients with acute and subacute myocarditis are at risk for lethal arrhythmia. If myocarditis is suspected from Covid-19 infection or Covid-19 mRNA vaccination, diagnostic tests should include biomarkers, ECG, and echocardiogram. ECG findings of ventricular tachycardia, low voltages, wide QRS duration, prolonged QTc, and Brugada pattern are associated with increased cardiac risk. Endomyocardial biopsy establishes histopathological data for diagnosing myocarditis by the presence of inflammatory infiltrate. The utilization of this invasive procedure is declining as the use of cardiac MRI is emerging. Cardiac MRI assesses the myocardium with mapping, strain techniques, and gadolinium enhancement imaging. Studies have indicated anteroseptal and mid-wall distribution associated with ventricular arrhythmia in children, and late gadolinium enhancement with patchy distribution is also associated with poor outcome.[23]

Multisystem inflammatory syndrome in children and cardiac arrhythmia

MIS-C-associated CA dilation or aneurysm increases the risk for demand ischemia and thrombotic events precipitating ventricular arrhythmia and risk of cardiac arrest. An echocardiogram is used for the primary evaluation of coronary arteries in patients with a clinical suspicion of MIS-C. CCTA and CAG are also options for assessing coronary anatomy but with considerations needing to be made regarding contrast and radiation exposure. Exercise stress testing is considered for pediatric patients with subacute myocarditis and a history of acute myocarditis and MIS-C to evaluate for adrenaline-sensitive arrhythmia prior to providing sports clearance.

Treatment

Management of cardiac arrhythmias associated with Covid-19 requires treatment of the underlying cause, including correction of electrolyte imbalance, heart failure medication optimization with ACEI, ARB, beta-blocker and diuretic, IVIG and glucocorticoids for treatment of MIS-C, intravenous anti-arrhythmic therapy, and ECMO support for unstable ventricular arrhythmias and ventricular collapse.

LONG QT AND CORONAVIRUS DISEASE 2019 ARRHYTHMIA PRECAUTIONS

There are proarrhythmic effects of several medications used to treat Covid-19, and they must be used with caution. Patients with LQTS are at an increased risk for ventricular arrhythmia, Torsade's de Pointes, and cardiac arrest if exposed to QT prolonging medications. Medications with pro-arrhythmic effects commonly used to treat Covid-19 include the antimalarial Hydroxychloroquine, antimicrobial azithromycin, and antiviral lopinavir-ritonavir. Close cardiac surveillance with rhythm monitoring and serial QTc measurements should be observed.

BRUGADA SYNDROME AND CORONAVIRUS DISEASE 2019 ARRHYTHMIA PRECAUTIONS

Brugada syndrome, a sodium channelopathy linked to mutations in the SCN5a gene, presents with ST segment elevation and right bundle branch block morphology in leads V1-V3. Patient with this syndrome are at risk for polymorphic ventricular tachycardia and SCD. Patients with Brugada may present without ECG abnormalities. When this concealed ECG pattern is unmasked, patients are at increased risk for death. Fever and sodium channel blockers such as flecainide, procainamide, and ajmaline are known to unmask the Brugada pattern with ST segment elevation and arrhythmogenesis. The use of these anti-arrhythmic medications warrants increased caution and surveillance with serial ECG. If a febrile patient with Covid-19 presents with Brugada pattern, aggressive fever management with antipyretics is imperative for preventing cardiac arrest.

POST CORONAVIRUS DISEASE 2019 AND POSTURAL ORTHOSTATIC TACHYCARDIA SYNDROME

POTS is a multisystem disorder that is often debilitating. It is characterized by an abnormal autonomic response. This causes many symptoms, including dizziness, lightheadedness, visual changes, tinnitus, sweating, flushing, palpitations or a rapid heart rate, headaches, and sometimes transient syncope. Symptoms are often exaggerated by an upright position. GI symptoms include nausea, early satiety, intermittent abdominal pain, and rarely vomiting. An autonomic neuropathy may also be demonstrated by numbness of the feet, legs, hands, or arms with an increased sympathetic tone. The etiology of this condition has not been fully defined. It is estimated to affect 0.2% −1% of the US population, which is about 1 to 3 million affected persons. It tends to affect more females than males, and the initiation of symptoms is common in the teen years.[24]

The exact cause of POTS is unknown. Additionally, the pathophysiology of the disorder is incompletely understood and likely multifaceted. Possible, but not exclusive or fully inclusive etiologies that may represent possible mechanisms of pathophysiology include: hypovolemia due to an altered renin-angiotensin aldosterone system, cardiovascular deconditioning and low stroke volume, inflammation mediators, inappropriate action of aortic arch baroreceptors, excessive central sympathetic activation, small fiber neuropathy, and connective tissue laxity.[24] Several triggers that often precede the onset of this syndrome have been identified and include trauma, autoimmune illness or other systemic disease (eg, diabetes, celiac, and multiple sclerosis), hormone changes or puberty growth, and a recent viral infection.[24]

In 2020, a new virus emerged and the world was changed. The SARS-Covid 19 virus also impacted the prevalence and recognition of POTS. The Covid virus is thought to cause immune-mediated damage to the autonomic nervous system. There are several hypotheses for how this happens, but an exact cause remains unknown. It is possible there is autoantibody production against one's own autonomic nerve fibers. There is another hypothesis that the syndrome results from a direct toxic effect of the virus. Lastly, there is a theory that the infection affects the stimulation/feedback of the autonomic nervous system.

POTS should be considered in patients with a history of Covid-19 infection within the last 6 to 12 months. A classic clinical presentation is a patient who has transient symptoms with position changes. Patients that have long covid may display extreme fatigue, palpitations, chest pain, shortness of breath both at rest and with light activity or climbing stairs, and dysautonomia. These patients usually struggle to get out of bed in the morning and express an extreme brain fog with difficulty focusing. It can be debilitating and affect daily functioning and the ability to meet educational or work expectations and requirements adequately.

The diagnosis of POTS is usually made clinically, and misdiagnosis is common. Vital signs are obtained supine and standing.

- A positive orthostatic vital sign is a drop in systolic blood pressure of at least 20 mm Hg with upright positioning. In POTS, typically, there is an absence of orthostatic hypotension.
- An increase of greater than 30 bpm in heart rate for patients more than age 19 years or an increase of 40 bpm in patients lesser than age 19 within 10 minutes of standing upright.
- Symptomatic orthostasis, including symptoms of dizziness, visual changes, tachycardia, presyncope, weakness, and fatigue.
- Duration of symptoms has been occurring for at least 3 months.
- The absence of other conditions that could cause or explain symptoms (eg, anorexia, anxiety, hyperventilation, hyperthyroidism, pheochromocytoma, or severe deconditioning)[24]

Autonomic testing is available, but seldom used in the pediatric population. A tilt table test may be performed. A complete set of blood work including a CBC, iron profile, CMP, TSH, T4, and vitamin D is often recommended to rule out other issues such as anemia, thyroid disease, or electrolyte disturbances. Cortisol levels and normetanephrine levels may be ordered to rule out secondary causes of orthostatic intolerance.

The management of patients with post-Covid POTS is similar to those whose POTS is of unknown etiology. The foundation of treatment is lifestyle changes and a nonpharmacologic approach. Aggressive oral hydration is recommended with a daily water goal of 64 to 90 ounces. The goal is to increase intravascular volume. Increased salt consumption is encouraged, which can be attained either by increasing dietary salt or consuming an over-the-counter encapsulated salt/electrolyte capsule. The daily goal is a sodium intake is 8 to 10 g.[25] Daily aerobic exercise is recommended to increase muscle contraction and encourage appropriate vasodilation/vasoconstriction. Often a gradual increase in exercise time is required. Recumbent stationary bike or floor exercises may need to be encouraged due to symptoms in the upright position. Compression socks or an abdominal binder may be used to prevent blood pooling in the lower extremities. A healthy sleep routine is recommended as well. Patients should attempt to sleep in sync with their circadian rhythm with the same bed and wake times daily. Pre-bedtime should be limited, especially up to 30 minutes prior to sleep. A daily activity to release thoughts and stress, such as journaling, yoga, meditation, or prayer, is encouraged. There is a high correlation of anxiety with POTS. Therefore, appropriate anxiety treatment is recommended, with cognitive behavioral therapy as first-line therapy.

In some patients, a nonpharmacologic approach may not be enough to eliminate or improve symptoms to a point where the patient is functional. Currently, there are no FDA-approved medications for POTS, but medications may be considered for symptomatic relief. If patients are hypovolemic or hypotensive, fludrocortisone or midodrine may be used. Fludrocortisone expands intravascular volume and temporarily increases peripheral vascular resistance. The recommended dose is 0.1 to 0.2 mg PO daily. Midodrine is a short acting alpha agonist that reduces peripheral blood pooling. The usual dose is 2.5 mg to 10 mg by mouth three times a day (PO TID). A beta-blocker is often helpful in patients with tachycardia. Beta blockers help reduce inappropriate tachycardia and improve orthostatic intolerance, exercise tolerance, and the hyperadrenergic state. Popular choices include atenolol, propranolol, and metoprolol. In some cases, ivabradine has been used for inappropriate tachycardia, but insurance coverage issues have limited the use of this medication. This medication works by blocking the channel responsible for cardiac pacemaker current and reduces heart rate. Pyridostigmine is a reversible ace cholinesterase inhibitor that improves orthostatic heart rates and clinical symptoms. Usual doses are 30 to 60 mg PO TID. Droxidopa is a medication typically used for Parkinson's disease and works on the neurotransmitter norepinephrine to cause vasoconstriction. Doses range from 100 mg PO TID to up to 600 mg PO TID based on blood pressures and symptoms. SSRIs are helpful both for the anxiety component of the syndrome but also to improve vasoconstriction by stimulating nerve communication. Common choices include fluoxetine and sertraline. For brain fog, methylphenidate, a long acting alpha agonist releases catecholamine in the synapses and may improve symptoms. Additionally, it improves fatigue and presyncope. Typical doses are 10 mg to up to 30 mg by mouth twice a day (PO BID).[25–27]

SUMMARY

Cardiac arrhythmia in pediatric patients with Covid-19 or post-Covid 19 condition requires accurate diagnosis and treatment for the prevention of tachycardia-induced cardiomyopathy, SCA, and death. Some patient populations are at increased risk for lethal arrhythmia, including those with Covid-19 myocarditis, MIS-C with coronary involvement, congenital heart disease, history of cardiac surgery, and IAS. Screening, surveillance, and prevention of SCD from arrhythmia in pediatric patients with a clinical history of Covid-19 starts in the office of the primary care provider/pediatrician with proper review of symptoms, family history, and physical examination.

CLINICS CARE POINTS

- Cardiac arrhythmias can occur because of coronavirus disease 2019 (Covid-19) and post-Covid-19 condition.
- Covid-19 associated arrhythmias in pediatric patients are related to multisystem inflammatory syndrome in children, myocarditis, congenital heart disease, and inherited arrhythmia syndromes (IAS).
- Pediatric patients may not present with typical respiratory symptoms of Covid-19, but Covid-19 may be considered in the pediatric patient with exercise induced chest pain, dyspnea with exertion, palpitations, or syncope.
- Special populations at risk for sudden cardiac arrest from Covid arrhythmias include student athletes with myocarditis and patients with undiagnosed IAS.
- Proper screening, diagnosis and treatment of Covid-19 arrhythmia are imperative to reduce risk of death from lethal arrhythmia.
- Some medications used to treat patients with Covid-19 are QT prolonging and pro-arrhythmic. They should be used with caution with close rhythm surveillance.
- Fever and some anti-arrhythmic medications may unmask Brugada pattern in patients with unknown SCN5A gene defects increasing risk of ventricular arrhythmia and death.

FUNDING

The authors have no funding sources related to the material presented.

DISCLOSURE

The authors do not have any financial or commercial conflicts.

REFERENCES

1. Kang M, Chippa V, An J. Viral myocarditis. [Updated 2023 nov 20]. In: StatPearls [Internet]. Treasure Island (FL): StatPearls Publishing; 2024. Available at: https://www.ncbi.nlm.nih.gov/books/NBK459259/.
2. Blauwet LA, Cooper LT. Myocarditis. Prog Cardiovasc Dis 2010;52(4):274–88.
3. Boehmer TK, Kompaniyets L, Lavery AM, et al. Association between COVID-19 and myocarditis using hospital-based administrative data - United States, March 2020-January 2021. MMWR Morb Mortal Wkly Rep 2021;70(35):1228–32.
4. Ammirati E, Lupi L, Palazzini M, et al. Prevalence, characteristics, and outcomes of COVID-19–associated acute myocarditis. Circulation 2022;145:1123–39.
5. Hajjo R, Sabbah DA, Bardaweel SK, et al. Shedding the light on post-vaccine myocarditis and pericarditis in COVID-19 and non-COVID-19 vaccine recipients. Vaccines (Basel) 2021;9(10):1186.
6. Fairweather D, Beetler DJ, Di Florio DN, et al. COVID-19, myocarditis and pericarditis. CircRes 2023.
7. Marchand G, Masoud AT, Medi S. Risk of all-cause and cardiac-related mortality after vaccination against COVID-19: a meta-analysis of self-controlled case series studies. Hum Vaccines Immunother 2023;19(2):2230828.
8. Boehmer TK, Kompaniyets L, Lavery AM, et al. Association between COVID-19 and myocarditis using hospital-based administrative data - United States, March 2020-January 2021. MMWR Morb Mortal Wkly Rep 2021;70:1228–32.
9. Altman NL, Berning AA, Mann SC, et al. Vaccination-associated myocarditis and myocardial injury. CIRCRESAHA 2023;132:1338–57.
10. Hviid A, Nieminen TA, Pihlström N, et al. Booster vaccination with SARS-CoV-2 mRNA vaccines and myocarditis in adolescents and young adults: a Nordic cohort study. Eur Heart J 2024;45:1327–35.
11. Rassi CE, Zareef R, Honeini R, et al. Multisystem inflammatory syndrome in children: another covid-19 sequel. Cardiol Young 2023;1–11.
12. Johnson PT, Fishman EK. CT angiography of coronary artery aneurysms: detection, definition, causes, and treatment. Am J Roentgenol 2010;195(4):928–34.
13. Lee YJ, Park KS, Kil HR. Change of coronary artery indices according to coronary dominance pattern in early childhood. Korean J Pediatr 2019;62(6):240–3.
14. Choi HJ. Importance of coronary artery dominance in children to determine coronary artery dilatation. Korean J Pediatr 2019;62(6):215–6.
15. Dionne A, Hanna B, Trinh Tan F, et al. Importance of anatomical dominance in the evaluation of coronary dilatation in Kawasaki disease. Cardiol Young 2016;27(5):877–83.
16. Aricatt DP, Prabhu A, Avadhani R, et al. A study of coronary dominance and its clinical significance. Folia Morphol 2023;82(1):102–7.
17. Dodge JT, Brown BG, Bolson EL, et al. Lumen diameter of normal human coronary arteries. influence of age, sex, anatomic variation, and left ventricular hypertrophy or dilation. Circulation 1992;86(1):232–46.

18. Choi JY, Yun YS, Noh CI, et al. Dimension of normal coronary arteries determined by cross-sectional echocardiography. J Korean Pediatr Soc 1992;35:1336–42.

19. Tan TH, Wong KY, Cheng TK, et al. Coronary normograms and the coronary-aorta index: objective determinants of coronary artery dilatation. Pediatr Cardiol 2003; 24(4):328–35.

20. Sakamoto S, Takahashi S, Coskun AU, et al. Relation of distribution of coronary blood flow volume to coronary artery dominance. Am J Cardiol 2013;111(10): 1420–4.

21. Acholonu C, Cohen E, Afzal SY, et al. Multisystem inflammatory syndrome in children. Pediatr Ann 2023;52(3).

22. Karki R, Sharma B, Tuladhar S, et al. Synergism of TNF-α and IFN-γ triggers inflammatory cell death, tissue damage, and mortality in SARS-CoV-2 infection and cytokine shock syndromes. Cell 2021;184(1):149–68.e17.

23. Beyerstedt S, Casaro EB, Rangel EB. COVID-19: angiotensin-converting enzyme 2 (ACE2) expression and tissue susceptibility to SARS-CoV-2 infection. Eur J Clin Microbiol Infect Dis 2021.

24. Liu X, Lou L, Zhou L. Molecular mechanisms of cardiac injury associated with myocardial SARS-CoV-2 infection. Front Cardiovasc Med 2022.

25. Williams J, Jacobs H, Lee S. Pediatric myocarditis. Cardiol Ther Jun 2023;12(2): 243–60.

26. Vernino S, Bourne K, Stiles L, et al. Postural orthostatic tachycardia syndrome (POTS): state of the science and clinical care from a 2019 National Institutes of Health Expert Consensus Meeting - Part 1. Auton Neurosci 2021;235:102828. ISSN 1566-0702.

27. Mallick D, Goyal L, Prabal C, et al. COVID-19 induced postural orthostatic tachycardia syndrome (POTS): a review. Cureus 2023;15(3):e36955.

The Great Cardiac Pretenders

Takotsubo Cardiomyopathy, Lyme Carditis, and Cryptogenic Stroke

Michael G. DePalma, DMSc, MHS, PA-C, DFAAPA

KEYWORDS

- Takotsubo cardiomyopathy • Lyme carditis • Complete heart block
- Cryptogenic stroke • Embolic stroke of undetermined etiology • Cardiology

KEY POINTS

- Takotsubo cardiomyopathy is a transient cardiomyopathy that can present as an acute coronary syndrome.
- Lyme disease can affect the atrioventricular node, resulting in a first, second, or complete heart block.
- Cryptogenic ischemic strokes in younger populations can be caused by a right-to-left shunt.

INTRODUCTION

Cardiac conditions present challenges for clinicians due to the extensive differential diagnoses that must be considered. After emergent and acute coronary protocols are followed and patients are stabilized, underlying causes are frequently attributed to known risk factors and common anomalies experienced by the general population. Although we consider more obscure causes for many cardiovascular conditions, several mechanisms are given less consideration due to their ability to closely mimic more common conditions. The following cases are examples of a few of the "great pretenders" in cardiology that present with classic clinical manifestations but have less common etiologies.

Patients presenting with clinical manifestations consistent with acute coronary syndrome (ACS) or cardiac arrhythmias often undergo a workup, including a diagnostic or therapeutic coronary angioplasty. When diagnostic findings are inconsistent with the typical cardiac causes, such as no occlusive vessel disease during heart

Master of Science in Biomedical Science Program, Department of Physician Assistant Studies, A. T. Still University – Arizona School of Health Sciences, 5850 E. Still Circle, Mesa, AZ 85206, USA
E-mail address: michaeldepalma@atsu.edu

Physician Assist Clin 10 (2025) 371–380
https://doi.org/10.1016/j.cpha.2024.11.009   physicianassistant.theclinics.com

Abbreviations	
ACS	acute coronary syndrome
AV	atrioventricular
BP	blood pressure
CT	computed tomography
CVA	cerebrovascular accident
ECG	electrocardiogram
ED	emergency department
EF	ejection fraction
ELISA	enzyme-linked immunosorbent assay
HR	Heart rate
IV	intravenous
LV	left ventricular
MI	myocardial infarction
PFO	patent foramen ovale
SILC	Suspicious Index in Lyme Carditis
TCM	Takotsubo cardiomyopathy

catheterization or no arrhythmias with telemetry, less common cardiac and noncardiac etiologies should be considered. The clinical presentation, diagnostic approach, and management of the conditions discussed are based on the cause. Takotsubo cardiomyopathy (TCM), Lyme carditis, and cryptogenic stroke were chosen to highlight atypical diagnoses because of their ability to mimic common cardiac anomalies. These cases are intended to increase awareness and review management after emergent or critical causes have been identified and treated.

CASE 1

A 64 year old female patient with a history of depression and hypertension presented to the emergency department with chest pain that began 30 minutes prior to arrival. She described the pain as midsternal, radiating to her neck and jaw, which started shortly after her primary care provider informed her that a recent biopsy following a colonoscopy was positive for cancer.

Medications: sertraline 100 mg daily, lisinopril 20 mg daily.

Allergies: no known allergies (NKA).

Past medical history: Hypertension and depression.

Family history: Coronary artery disease, hypertension, colon cancer, and diabetes mellitus.

Surgical history: Colonoscopy 1 week ago, tubal ligation.

Social history: Married with 2 sons in good health. Plays pickleball 3 times per week and walks 3 to 5 miles, 3 times per week. Drinks 1 to 2 glasses of wine 2 to 3 days per week. Denies tobacco or recreational drug use.

Cardiac Workup

- *EKG*: ST-segment elevation in leads V2 to V4, T-wave inversion in leads I, AVL, and V5 to V6
- *Chest radiography*: No acute radiographic cardiopulmonary processes
- *Serum troponin*: 3.2 ng/mL (normal range <0.04)
- *N-terminal pro-B-type natriuretic peptide (NT-proBNP)*: 750 pg/mL (normal <125 pg/mL for people aged under 75 years)

Cardiology was consulted, and the patient underwent a heart catheterization.

- *Coronary angiography with left ventriculography*: Significant mid-anterior and apical segment akinesis. Ejection fraction (EF) 30%. Coronary arteries are unremarkable, with no evidence of plaque or luminal stenosis.

Diagnosis: Takotsubo cardiomyopathy

Introduction. TCM is a stress-induced cardiomyopathy that is often referred to as "broken heart syndrome" and is characterized by an acute transient left ventricular (LV) systolic dysfunction.[1] Commonly triggered by emotional or physical stress, TCM can cause symptoms of chest pain, ST-segment elevation on electrocardiogram (ECG), and elevated cardiac biomarkers often associated with ACS.[2,3] Despite the similarity with ACS findings, cardiac angiography in patients with TCM finds no evidence of coronary stenosis or occlusion as a cause for the symptoms.[4] The transient LV dysfunction caused by TCM is often reversible; however, clinicians should be familiar with the potential complications and management strategies for patients with TCM.

EPIDEMIOLOGY

The actual incidence of TCM is unknown, but 1% to 2% of patients with TCM are suspected of having ACS. TCM can occur in any age group; however, it is more predominant in postmenopausal female individuals.[1,5,6] Common triggers contributing to TCM include emotional (eg, natural disasters, loss of a loved one, and traumatic event) and physical triggers (surgical procedures, motor vehicle crashes, and critical illness), which are thought to be associated with an increase in catecholamine.[3,5] Although emotional stressors contribute to a small number of cases of TCM, the overall incidence is increasing, purported to coincide with rising rates of stress and anxiety in society.[1] Individuals with a history of anxiety and depression have a higher risk for TCM, although there has been no association with genetic predisposition.[1,5]

CLINICAL MANIFESTATIONS AND DIAGNOSTIC APPROACH

The clinical presentation of TCM is chest pain, often similar to myocardial infarction (MI) location and distribution, requiring ACS protocols to be followed.[2] In the acute setting, the ECG often indicates widespread ST-segment elevation, moderate cardiac troponin elevation, and marked B-type natriuretic peptide (BNP) elevation.[1] The bloodwork of patients presenting with MI often reveals markedly elevated serum troponin and moderately increased BNP, which remains elevated longer than TCM.[4] Patients undergo coronary angiography for a definitive diagnosis, whereby TCM can be confirmed by findings consistent with a lack of coronary obstruction, the presence of midanterior or apical segment akinesis, and decreased EF.[3,5] In the absence of coronary angioplasty, transthoracic echocardiography performed acutely demonstrates apical and mid-ventricular wall motion hypokinesis or akinesis and decreased LV function, as well as identification of potential thrombus formation from apical dysfunction.[3]

COMPLICATIONS

The risk of complications in hospitalized patients with TCM is similar to that of acute MI.[6] Although LV dysfunction improves in most patients with TCM, and treatment mostly requires supportive care, approximately 20% of patients with TCM can have acute and potentially life-threatening complications.[3,5] These include hypotension and cardiogenic shock from a decrease in cardiac output and systolic function.[5]

Cardiac arrhythmias, including ventricular arrhythmias (eg, torsades de pointes and ventricular fibrillation) and atrial fibrillation, can occur in up to 25% of patients with TCM and are managed based on arrhythmia treatment protocols.[5] TCM patients with hypokinesis or akinesis of the apex have an increased risk of thromboembolic development, requiring short-term anticoagulation therapy.[5]

MANAGEMENT

As TCM is a transient condition, management is supportive and primarily based on treating complications arising from cardiogenic shock, LV thrombus, or acute heart failure.[3] Outpatient continuation of angiotensin-converting enzyme inhibitors, angiotensin II receptor blockers, beta blockers, and/or diuretics is recommended for 3 months or until the LV function has recovered.[3,5] Anticoagulation for a confirmed LV thrombus should be continued for 3 months or until the thrombus resolves.[3] In patients with known coronary artery disease, statin and aspirin therapy should be used for secondary prevention.[3]

PROGNOSIS AND RECURRENCE

Although TCM is more prevalent in postmenopausal women, male individuals with TCM have a worse prognosis.[6] The prognosis of patients with TCM is dependent on the underlying cause and is worse when associated with physical triggers in a hospital setting and dependent on the occurrence of complications.[6] Additionally, the presence of LV thrombus is associated with an increased mortality and a poorer prognosis.[5] Recurrence of TCM is uncommon but occurs between 3 months and 13 years and follows similar triggers with a different morphology.[5]

CASE DISCUSSION

The patient presented to the emergency department (ED) with chest pain, and the initial workup for ACS included an ECG with ST-elevation in anterior leads. Cardiac markers revealed a slight elevation of serum troponin with a marked elevation of BNP, which is more consistent with TCM than MI. Coronary angiography confirmed the diagnosis of TCM; however, clinician suspicion should be raised based on the patient recently undergoing a physical trigger (ie, colonoscopy) and an emotional trigger when she received the biopsy results. Additional risk factors for this patient that support TCM include a postmenopausal female individual with a history of anxiety and depression.

CASE 2

A 28 year old male individual with no previous medical history presents to the ED following a near syncopal episode that occurred prior to arrival. The patient admits to having mild chest pressure, palpitations, shortness of breath, fatigue, joint aches, and lightheadedness that began that morning. He states he is in good physical shape overall and was camping 2 weeks ago in Pennsylvania. He denies any recent illnesses, recreational drug use, or tobacco products. On examination, the patient is diaphoretic and appears anxious; a concentric rash with central clearing is noted on the back of the patient's neck.

Vital signs: Heart rate (HR) 40 beats per minute, blood pressure (BP) 90/60 mm/Hg, T 102.6 F.

Medications: None.

Allergies: NKA.

Past medical history: Denies past medical history, including cardiac.
Family history: No history of cardiac conditions or early death.
Surgical history: None.
Social history: Physically active. Occasional alcohol use (1–2 times per week). Denies tobacco products or recreational drug use. Enjoys outdoor activities, including camping, fishing, and hiking.

Cardiac Workup

- *EKG*: Third degree heart block
- *Chest radiography*: No active disease
- *Serum troponin*: 0.12 ng/mL

Treatment

ACS protocol was initiated, and no cardiac etiology was identified. Cardiology was consulted for a temporary pacemaker. An immunoglobulin M/immunoglobulin G enzyme-linked immunosorbent assay (ELISA) was obtained. Ceftriaxone 2 g intravenous (IV) daily was ordered.
Diagnosis: Complete heart block secondary to presumptive Lyme carditis.

INTRODUCTION

The most common vector-borne disease in the United States is Lyme disease, caused by infection with the spirochete *Borrelia burgdorferi*.[7] Early disease often presents with an annular rash with central clearing, known as *erythema migrans*, fever, and fatigue.[7] However, the spirochete responsible for Lyme disease can cause multisystem disease, including carditis.[8] During a systemic infection, *B burgdorferi* can directly penetrate myocardial tissue, causing a subsequent exaggerated inflammatory response.[9] Although Lyme carditis can cause myocarditis, pericarditis, endocarditis, and dilated cardiomyopathy, the most common manifestation involves the conduction system, with the atrioventricular (AV) node being the most prominent location affected.[8,9] The incidence of Lyme carditis had previously been estimated between 4% and 10% in the United States; however, earlier recognition and prompt treatment of Lyme disease is thought to be decreasing the occurrence of Lyme carditis.[10] Despite a low incidence of carditis, cases of Lyme disease continue to rise annually, which necessitates clinician awareness. Revised surveillance definitions by the Centers for Disease Control and Prevention revealed a greater than 68% increase in Lyme disease cases in 2022, with 62,551 compared with the annual average number of cases reported from 2017 to 2019, 37,118.[7] Therefore, cardiac complaints in patients presenting with clinical signs and symptoms consistent with Lyme disease (ie, fever, arthralgia, and rash), the patient's geographic location, and consideration of outdoor activities should raise provider suspicion to include Lyme carditis in the cardiac differential diagnosis.

CLINICAL MANIFESTATIONS AND DIAGNOSTIC APPROACH

The constitutional symptoms often associated with Lyme disease include fever, malaise, and arthralgia, corresponding with a history of a tick bite and a rash with central clearing.[11] In addition, patients who develop Lyme carditis most commonly experience an AV block that may cause syncope, presyncope, palpitations, chest pressure, and dyspnea.[11] In addition to the ACS workup that patients with chest pain typically undergo, in the presence of Lyme constitutional symptoms, the Suspicious Index in Lyme Carditis (SILC) tool can be used by a clinician to determine the likelihood of a high-degree heart block being caused by Lyme carditis.[11] A single point is given for age less than 50 years, male sex, associated outdoor activity, or location in an endemic area. Any Lyme constitutional symptom scores 2 points, the presence of a tick bite scores 3 points, and the presence of an erythema migrans scores 4 points.[11] The total score is associated with the suspicion of Lyme carditis: 0 to 2 is low, 3 to 6 is intermediate, and 7 to 12 is high.[11] Lyme ELISA is reliable for detecting the antibodies for B burgdorferi; however, the initiation of antibiotic therapy should not be delayed while awaiting the results of confirmatory tests.

MANAGEMENT

In the acute presentation of Lyme carditis, AV block is present in 90% of cases and may resolve spontaneously.[9,12] Despite this, empiric IV antibiotics should be initiated in patients with an intermediate or high SILC score in the presence of high-degree AV block and constitutional symptoms while awaiting serologic testing.[12] Ceftriaxone is the first-line IV therapy, and if serologic testing confirms Lyme disease, oral treatment includes doxycycline, amoxicillin, or cefuroxime for 14 to 21 days of total antibiotic therapy.[12] Patients presenting with lower degree AV block can rapidly progress to a third-degree heart block or asystole; therefore, like patients with high-degree AV block, they should be admitted with cardiac monitoring.[12] Symptomatic bradycardia or hemodynamic instability associated with high-degree AV block are generally considered reversible and should be treated with a transvenous temporary pacemaker, which is required in approximately one-third of patients with Lyme carditis.[9,11]

PROGNOSIS AND RECURRENCE

High-degree AV block due to Lyme disease most often resolves with early recognition and appropriate antibiotic therapy, and patients do not usually experience recurrent conduction abnormalities.[9] The persistence of AV conduction abnormalities has rarely been described after treatment and reversal of the AV block.[11] Although little data regarding long-term outcomes have been reported, prompt treatment suggests the restoration of normal AV function, and patients with Lyme carditis have an excellent prognosis.[11]

CASE DISCUSSION

Proper ACS protocols should always be followed when patients have AV block and present with constitutional symptoms. However, a concurrent consideration for the cause should include Lyme carditis when patients experience associated fever, myalgias, arthralgias, erythema migrans, or a confirmed tick bite. Although the patient did not present with the complaint of a fever, a review of vital signs indicates an elevated temperature. The history of outdoor activities in an area endemic for Lyme disease should also raise suspicion for Lyme carditis. As the AV block associated with Lyme disease is reversible, an early initiation of antibiotics can effectively treat Lyme carditis without long-term complications.

CASE 3

A 29 year old male patient presents to the office for follow-up after discharge from the hospital for an ischemic cerebrovascular accident (CVA). The patient states he is currently training for a triathlon and prior to his admission, he was lifting weights at the gym when he experienced a sudden onset of left-sided weakness and facial drooping, slurred speech, and partial vision loss in both eyes. He denied a headache or neck pain before the onset of symptoms and has never experienced similar symptoms in the past. He also denied chest pain, palpitations, or fluttering.

Hospital course: The patient was transported to the ED from the gym via advanced life support. A computed tomographic (CT) scan on arrival was negative for intracranial hemorrhage and, with all criteria appropriately met, the patient received thrombolytic therapy. Continuous telemetry monitoring during the admission showed normal sinus rhythm without atrial or ventricular arrhythmia. A transesophageal echocardiogram performed during the hospitalization revealed a patent foramen ovale (PFO) with a right-to-left shunt and no identifiable thrombus. Anticoagulation and antiplatelet therapies were coordinated at discharge, and the patient is continuing both medications.

Vital signs: HR 54 bpm, BP 116/62 mm/Hg, T 98.6 F, respiratory rate (RR) 16 PM, oxygen saturation (SpO$_2$) 99%

Medications: None.

Allergies: NKA.

Past medical history: Denies past medical history.

Family history: No history of CVA.

Surgical history: None.

Social history: Physically active. Currently training for a triathlon. Denies tobacco products or recreational drug use.

Diagnosis: Cryptogenic stroke likely secondary to PFO.

INTRODUCTION

According to the American Stroke Association, ischemic strokes account for approximately 87% of all strokes, and roughly 1 in 3 ischemic strokes has no definitive identifiable cause.[13,14] Strokes of unknown origin for which no cause can be identified after a thorough diagnostic workup (ie, echocardiography, cardiac monitoring, CT/MRI, or angiography) are known as cryptogenic strokes.[15,16] Approximately 10% to 15% of all strokes occur at younger ages, and the rate of strokes among individuals 25 to 44 years has been rapidly increasing.[17,18] Most cryptogenic ischemic strokes are associated with right-to-left shunts, and up to half of young adults with cryptogenic stroke have been found to have a PFO.[16] Early recognition of potential causes and identification of risk factors of cryptogenic stroke is essential in reducing reoccurrences and optimizing treatment.[17]

RISK FACTORS AND DIAGNOSTIC APPROACH

In addition to overall risk factors for atherosclerotic disease, younger populations experiencing cryptogenic ischemic strokes should be screened for arrhythmia (eg, atrial fibrillation), cardiac embolism (eg, septal abnormalities and PFO), hypercoagulable conditions (eg, malignancy and antiphospholipid syndrome), and intravenous drug use.[16] As cryptogenic strokes are essentially a diagnosis of exclusion, a detailed history and physical examination can guide the strategy for the diagnostic approach.[16] Without an identifiable cause of cryptogenic stroke, the approach to the workup should include a transesophageal echocardiogram, which is important for evaluating potential sources of right-to-left shunt, such as a PFO or atrial septal defect.[15] A Holter monitor or long-term outpatient cardiac telemetry should also be ordered to screen for paroxysmal atrial fibrillation or flutter.[15] Laboratory analysis should focus on hypercoagulability studies and infectious, autoimmune, and inflammatory causes of vasculopathy.[15] As cryptogenic strokes have a high rate of recurrence, the differential diagnosis should be broad and thorough for appropriate treatment and prevention.[19]

MANAGEMENT

Treatment of cryptogenic ischemic strokes should focus on secondary stroke prevention and reduction of risk factors. Antiplatelet therapy continues to be the preferred treatment; however, multiple clinical trials suggest that anticoagulation may be preferential due to its efficacy with venous thromboembolism and atrial fibrillation.[20] Antiplatelet and/or anticoagulation therapy should be continued while awaiting the results of long-term cardiac monitoring.[21] In younger patients in whom a PFO is detected, PFO closure should only be considered after a thorough evaluation has eliminated alternative mechanisms of cryptogenic stroke.[20]

CASE DISCUSSION

The young patient presenting for follow-up from a cryptogenic ischemic stroke is at high-risk for a secondary event. Although PFO is common in younger populations, the presence of a PFO should not bias the clinician as to the potential cause of the cryptogenic stroke. Following hospital discharge, the patient requires an extensive evaluation and workup to determine modifiable risk factors. A thorough review of medical, family, and social histories should focus on intravenous drug use, malignancies, coagulopathies, and vasculopathies. In addition, the lack of atrial or ventricular arrhythmia does not exclude the possibility of occult paroxysmal atrial fibrillation, which should be evaluated with a long-term event recorder or telemetry monitoring. Antiplatelet and/or anticoagulation therapy should be continued, and PFO closure may be considered for this patient if a cause is not identified.

SUMMARY

Patients presenting with common cardiac complaints should receive emergent medical treatment as appropriate. However, when diagnostic findings do not support a common etiology, clinicians should be aware of many conditions that can mimic classic presentations. Takotsubo cardiomyopathy, Lyme carditis, and cryptogenic stroke are 3 cases that can "pretend" to present as different cardiac etiologies. Increased awareness of their clinical presentations, epidemiologic characteristics, and prognosis can lead to earlier recognition and appropriate management.

CLINICS CARE POINTS

- Takotsubo cardiomyopathy is more prevalent in post-menopausal females, and increasing rates are thought to be associated with emotional and physical triggers.
- Atrioventricular block caused by Lyme carditis is transient; early recognition and treatment can restore normal atrioventricular function.
- The risk of secondary events in patients with an initial cryptogenic ischemic stroke is high and requires a work-up and determination of modifiable risk factors.

DISCLOSURE

No disclosures.

REFERENCES

1. Singh T, Khan H, Gamble DT, et al. Takotsubo syndrome: pathophysiology, emerging concepts, and clinical implications. Circulation 2022;145(13): 1002–19. Accessed April 15, 2024.
2. Templin C, Ghadri JR, Diekmann J, et al. Clinical features and outcomes of takotsubo (stress) cardiomyopathy. N Engl J Med 2015;373(10):929–38. Accessed April 15, 2024.
3. Assad J, Femia G, Pender P, et al. Takotsubo syndrome: a review of presentation, diagnosis, and management. Clin Med Insights Cardiol 2022;16. https://doi.org/10.1177/11795468211065782. Accessed April 15, 2024.
4. Merchant EE, Johnson SW, Nguyen P, et al. Takotsubo cardiomyopathy: a case series and review of the literature. West J Emerg Med 2008;9(2):104–11. Available at: https://www.ncbi.nlm.nih.gov/pmc/articles/PMC2672240/. Accessed April 15, 2024.
5. Lynch M, editor. Takotsubo cardiomyopathy: risk factors, management and long-term Outlook. Nova Science Publishers; 2016.
6. Ahmad SA, Brito D, Khalid N, et al. Takotsubo cardiomyopathy. In: StatPearls. Treasure Island. StatPearls Publishing; 2024. Available at: https://www.ncbi.nlm.nih.gov/books/NBK430798/. Accessed April 15, 2024.
7. Kugeler KJ, Earley A, Mead PS, et al. Surveillance for Lyme disease after implementation of a revised case definition – United States, 2022. MMWR Morb Mortal Wkly Rep 2024;73:118–23. Accessed April 15, 2024.
8. Rivera OJ, Nookala V. Lyme carditis. In: StatPearls. Treasure Island. StatPearls Publishing; 2023. Available at: https://www.ncbi.nlm.nih.gov/books/NBK546587. Accessed April 15, 2024.
9. Baranchuk A, Wamboldt R, Want CN. Lyme carditis: from A to Z. Springer Publishing; 2023.
10. Radesich C, Del Mestre E, Medo K, et al. Lyme carditis: from pathophysiology to clinical management. Pathogens 2022;11(5):582. PMID: 35631104; PMCID: PMC9145515. Accessed April 15, 2024.
11. Yeung C, Baranchuk A. Systemic approach to the diagnosis and treatment of Lyme carditis and high-degree atrioventricular block. Healthcare 2018;6(4):119. Accessed April 15, 2024.
12. Radesich C, Baranchuk A. Diagnosis and treatment of Lyme carditis. J Am Coll Cardiol 2019;73(6):717–26. Accessed April 15, 2024.
13. Ischemic Stroke. American stroke association. 2024. Available at: https://www.stroke.org/en/about-stroke/types-of-stroke/ischemic-stroke-clots. Accessed April 15, 2024.
14. Cryptogenic Stroke or Stroke of Unknown Cause. American stroke association. 2024. Available at: https://www.stroke.org/en/about-stroke/types-of-stroke/cryptogenic-stroke. Accessed April 15, 2024.
15. Yaghi S, Elkind MSV. Cryptogenic stroke. Neurol Clin Pract 2014;4(5):386–93. Accessed April 15, 2024.
16. Saver JL. Cryptogenic stroke. N Engl J Med 2016;374(21):2065–74. Accessed April 15, 2024.
17. Ekker MS, Verhoeven JI, Schellekens MMI, et al. Risk factors and causes of ischemic stroke in 1322 young adults. Stroke 2023;54(2):439–47. Accessed April 15, 2024.
18. Bhatt N, Malik AM, Chaturvedi S. Stroke in young adults. Neurol Clin Pract 2018; 8(6):501–6. Accessed April 15, 2024.

19. Serhal M. Evaluation of cryptogenic stroke. American College of Cardiology 2019. Available at: https://www.acc.org/Latest-in-Cardiology/Articles/2019/10/10/23/20/Evaluation-of-Cryptogenic-Stroke#:~:text=Cryptogenicstrokesaccountfor%2015, diagnosedwithanewstroke. Accessed April 15, 2024.
20. Messe SR, Gronseh GS, Kent DM, et al. Practice advisory update summary: patient foramen ovale and secondary stroke prevention. Neurology 2020;94(20): 876–85. Accessed April 15, 2024.
21. Zhang C, Kasner S. Diagnosis, prognosis, and management of cryptogenic stroke. F1000Res 2016;5. F1000 Faculty Rev-168. Accessed April 15, 2024.

Social Determinants of Health

Let's Get to the Heart of the Matter

Camille J. Dyer, DMSc, PA-C, AACC, DFAAPA

KEYWORDS

- Health disparities • Health equity • Racial inequities
- Social determinants of health (SDOH) • Hypertension • Cardiovascular mortality
- Social construct of race • Black and hispanic health disparities

KEY POINTS

- Health disparities refer to the differences in health outcomes and their fundamental causes among different groups of people, as it relates to disease prevalence, mortality rates, and access to care.
- Regardless of race, background, or social status, health equity is enables everyone to have the opportunity to achieve their full health and well-being potential.
- Barriers such as economic inequalities, social disadvantages, and discrimination must be eradicated to achieve health equity and improve health care access.
- For justice in health care to be achieved, systemic barriers that create inequities need to be removed, and underlying causes of disparities need to be addressed.
- Social determinants of health include economic stability, educational access and quality, health care access and quality, neighborhood and built environment, and social and community context.

INTRODUCTION

According to the Census Bureau, minority groups are 38% of the US population and it is anticipated by 2045 these groups will dominate. The largest members of this group are Blacks and Hispanics/LatinX. There is a discrepancy in life expectancy among minorities, and this is due to differences in cardiovascular mortality between the populations. Disparities in cardiovascular disease as well as cardiovascular disease are the leading cause of morbidity and mortality globally. It is a constant reminder of the impact social injustices and racial inequities have on physical and psychological well-being.

Constituent Organization, African Heritage PA Caucus, PO Box 741432, Boynton Beach, FL 33474, USA
E-mail addresses: camidyer@yahoo.com; camid10@gmail.com

Physician Assist Clin 10 (2025) 381–398
https://doi.org/10.1016/j.cpha.2024.11.013   physicianassistant.theclinics.com
2405-7991/25/© 2024 Elsevier Inc. All rights reserved, including those for text and data mining, AI training, and similar technologies.

Abbreviations	
ACC	American College of Cardiology
AMI	acute myocardial infarction
CABG	coronary artery bypass graft
CHAT	Community Health Advocate Training
CVD	cardiovascular disease
FIW	Federal Interagency Workgroup
HF	heart failure
HIV	human immunodeficiency virus
IT	information technology
MI	myocardial infarction
PTCA	percutaneous transluminal coronary angioplasty
SAVR	surgical aortic valve replacement
SDOH	social determinants of health
SES	socioeconomic status
SRH	self-rated health
TAVR	transcatheter aortic valve replacement

Since the George Floyd murder in the setting of the coronavirus disease 2019(COVID-19) pandemic, which disproportionately affected underrepresented communities, there has been an unprecedented reckoning on racism and social injustice. As a result, there has been a focus on disparities in health and health care. The social, cultural, and demographic constructs are important to this evaluation as providers strive to achieve health equity. Disparities in cardiovascular care must be addressed.

WHY IT MATTERS

"Health disparities are the differences in health outcomes and their causes among one group of people relative to another group of individuals."[1] Health equity is "when everyone can attain their full potential for health and well-being."[1]

Diversity, equity, and inclusion are the idea that all people should have equal rights and treatment.[2] All should be welcomed and included to avoid experiencing any disadvantage because of belonging to a particular group and each individual should be given the same opportunities as others according to their needs.[2]

Health equity is the state in which everyone has a fair and just opportunity to attain the highest level of health.[2] Achieving this requires focused and ongoing societal efforts to address historical and contemporary injustices to overcome economic, social, and other obstacles to health and health care and to eliminate health disparities.[2]

Equality is the assumption that everyone benefits from the same support. This is equal treatment.[2] However, everyone getting the support they need is equity and the goal of "affirmative action." Justice is the removal of systematic barriers and/or the removal of the etiology of the inequities.[2]

In addressing health care disparities, it is important to remember that race is a social construct.[3] Race is not a biological determinant of disease.[3] Furthermore, race and ethnicity are essentially a proxy for socioeconomic status (SES).[3] Drivers of disparities include implicit bias, stereotyping, and prejudice.[3] The impact of these issues within society influences health care outcomes across the lifespan.[3]

DISCUSSION

Upon close examination of working-age adults from 1990 to 2017, research suggests there have been over 4.8 million deaths attributed to cardiometabolic diseases.[4] Since

2010, all-cause mortality has increased, and it is believed that cardiometabolic diseases have significantly increased.[4] Members of underrepresented groups have additional barriers to cardiovascular disease (CVD) diagnosis and care, have implementation of suboptimal treatment strategies, and have more significant adverse outcomes than their White counterparts.[5] Mortality difference between Blacks and Whites is evident for both women and men.[3] Studies suggest there is about a 40% difference in mortality for Black women compared to White women and a 30% mortality difference between Black men and White men.[3] The difference is attributed to the disparities identified in CVD outcomes.[3] Although tremendous progress regarding the assessment and treatment of cardiovascular disease has occurred over the years, disparities persist, resulting in outcomes that are below expectations.

The Atherosclerosis Risk in Communities study was a prospective evaluation of atrial fibrillation.[5] The study revealed that Black individuals with atrial fibrillation had a higher incidence of not only stroke but heart failure, coronary heart disease, and mortality in comparison to the White study participants.[5]

In a study by Agarwal and colleagues, which explored familial hypercholesterolemia and racial differences in predictors of CVD, it became evident that Black individuals had an increased prevalence of modifiable risk factors such as smoking and hypertension.[3] This increase was not only due to the increased prevalence of obesity but also the increase in health disparities that can be attributed to the (SDOH which are influenced by an individual's social and environmental conditions.[4]

Hypertension is the leading preventable risk factor for heart disease and stroke, thus a major contributor to ethnic disparities in cardiovascular health. Additionally, pre-pregnancy hypertension and hypertensive disorders of pregnancy show an increased risk of maternal heart failure within 5 years of delivery.[3,5] The impact of cardiovascular disease risk burden significantly affects women of childbearing age.[3] It not only affects the mother, but there are long-term implications for the children who may also experience earlier onset of CVD.[3]

Nonischemic cardiomyopathy has a higher incidence and lower survival in Black individuals, yet fewer of those individuals are referred to transplant. Black patients with hypertrophic cardiomyopathy are more likely to present with heart failure (HF) but are less commonly referred for evidence-based interventions that increase survival. An understanding as to why Black adults have the highest risk of HF, typically present with an earlier onset of disease and have the highest risk of hospitalizations and death compared to White patients, is imperative. In 2017, the age-adjusted heart failure -cardiovascular deaths (HF-CV) deaths were 2.60-fold higher in Black men and 2.97-fold higher in Black women. Hispanic/LatinX patients were also noted to have a higher risk of HF.

Published data show Black patients are less likely to receive guideline-concordant care before an acute myocardial infarction (MI) and after coronary revascularization, and are at high risk for adverse outcomes, including recurrent MI, rehospitalization, and, in most studies, sudden death.[6] A study posed the question of whether race serves as a surrogate for socioeconomic status and, if adjusted for, would the discrepancy seen in the mortality of Black and White patients following an acute MI still be evident.[6] This is often referred to as propensity scoring. The study was limited to self-identified Black and White individuals.[6] Patient characteristics were assessed and divided into 8 domains.[6] The study attempted to determine what patient characteristics are associated with racial disparities.[6] Propensity scoring is routinely used in comparative effective research to statistically balance the characteristics of patients treated with one strategy versus another.[6] The analysis here is done using 2 observational registries (Prospective Registry Evaluation MI: Events and Recovery and

Translational Research Investigating Underlying Disparities in Acute MI Patients' Health Status) which prospectively collected data on patient's socioeconomic health, social support, psychological status, and treatment and examined how these characteristics differ by race.[6]

Black and White patients in the study were different in almost every domain.[6] The greatest difference was in socioeconomic status, followed by social history and medical history.[6] Once the propensity to be Black was identified, it revealed an overall 1-year mortality of 10.6% for Black patients and 5.8% for White patients.[6] The 5-year mortality was 28.9% for Black patients and 18.0% for White patients.[6] Essentially, there was a strong association between being a Black individual and increased risk of mortality regardless of patient race[6] Eradicating racial disparities in survival after MI must remain a national priority.[6]

Many studies show that SDOH can account for 30% to 35% of the health outcomes in patients. The risk of complications associated with coronary angiography is typically 1% to 3%. Imagine the impact if the risk from SDOH were reduced to 1% to 3%. These social constructs adversely affect many communities, and it is amazing how these constructs are so intimately intertwined.

The sequelae of health disparities can last for generations and are often perpetuated by personal and institutional discrimination and income inequality. Differences in health outcomes have been linked to social or economic disadvantages. To close the gap, the health care industry must address SDOH.

Implementing evidence-based care will not only improve health equity but will also impact other conditions that are of high cost to the health care system, such as repeat admissions for HF.[7] It has been shown that cardiovascular-attributable death rates have declined by 25.3% and cardiovascular deaths have decreased by 6.7%.[7] However, according to the Centers for Disease Control and Prevention, the decline in cardiovascular-related mortality has declined more slowly for the Black community than the White community. Data suggest a decline by 2.2% per year for Blacks and 2.4% per year for Whites.[7] Before 2010, the decline was 3.9% for Whites and 3.4% for Blacks.[7]

Disparities in cardiovascular care are seen in invasive cardiovascular medicine, with Black individuals less likely to undergo invasive procedures.[7] In 2002, the Institute of Medicine released a report examining the disparities in cardiac care and although subsequent evaluation from 2004 to 2014 has shown improvement for all populations, at the time of the report, it was noted that there was an approximately 50% lower rate of "necessary cardiovascular procedures in Blacks."[7] Invasive cardiac procedures in this reference are defined as cardiac catheterization, percutaneous transluminal coronary angioplasty (PTCA), coronary artery bypass graft (CABG), and implantation of defibrillators.[7] When evaluating PTCA amongst the different populations, the disparities persist. In an analysis by Pegus and colleagues, for those individuals with acute myocardial infarction (AMI) per 1000 patients per year, the procedure rate for White individuals was 83.03[7]; however, for Black individuals, it was 68.90.[7] Based on the extrapolation, the rate ratio is 1:21, which suggests there was a 21% higher procedure rate for Whites than Blacks.[7] To normalize the rate in the Black community to that of the White community, 20.5% more procedures would need to be performed on Black patients.[7] Pegus and colleagues not only evaluated this as it relates to AMI but also for individuals with intermediate coronary syndrome.[7] In this group, it was noted that the procedure rate per 1000 patients per year was 73.97 for White patients and 63.17 for Black patients.[7]

According to a study by Cram and colleagues, there is a 30% lower rate of coronary revascularization in Blacks hospitalized with acute myocardial infarction; furthermore,

Black patients are 50% less likely to undergo CABG.[7] These findings are evident despite controlling for age, disease severity, comorbidities, insurance status, and site of care.[7] Exploring the differences is imperative to continue to improve the care provided to patients.

Although there are limited data exploring the impact of disparities in care, there is evidence of a discrepancy in the care with aortic stenosis.[7] Studies suggest the prevalence of aortic stenosis is less in Black individuals, but this does not mean those individuals should not be entitled to the same care as members of other communities.[7] A study that evaluated surgical aortic valve replacement (SAVR) noted that 40.3% of White patients underwent the procedure whereas only 26.6% of Black patients underwent the procedure from 1999 to 2013.[7] Subsequent analysis from 2004 to 2010 revealed that 39% of Blacks underwent SAVR compared to 53% of White patients.[7]

The treatment strategy discrepancy persists when evaluating individuals who undergo transcatheter aortic valve replacement (TAVR).[7] A study by Holmes and colleagues revealed that 93% of Whites underwent TAVR and only 3.8% of Black patients underwent TAVR from 2012 to 2015.[7] It is important to note that even though members of the Black community are often deemed as higher risk, treatment with aortic valve replacement has shown similar 1-year and 3-year survival between both communities.[7]

A study that examined health and health care measures among racial and ethnic minorities identified differences in multiple measures.[8] In comparison to the White population, Blacks had 55 measures that were worse than their White counterparts and 12 measures that were better.[8] In looking at the Hispanic/LatinX community, 44 measures were worse and 22 were better. Examination of the Asian community identified 15 measures that were worse and 42 measures that were better.[8] Forty-three measures were worse, and 12 measures were better when the American Indian and Alaska Native community was assessed.[8] The final community explored was the Native Hawaiian and Other Pacific Islander community, in which 25 measures were worse and 5 were better.[8]

Low-income White people have health outcomes similar to high-income Black people.[1] Black women with college degrees have the same chance of having underweight or premature babies as White women without a high school education.

The impact of adversity on the health of patients continues to be studied, but it is suggested that there is a significant influence on the pathways that contribute to chronic inflammation.[4] Poverty/low socioeconomic status, increased noise exposure, food insecurity, unsafe housing, neighborhood violence, lack of educational opportunity, limited health care access, and decreased sleep quality are just a few of the chronic stressors that influence overall health.[4] These stressors enhance the production of catecholamines, dopamine, norepinephrine, and epinephrine as well as glucocorticoids.[4] The involved inflammatory pathways include impaired nuclear translocation of the glucocorticoid receptor as well as decreased antiinflammatory gene transcription.[4] The hypothalamic-pituitary-adrenal axis and the sympathoadrenomedullary axis can also be disrupted by chronic stress.[4] The disruption of these pathways also increases the signaling of the B-adrenergic receptors increasing the production of inflammatory cytokines.[4] There is also upregulation of B3 receptors which may contribute to the development of atherosclerotic plaque.[4] By default, these disrupted pathways impact obesity, hypertension, diabetes mellitus, and atherosclerosis thereby contributing to major adverse cardiovascular events and CVD mortality.[4]

Healthy People 2030

There are 359 core or measurable objectives as well as developmental and research objectives that comprise the components of Healthy People 2030.[9] The initiative consists of national objectives developed by subject matter experts, driven by data, and designed to improve health and well-being over the next decade.[9]

The *core objectives* focus on high-priority public health issues and have evidence-based interventions associated with them.[9] Their key components include that baseline statistics used are from 2015 onward to provide data for at least 3 time periods through the decade.[9] To assess the progress of these objectives, they are evaluated as baseline only, target met or exceeded, improving, little or no detectable change, and getting worse.[9]

Developmental objectives include high-priority public health issues that have evidence-based interventions, but reliable baseline data are not available.[9] These objectives are evaluated throughout the decade by the Federal Interagency Workgroup (FIW) to determine if baseline data become available, at which time they would be transitioned into core objectives.[9] The ability to transition is often evaluated in the context of how a developmental objective relates to core objectives.[9]

The *research objectives* are those that do not yet have evidence-based interventions but have either a high economic or high health burden on society or those with marked disparities between population groups.[9] A research objective will not become a core objective until there is reliable baseline data and evidence-based interventions.[9] The process involves the Healthy People workgroup making a formal recommendation to the FIW for the research objective to become a core objective.[9] The FIW will then consider how the research objective relates to the existing core objectives and then make a final decision.[9]

Changes to the objectives are identified as new, revised, archived, moved, or recategorized.[9] Objectives identified as new means that it was added to the Healthy People 2030 within the last year.[9] If an objective has been revised, it will be labeled as such and if it is archived, it means that it was retired from Healthy People 2030.[9] Objectives marked as moved now fall under the auspices of a different workgroup.[9] An objectives history can be reviewed in the Data Methodology and Measurement page.[9]

To assess the impact of SDOH, it is important to understand the lived personal experiences of vulnerable populations, which include not only ethnic minorities but those individuals who qualify as disabled, chronically ill, elderly, women, transgender, lesbian, gay, bisexual, and queer.[4] Lived experiences take into consideration implicit bias, and everyday discrimination, which not only includes racism but also sexism, homophobia, and stigma.[4] One's lived experience is also influenced by the neighborhood and perceptions of the neighborhood, health literacy, and social needs.[4] An individual may suffer social isolation and exclusion from these experiences thereby affecting not only psychological health but also physical health.[4]

A history of discrimination enables policies, laws, and practices to become part of society resulting in structural racism.[4] Structural racism essentially becomes a society's norm.[4] Analysis of these factors affects an individual's and/or community's access to resources.[4] State-level structural racism is influenced by political participation, judicial treatment, employment status, and educational achievement.[4] Research suggests that individuals who reside in states with significant amounts of structural racism are more likely to suffer from myocardial infarction than Black individuals who live in states that do not have as much structural racism.[4] This finding exists even after accounting for age, sex, education, household income, medical insurance, and state-level poverty.[4]

Residential segregation, also known as *redlining*, is just 1 form of structural racism. It was a program established by the government in the 1930s and enabled financial institutions to not provide lending options to those homes deemed in dangerous or hazardous neighborhoods. Many of these homes were in Black communities.[4] Studies suggest that individuals living in these neighborhoods have a 12% higher incidence of cardiovascular disease.[4]

Assessment of White populations compared to black individuals elucidated that there was 12% lower CVD for the White individuals even when adjustments were made for characteristics of the neighborhood. This includes poverty as well as residential segregation.[4] Redlining not only reduces employment opportunities which impacts economic status, but it also influences educational opportunities and access, as well as poverty, violence, and crime in the neighborhoods.[4] This does not even take into account the impact on intergenerational wealth.

In the Hispanic/LatinX community, segregation seemed to promote better health outcomes in those who are foreign-born but worse for those who are born in the United States.[4] It is believed this difference may be due to the foreign-born Hispanic/LatinX having more community/social support thereby providing some indirect protection from discrimination. US-born Mexicans and Puerto Ricans are more impacted by segregation than other Hispanic communities.[4] These findings are based on self-rated health (SRH) and suggest that social isolation in addition to segregation may have negative impacts on health.[4] Differences exist even within the Hispanic/LatinX community, and it is suggested that US-born Mexicans and Puerto Ricans are more impacted by segregation than other Hispanic communities.

Further examination of sub-groups elucidated differences within the Caribbean community as well.[4] Those individuals of Afro-Caribbean descent are more likely to have an improved SRH with increased residential concentration.[4] However, this is not the finding for the African Americans for whom an increased residential concentration resulted in a lower SRH score.[4]

Many studies suggest that SDOH can account for 30% to 35% of health outcomes.[1] These key influential factors include economic and social conditions that influence the health of people and their communities. Economic stability, educational access and quality, health care access and quality, neighborhood and built environment, and social and community context are instrumental in patients' and communities' physical and mental health. More specifically, these factors include the impact of early childhood development, social inclusion, and nondiscrimination, structural conflict. Also included are income and social protection, education, unemployment, job insecurity, working life conditions, food insecurity, housing with basic amenities, and environment.[1]

Social Determinants of Health

Economic stability

Economic stability includes employment, food insecurity, housing instability, and poverty. Employment status and occupational categories are important predictors of physical and psychosocial well-being. Negative impacts of these factors influence depression, hypertension, and diabetes mellitus.[10] Additionally, the consequences of poverty on brain development and performance in school are well known.

Studies suggest the impact of low socioeconomic status (SES) as a child influences the likelihood of cardiovascular events as an adult.[4] It is believed that chronic stress from an individual's financial situation creates a proinflammatory environment thereby leading to cardiovascular events.[4]

Further exploration of job security noted that Black and Hispanic/LatinX individuals are more likely to experience job insecurity and are also more likely to experience psychosocial occupational stressors such as low job control and high demands.[11]

It has been well established that the experience in the labor market for Black individuals has been very different from the experience of their White counterparts. The depth extends back to a time were Black-owned businesses were destroyed in 1921 with the riots on the Black Wall Street in Tulsa, Oklahoma, segregation, the Reconstruction period during the Civil Rights Era, the continued intentional exclusion of blacks from more secure jobs, and occupational segregation.[12] This is fostered by the higher unemployment rates in the Black community which can be attributed to discrimination, and limited educational opportunities thus fewer Black individuals graduating from college which can partially be attributed to challenges in obtaining the financial resources to attend college thus Black students often have more debt upon graduation.[12] Even in 2019, when the unemployment rate for both Black and White individuals significantly improved, for Black individuals over the age of 16, the unemployment rate was 5.5% whereas for White individuals, it was 3.2% which was a 50-year low.[12] These figures represent the lowest rate for those who identify as Black since 1973 and for Whites since 2000.[12] A difference is maintained regardless of the educational achievement of the worker. Evaluation between November 2018 and October 2019 revealed that Black college graduates had an unemployment rate of 2.8% and 2.0% for White college graduates, essentially representing a 40% difference.[12] Additionally, despite educational achievement, Black workers are subject not only to unequal pay but also experience "employment discrimination and occupational segregation."[12] The racial gap in economic security becomes even more evident when the wages and benefits are closely examined. In a study, those Black workers with full-time employment earned a median weekly salary of $727.00. In contrast, White individuals earned $943.00 during the same period in 2019. This contributes to less savings thereby affecting not only retirement opportunities but intergenerational wealth as well as less discretionary income.[12] Examination of benefits also revealed that Black workers had private health insurance at a rate of 55.4%. Whites were insured at a rate of 74.8%.[12] Additionally, Black individuals often worked in occupations that were less stable or part of the health care system in roles such as home health aides and/or nursing home employees.[12] During the assessed period from September 2018 through September 2019, White unemployed individuals were out of work for approximately 20.8 weeks and the Black individuals during the same time frame were not working for approximately 25.5 weeks.[12]

In a study that evaluated the impact of socioeconomic status in low-income and middle-income countries, it was seen that being unemployed was associated with depression in diabetic patients.[13] "Depression was also more likely to be associated with those individuals who had less income and fewer assets."[13]

The Healthy People 2030 goal for economic stability is to help people earn steady incomes to meet their health needs.[14] For the objectives set, none of the targets have been met or exceeded.[12] There are 3 areas of improvement including increased employment of working-age people.[12] An increase in the number of children living with at least 1 parent who works full-time has also seen an improvement.[14] A reduction in work-related issues resulting in missed days of work is another objective that has seen improvement.[14]

The objective of reducing household food insecurity and hunger has worsened. The target is 6.0%.[14] However, in 2018, 11.1% of households were food insecure and in 2022, it increased to 12.8%.[14] The goal to eliminate very low food security is 0%.[14] The data from 2022 reveal 1.02% of households with children under 18 years had very low food security which is an increase from the baseline of 0.59% in 2018.[14]

Housing instability is another component of economic stability. To support the economy during the New Deal Era, government-insured mortgages were established.[13] The government subsequently established maps of different properties and areas. These maps were then color-coded to represent the worthiness of the neighborhood.[13] Red represented areas deemed not worthy of inclusion in homeownership programs.[13] Most of the homes in red areas were occupied by Black residents.[13] This program was established by the US government's homeownership programs in the 1920s to 1930s and existed in Atlanta, Georgia, as recently 1981 to 1986.[13] It is the discriminatory and systematic denial of services such as mortgages, insurance loans, and other financial services to residents of certain areas based on their race and ethnicity.[13] It disregards an individual's qualifications and credit worthiness.[13] It was typically based on the residency of the individual and often involved minority neighborhoods, which were perceived to be "hazardous and dangerous."[13]

Residential segregation influences more than just where a person lives. It is often tied to reduced employment opportunities, decreased economic status, and restricted access to quality education.[4] This then indirectly influences violence and crime in a neighborhood. Further complicating the picture is its manifestation in intergenerational trauma from these experiences and its effects.[4]

Additionally, research suggests that the lower SES of a neighborhood has been associated with incident coronary heart disease as well as incident heart failure.[4] The deprivation index is used to assess socioeconomic status.[4] People with a higher index appear to be more vulnerable to mortality attributed to CVD.[4] This impact seems to be most pronounced in the younger age group, those less than 50 years of age.[4]

Educational access and quality
Educational access encompasses literacy, language, early childhood education, vocational training, and higher education. Individuals with high levels of education are healthier and live longer.[15,16] Low-income families are more likely to struggle with reading and math. These families are also more likely to experience routine social discrimination such as bullying and are less likely to graduate from high school or attend college.[15,16] People with lower levels of education are less likely to have safe jobs, less likely to have high-paying jobs, and more likely to have heart disease, diabetes mellitus, and depression.[17] The goal for Healthy People 2030 is to increase educational opportunities and help children and adolescents do well in school.[15]

Unfortunately, none of the educational access and quality objectives had targets met or exceeded.[15] There were 2 areas in which there is some improvement.[15] There has been an improvement in the proportion of high school students who graduate in 4 years.[15] Improvement has also been seen in the proportion of students with disabilities who are usually in regular education programs.[15]

An area where the objective is worse is increasing the proportion of high school graduates in college the October after graduating.[15] The target set by the committee is 73.7%.[15] In 2018, 69.1% were enrolled in college in October immediately after completing high school.[14] In 2022, the number dropped to 62%.[15] Another objective that has become worse is the target of 41.5% to increase the proportion of fourth graders with reading skills at or above the proficient level.[15] In 2017, the percentage of fourth-grade students who attended both public and private schools and had reading levels above the proficient level for their grade was 36.6%.[15] This number was 33.3% in 2022.[15] It is noted that those who struggle with reading proficiency are more likely to struggle in school and have been noted to be more likely to participate in risky behaviors as adolescents.[15] Studies suggest intervening early can improve school performance, leading to more healthy behaviors.[15] There is also a drop in the percentage of students in both public and private schools whose mathematical skills are at the proficient level for fourth graders.[15] The target number is 43.1%, and the most recent data for 2022 was 36.3%, whereas it was 40.2% in

2017.[15] Strong performance in school is linked to doing well in math and overall better health outcomes.[15]

Health care access and quality

Health care access encompasses health coverage, provider availability, appropriate linguistics, cultural competency, and quality of care.[18] Individuals who belong to underrepresented groups often face barriers not only to CVD diagnosis but also care, receive less optimal care, and experience overall worse adverse outcomes.[3] One in ten people in the United States are uninsured.[18] Uninsured individuals are less likely to have a primary care provider, participate in preventive care services, and seek treatment for chronic illnesses.[18] The goal for Healthy People 2030 is to increase access to comprehensive, high-quality health care services.[17]

In 2015, 8.5% of adults over or equal to age 35 received all of the recommended high-priority appropriate clinical preventive services.[18] The number of adults who received the recommended evidence-based preventive health care decreased in 2020 to 5.3%.[18] Factors influencing health care access and quality include the distance from health care services, as well as communication options such as the ability to participate in remote access.[18]

There were 4 areas in which the targets were met and/or exceeded.[18] There has been a reduction in the proportion of people who cannot get prescription medications when they need them and an increase in the use of the oral health care system.[18] An increase in the proportion of adults offered online access to their medical records has also met or exceeded targets.[18] Additionally, there has been a reduction in the proportion of people who cannot get the dental care needed when it is needed.[18]

Areas of improvement include reducing the number of individuals who cannot get medical care when needed.[18] There has also been an increase in the proportion of people with health insurance and the proportion of individuals with prescription drug insurance.[18] Additional improvements have occurred in reducing the number of new human immunodeficiency virus (HIV) diagnoses, increasing the linkage to HIV medical care, and reducing the rate of mother-to-child HIV transmission.[18]

Compared to prior, the areas in which health care access and quality are worsening include increasing the proportion of adults who get recommended evidence-based preventive health care.[18] The target is 11.5% and it was noted to be 8.5% for those adults aged 35 and above who received all of the recommended high-priority appropriate clinical preventive services in 2015.[18] The number declined to 5.3% in 2020.[18] This area also worsens in adolescents.[18] The target has been set at 82.6% but in 2016 to 2017 for those aged 12 to 17, the baseline was 78.7% and received 1 or more preventive health care visits within 12 months.[18] That number was only 69.6% in 2020 to 2021.[18] Preventive services are important to prevent disease and reduce the risk of premature death.[18] It is especially important in this age group as behaviors that can have long-term effects on health begin at an early age.[18] Evaluation of the other health objectives such as increasing the proportion of low-income youth who have preventive dental visits has also worsened.[18] The target for this measure is 79.9%.[18] The most recent data are 68.7% in 2020 to 2021, which were less than the baseline of 75.8% that was established in 2016 to 2017.[18] This number refers to children aged 1 to 17 whose household income is less than 200% of the federal poverty level who received preventive dental services.[18] It is the hope that nondental providers will do more oral screenings, speak to caregivers about oral health, and refer patients to dental care.[18] The impact of oral health on overall health is important and the effects on cardiovascular health are well established.[18] The evaluation also shows that the increased proportion of pregnant women who receive early and adequate prenatal care has worsened.[18] In 2018, 76.4% of pregnant females received early and adequate prenatal care which fell to 74.9% in 2022[18] The target set by Healthy People 2030 is 80.5%.[17] Although it must be acknowledged that some of these findings may be secondary to the COVID-19 pandemic, there is still some concern.[18]

Neighborhood and built environment

Numerous factors influence the health and safety of where people are born, live, learn, work, play, worship, and age.[19] In assessing one's neighborhood, its components include transportation, safety, parks, playgrounds, and walkability.[20] Environments that promote physical activity appear to have an important connection to type II diabetes mellitus in that there is a lower risk of developing the disease state.[4] Additionally, those areas with homes that are close to the roads as well as high-traffic areas were associated with incident coronary heart disease.[4] Noise and air pollution appear to be associated with a higher risk of developing type II diabetes mellitus.[19] Occupational hazards such as loud noises and air pollutants such as secondhand smoke also impact health and well-being.[19] The presence of green spaces helps to negate the negative Impacts from climate change such as heat exposure, noise pollution, and mitigation of air pollution.[4]

Marginalized individuals are more likely to live in neighborhoods with high rates of violence and unsafe air and/or water.[8] Both increasing the proportion of people whose water supply meets safe drinking water regulations and reducing the number of toxic pollutants released into the environment have met or exceeded the targets.[19] Reducing health and environmental risks from hazardous sites, increasing the proportion of homes that have an entrance without steps, and increasing the proportion of smoke-free homes have also shown improvement since Healthy People 2030.[19]

However, since implementation, the proportion of adults with broadband internet has worsened.[19] The target set by Healthy People 2030 is to have 60.8% of individuals with broadband internet.[19] However, in 2020, it was noted to be 41.5%, which was markedly lower than the numbers in 2017 which was 55.9%.[19] The deaths from motor vehicle crashes have also worsened.[18] Data from 2021 show 13.3 motor vehicle traffic-related deaths whereas in 2018 the baseline was noted as 11.2 per 100,000.[19] The target had been set at 10.1 per 100,000.[19] This is important in that compared to other high-income countries, the deaths from motor vehicle crashes are twice that in the United States.[19] The second leading cause of death from unintentional injuries is motor vehicle crashes in the United States.[19]

Social and community context

When evaluating social and community context, there is an emphasis on understanding personal relationships, which include not only family and friends but also relationships with coworkers and members of the community.[20] The goal is for individuals to have support in the places where they are "born, live, learn, work, play, worship, and age."[20] It has been well established that positive relationships help lessen the negative impact of some of the factors for which people do not have control.[20] They include unsafe neighborhoods, discrimination, and affording necessities.[20] To improve health and well-being, it is important to provide interventions that will provide these important social and community supports."[20]

The Health Information Technology (IT) target has been met or exceeded and refers to increasing the proportion of adults who use IT to track health care data or communicate with providers.[21]

There has been improvement in 2 other areas, one of which includes reducing the proportion of people with intellectual and developmental disabilities who live in situational settings with 7 or more people.[21] The other area of improvement is reducing the proportion of children with a parent or guardian who has served time in jail or prison.[21]

Some areas have worsened since the implementation of Healthy People 2030.[21] Included in those objectives is an increase in the proportion of citizens of voting age who vote.[21] The set target by Healthy People 2030 is 58.4%.[21] In 2022, 52.2% and the baseline from 2018 was 53.4% of US citizens 18 years and older.[21] Another set objective is to increase the proportion of children and adolescents communicating positively with their parents. Positive communication refers to having the opportunity to discuss one's feelings, one's experiences, and one's beliefs.[21] Assessment was based on children and adolescents aged 6 to 17 whose parents reported the ability to share and talk about meaningful things which supports the idea of positive communication and had a target set at 73%.[21] However, the most recent data revealed 62.0% in 2020 to 2021 and the established baseline was 68.5% in 2016 to 2017.[2] Thus, in this area, there has been a decline instead of an improvement. It is believed that the ability to communicate not only influences performance in school but also fosters the development of healthy habits.[21] Increasing the proportion of children whose families read to them at least 4 days per week also worsened in this period.[21] The target set is 63.2%.[21] However, in 2020 to 2021, it is noted to be 55.1% and the baseline mark is 58.3% from 2016 to 2017.[21] Additionally, the data suggest increasing the proportion of adults who talk to friends or family about their health has worsened.[21] In 2017, it was noted that 86.9% of adults, 18 years and older, reported having family or friends with whom they discuss health issues.[21] However, the data from 2022 showed a decrease of 79.6%.[21] Food security is defined as the "assured availability of nutritionally adequate foods acquired in socially acceptable ways."[4] These opportunities not only influence dietary behaviors but also CV risk factors.[4] It has also been established that the quality of dietary choices is related to the number of supermarkets compared to smaller chain grocery stores, fast-food restaurants, as well as traditional restaurants. Additionally, food selections are often impacted by a person's social network as well as one's occupation.[4]

Finally, there is a worsening of elimination of very low food insecurity in children.[21] The goal was to reduce very low food insecurity to 0%.[21] In 2018, 0.59% of the homes with children under the age of 18 had very low food insecurity and it increased to 1.02% in 2022.[21] The negative impact of not having enough food to eat is well known and impacts not only performance in school but the health of children.[21] Combating this involves nutrition assistance programs, increased benefit amounts, and reducing unemployment.[21]

THE ROLE OF HEALTH CARE PROVIDERS

All of these SDOH are interconnected with lower SES. In an assessment of SES, lower SES considered those individuals whose household income was less than 150% of the federal poverty level or an education level less than a high school diploma.[22] As the research continues to occur, it becomes more evident that SDOH also known as fundamental causes of disease have a synergy with lower SES that has a significant impact of approximately one-quarter of the US population.[22] Race and ethnicity are intertwined with SES in the United States.[22] Chronic poverty appears to be linked to those pathways that are atherogenic in addition to its impact on allostatic load which results from chronic stress and is affected by weathering which is known as a premature deterioration of health.[22] Access to quality health care, quality food, and quality education is an important factor affecting those who are in the lower SES groups. Those with higher SES also appear to have enhanced cognitive ability and are more likely to make better decisions as it relates to healthy lifestyles.[22] Risk factors for coronary heart disease are impacted by all of these and even impact intergenerational health and wealth.[22]

Research suggests that depression is more prevalent among Black and Hispanic/LatinX individuals due to both cultural barriers and the paucity of tailored services.[23] Establishing and promoting culturally sensitive mental health services can enhance utilization and improve cardiovascular outcomes.[23] Health care providers (HCPs) can encourage the acknowledgment of mental health disorders and help patients and their communities navigate the health care system.[23] Ensuring policies that consider all of the influences in cardiovascular disease is imperative to enhancing health equity.

The bidirectional relations between mental and physical health have been well established. Mental health conditions such as depression, anxiety, and posttraumatic stress disorder can result from cardiovascular diseases which include coronary artery disease, cerebrovascular disease, heart failure, peripheral artery disease, and other associated conditions.[23] Additionally, these states can result in unhealthy behaviors such as smoking, medication nonadherence, and sedentary lifestyles, all of which contribute to the aforementioned cardiovascular diseases and their associated complications.[23]

HCPs can impact the role of SDOH on mental health and physical health, specifically those conditions that impact cardiovascular disease by having compassion and empathy in every patient encounter. Compassion is defined as the ability "to recognize the suffering of others and then take ACTION to help."[24] There are 3 types of COMPASSION: familial compassion applies to family member who is suffering, familiar compassion—compassion for people with whom there is a relation, and stranger compassion—compassion for people not known.[24] EMPATHY can be defined as the ability to understand and share the feelings of another.[25] Three types of empathy include cognitive empathy—being aware of the emotional state of another person, emotional empathy—engaging with sharing those emotions, and compassionate empathy—taking action to support other people.[25]

Compassionate empathy is important as it tries to balance the emotional and cognitive impact of an event. The cornerstones of compassionate empathy include connecting with the other person, exhibiting a genuine curiosity about the individual, acknowledging and validating the other person's emotions, creating an environment where the individual feels safe to share and resolve their struggle, helping to find their inner strength and wisdom, and helping them connect with themselves or their own heart and logic which provides the necessary insight and courage to act.[25]

To further complicate the intertwined nature of one's lived experience, research suggests that even experiences from early in one's life can impact their morbidity and the age at which mortality occurs. Therefore, it is important that as health care providers the individuals' experience across the lifespan is considered in their evaluation.[26]

"The evidence has become clear that the current cardiovascular risk models underpredict risk in those populations with very high social risk."[23] One of the greatest challenges faced by health care providers is time. Yet, HCPs must spend the time to ask key questions that envelop the SDOH. This will require the development of screening tools to take into account those factors that continually influence one's psychological and physical health with the understanding this may trigger the need for additional appointments for more extensive assessments.[23]

Providers can assist by facilitating timely access to diagnostic tests such as echo-cardiograms, stress testing, coronary artery calcification/CT coronaries, and invasive cardiac testing. Increasing referrals to new treatment modalities such as TAVR and minimally invasive approaches to coronary revascularization.

Additionally, HCPs can encourage and assist patients with acknowledging their responsibility.[4] Emphasizing the importance of awareness of health issues, managing their medications, and engaging in healthy lifestyles.[4] Patient education is an area where HCPs can truly make a difference. A commitment to understanding each patient's health literacy will foster a mutually beneficial environment.

Engaging with legislative leadership not only on a federal level but also within the state and local arenas is important. HCPs have the opportunity to support and advocate for a wide array of policy interventions. These interventions can influence community planning and investment, access to education, and access to health insurance. Advocating for policies and interventions to reduce poverty is paramount. Poverty affects the brain's growth, especially in the first 4 years of life.[27] It is believed that this impact with a decrease in the gray matter volume in the frontal and parietal lobes can impact children both academically in their ability to learn as well as socially and how they engage with others.[27] Those living in poverty have multiple environmental stressors such as noise, crowding, crime, and violence, thus creating an environment with a lack of emphasis on academic stimulation.[27]

Additionally, those parents in that environment are often exposed to different parenting styles than those in more affluent neighborhoods.[27] Providing nurse visitation programs reduced the amount of abuse, and neglect, and improved outcomes into adolescence.[27] Establishing policies that will help reduce poverty will indirectly impact cardiovascular health. As HCPs, promoting policies that support income such as the Earned Income Tax Credit and increasing the minimum wage can help increase the income of low-income families thereby reducing poverty and potentially enhancing achievement.[27] Early education programs have also been shown to improve both short-term and long-term outcomes.[27] Supporting those initiatives that create better job opportunities and close the wealth gap are critical in improving cardiovascular health in patients of marginalized groups.[26] Advocating for programs to assist with loan relief will also help diversify health care.[23]

Working with strategic partners and key stakeholders such as health care organizations/health care systems, local policymakers, national policymakers, churches, retailers, and pharmacies is vital. The development of effective partnerships is paramount to the success and advancement of equitable cardiovascular outcomes and is a critical way HCPs can use their platform for change. Health care providers can actively engage with organizations that have committed to advocating for underrepresented minority groups. Those who have committed to this work included the Association of Black Cardiologists, the American College of Cardiology (ACC), the American Heart Association, and the Cardiovascular Research Foundation. Through working with these organizations, educational opportunities can be distributed to large numbers of individuals.

HCPs can use examples set by professional organizations such as ABC through encouraging the identification of community health advocates and training of community health workers.[28] Through a venture with the National Institutes of Health/National Heart, Lung, and Blood Institute, a program known as the Community Health Advocate Training (CHAT) Program was established in 2020.[28] In the training of community health workers, individuals learn to promote cardiovascular health, lifestyle, risk factors, and prevention.[28] Workers are then able to go into the community and provide monthly health education sessions and provide at least 2 community outreach or health promotion activities annually.[28] Programs like CHAT will increase awareness of CVD and the associated risk factors, provide community leaders with knowledge and skills to provide consistent education to members of the community about lifestyle changes that can be tailored to their neighborhood/environment, and serve as liaisons between the community, local health care systems, and professional societies.[28] These services can prove beneficial to marginalized communities.[28]

The importance of leveraging community partnerships has never been more important to reduce the disparities that exist in CVD and its care. Establishing sustainable relationships within the community is critical to achieving health equity. Key stakeholders can identify the importance of engagement. Once the target population has been identified, individuals can work together to build trust, which requires transparency and authenticity.[28] Evaluation of the assets available specific to the target community is important and will impact the program's development and working together to develop culturally appropriate programs will enhance the likelihood of success of the program. Integrating community health care workers can help provide the necessary resources. The intent and ideal are to provide services unique to the target community. The use of focus groups will enable community-specific content to be included. Ideas formulated here can then be used to help all members of the community advocate for policies that will promote the needs of their individuals.[28]

Striving to create a culture of health, eliminating CVD disparities, and advancing health equity are key pillars to improving care. Encouraging organizations to embrace and integrate the establishment of community partnerships as part of their core mission will contribute to reducing pervasive disparities.

Community engagement is an ongoing process that requires continued evaluation and evolving priorities, nurturing relationships, and allocation of funding and resources.[28] Through this type of advocacy, trust is built with those who have similar interests and circumstances providing an inherent understanding.[28,29]

Encouraging continued research on the impact of SDOH on cardiovascular disease and its risk factors will only enhance the ability to care for cardiovascular patients. Participation in research endeavors and encouraging members of the various communities to engage in research to ensure study results are as expected is essential. It is well established that there is underrepresentation of racial and ethnic groups in clinical trials.[3] The All of US research program is a national program attempting to address this issue by enrolling participants who agree to share electronic health record data, complete surveys, and provide biospecimens as indicated to increase the numbers of historically underrepresented groups.

To be seen and have members of the health care team look like their patients is also an integral part of impacting change and enhancing trust in the health care system. Health care providers of all backgrounds can advocate for diversifying the medical profession and all members of the health care team. All stakeholders must actively participate in efforts to reduce the impact of SDOH on CVD and the care provided to all communities.

WHAT THE FUTURE HOLDS

Continued research to understand the impact of structural racism, which may manifest through lending practices, residential segregation, occupational opportunities, access to education, and racial profiling, is imperative to further understand the impact on psychological and physical health.[4] Examination of the role adversity plays in the activation of the sympathetic nervous system and its impact on cardiovascular health warrants further exploration. Additionally, further evaluation of the impact of the immune response to chronic stress is also important and may impact future work in this field. Job-related stressors, food insecurity, neighborhood violence, lack of social support and isolation, as well as discrimination and micro/macroaggression all fall under the umbrella of adversity and affect an individual's physical and psychological health.[4]

SUMMARY

Guideline concordant health care delivery is necessary and can be achieved by examining how to provide more effective and equitably distributed evidence-based health care and address the drivers of disparities in health and health care outcomes.

SDOH are the economic and social conditions that affect an individual's health both physically and mentally. Disparities in cardiovascular care disproportionately affect racial and ethnic minority patients. Providing consistent evidence-based care is at the pinnacle of achieving the desired health care outcomes for all communities. Effectively optimizing treatment, assessment, and acknowledgment of SDOH are integral to the success of proposed treatment plans. Our most important role, as stated by ACC Dr Itcchaporia, is "Never has there been a better time to increase our efforts to actualize health equity."

CLINICS CARE POINTS

- To remain cognizant of the disparities in society and health care locally and nationally.
- To maintain a keen awareness of the importance of emotional health and its impact on physical well-being.
- To help patients understand the value of understanding the impact of SDOH on their overall health.
- To tailor questions related to the social determinants of health to the individual.
- To gauge an understanding of the patient's awareness of their health status.
- To ask questions with the compassion and dignity that each unique patient deserves.
  - Can you share your current living situation?
  - Are there any concerns about your ability to obtain food and do you often choose healthy food options?
  - In your neighborhood are there challenges to accessing transportation?
  - How do you feel about education? Do you think education is valuable?
  - Do you enjoy your current job? Do you have any concerns about your current position?
  - Have you had any recent unexpected financial constraints?
  - When you experience life's challenges who provides the needed support?
- To encourage patients to pursue achieving goals that will improve specific areas related to their SDOH.
- To be prepared to provide resources to address issues that may arise from the patient's responses to questions such as housing resources, food insecurity options, educational support, medical-legal partnerships, and interpersonal security resources.
- To advocate for social policies that will benefit a majority of the patients.

DISCLOSURE

There are no financial conflicts of interest to disclose.

REFERENCES

1. WHO, Available at: who.int/health-topics/social-determinants-of-health (Accessed 7 May 2024).

2. CDC, Available at: cdc.gov/oralhealth/about/healthy-people.html (Accessed 7 May 2024).

3. Lewsey SC, Breathett K. Racial and ethnic disparities in heart failure. Curr Opin Cardiol 2021;36(3):320–8. https://doi.org/10.1097/HCO.0000000000000855.

4. Powell-Wiley TM, Baumer Y, Osei Baah F. Social determinants of cardiovascular disease. Circ Res 2022;130:782–99.

5. Mazimba S, Peterson PN. JAHA spotlight on racial and ethnic disparities in cardiovascular disease. J AM Heart Assoc 2021;10:e023650. https://doi.org/10.1161/JAHA.121.023650.

6. who.int/health-topics/social-determinants-of-health. Available at: https://www.who.int/health-topics/health-equity#tab=tab_1 https://www.kff.org/racial-equity-and-health-policy/issue-brief/disparities-in-health-and-health-care-5-key-question-and-answers/#:~:text=A%20%E2%80%9Chealth%20disparity%E2%80%9D%20refers%20to%20a%20higher%20burden,and%20use%20of%20care%2C%20and%20quality%20of%20care" [Accessed 7 May 2024].

7. Graham GN, Jones PG, Chan PS, et al. Racial disparities in patient characteristics and survival after acute myocardial infarction. JAMA Network 2018;1(7):e184240. https://doi.org/10.1001/jamanetworkope.2018.4240.

8. Pegus C, Duncan I, Greener J, et al. Achieving health equity by normalizing cardiac care. Health Equity 2018;2(1):404–11. https://doi.org/10.1089/heq.2018.0067.

9. Javed Z, Maqsood MH, Yahya T, et al. Race, racism, and cardiovascular health: applying a social determinants of health framework to racial/ethnic disparities in cardiovascular disease. Circ Cardiovasc Qual Outcomes 2022;15:e007917. https://doi.org/10.1161/circoutcomes.121.0079.17.

10. Healthy people 2030, U.S. Department of health and human services, office of disease prevention and health promotion. Available at: https://health.gov/healthypeople. Accessed May 30, 2024.

11. Commodore-Mensah Y, Turkson-Ocran RA, Foti K, et al. Associations between social determinants and hypertension, stage 2 hypertension, and controlled Blood pressure among men and women in the United States. Am J Hypertens 2021;34(7):707–17.

12. National Health Research Council, American progress, Available at: https://www.americanprogress.org/article/african-americans-face-systematic-obstacles-getting-good-jobs/ (Accessed 15 June 2024).

13.. Borkowski P, Borkowska N, Mangeshkar S, et al. Racial and Socioeconomic Determinants of Cardiovascular Health: A Comprehensive Review. Cureus 2024;26(5):e59497. https://doi.org/10.7759/cureus.59497.

14. Healthy people 2030. Economic stability. Available at: https://health.gov/healthypeople/objectives-and-data/browse-objectives/economic-stability (Accessed 7 May 2024).

15. Law.cornell.edu/wex/redlining, Available at: https://www.law.cornell.edu/wex/redlining (Accessed 9 May 2024).

16. Healthy people 2030. Educational access and quality. Available at: https://health.gov/healthypeople/objectives-and-data/browse-objectives/education-access-and-quality (Accessed 7 May 2024).

17.. Raghupathi V, Raghupathi W. The influence of education on health: an empirical assessment of OECD countries for the period 1995-2015. Arch Publ Health 2020;78(20):1–18. https://doi.org/10.1186/s13690-020-00402-5.

18. Healthy people 2030. Healthcare access and quality. Available at: https://health. gov/healthypeople/objectives-and-data/browse-objectives/health-care-access-and-quality (Accessed 7 May 2024).
19. Healthy people 2030. Neighborhood and built environment. Available at: https:// health.gov/healthypeople/objectives-and-data/browse-objectives/neighborhood-and-built-environment (Accessed 7 May 2024).
20.. Brennan Ramirez LK, Baker EA, Metzler M. Promoting Health Equity: a resource to help communities address social determinants of health. Atlanta, GA: CDC; 2008.
21. Healthy people 2030. Social and community context. Available at: https://health. gov/healthypeople/objectives-and-data/browse-objectives/social-and-community-context (Accessed 9 May 2024).
22. Hamad R, Penko J, Kazi DS, et al. Association of low socioeconomic status with premature coronary heart disease in US adults. JAMA Cardiol 2020 (Epub ahead of print).
23. American College of Cardiology. Available at: acc.org/Latest-in-Cardiology/Articles/202006/01/12/42/Cover-Story-Health-Disparities-and-Social–Determinants-of-Health-Time-for-Action (Accessed 30 May 2024).
24. Eckman P, Compassion. Available at: https://www.paulekman.com/what-does-compassion-mean/ (Accessed 30 May 2024).
25. Williams JA, The three kinds of empathy: emotional, cognitive, compassionate. 2018. Available at: https://blog.heartmanity.com/the-three-kinds-of-empathy-emotional-cognitive-compassionate?hs_amp=true (Accessed 30 May 2024).
26. National Research Council (US) Panel on Race, Ethnicity, and Health in Later Life. Understanding racial and ethnic differences in health in late life: a research agenda. (US): National Academies Press; 2004.
27. Institute for research on poverty, *Acad Pediatr*, 16, 2016, S30, Available at: https://morgridge.wisc.edu/wp-content/uploads/sites/4/2017/02/Brain_Drain_A_Childs_Brain_on_Poverty.pdf (Accessed 15 June 2024).
28.. Bess C, Ferdinand D, Underwood P, et al. Promoting cardiovascular health equity. Association of Black Cardiologists practical model for community-engaged partnerships. J Am Coll Cardiol 2024;83(5):632–6.
29. Leone T, Coast E, Narayanan S, et al. Diabetes and depression comorbidity and socioeconomic status in low- and middle-income countries (LMICs): a mapping of the evidence. Glob Health 2012;8:39.

Moving?

Make sure your subscription moves with you!

To notify us of your new address, find your **Clinics Account Number** (located on your mailing label above your name), and contact customer service at:

Email: journalscustomerservice-usa@elsevier.com

800-654-2452 (subscribers in the U.S. & Canada)
314-447-8871 (subscribers outside of the U.S. & Canada)

Fax number: 314-447-8029

Elsevier Health Sciences Division
Subscription Customer Service
3251 Riverport Lane
Maryland Heights, MO 63043

*To ensure uninterrupted delivery of your subscription, please notify us at least 4 weeks in advance of move.

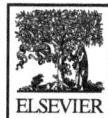

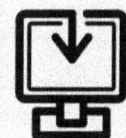

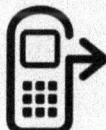

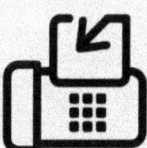

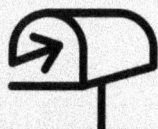

ELSEVIER

www.ingramcontent.com/pod-product-compliance
Lightning Source LLC
Chambersburg PA
CBHW071203210326
41597CB00016B/1657